Immunology of Neuromuscular Disease

IMMUNOLOGY AND MEDICINE SERIES

IMMUNOLOGY
SERIES · SERIES · SERIES · SERIES · SERIES AND SERIES · SERIES · SERIES · SERIES · SERIES
MEDICINE

Volume 24

Immunology of Neuromuscular Disease

Edited by
R. Hohlfeld
Department of Neurology, Klinikum Großhadern,
Ludwig-Maximilians University, Munich,
and
Department of Neuroimmunology,
Max-Planck Institute, Martinsried, Germany

Series Editor: K. Whaley

KLUWER ACADEMIC PUBLISHERS
DORDRECHT/BOSTON/LONDON

Distributors

for the United States and Canada: Kluwer Academic Publishers, PO Box 358, Accord Station, Hingham, MA 02018-0358, USA
for all other countries: Kluwer Academic Publishers Group, Distribution Center, PO Box 322, 3300 AH Dordrecht, The Netherlands

A catalogue record for this book is available from the British Library.

ISBN 0-7923-8844-5

Published in the United Kingdom by Kluwer Academic Publishers, PO Box 55, Lancaster, UK.

Kluwer Academic Publishers BV incorporates the publishing programmes of D. Reidel, Martinus Nijhoff, Dr W. Junk and MTP Press.

Typeset by Lasertext Ltd., Stretford, Manchester, U.K.
Printed and bound in Great Britain by Hartnolls Ltd., Bodmin, Cornwall.

Contents

Series Editor's Note

The interface between clinical immunology and other branches of medical practice is frequently blurred and the general physician is often faced with clinical problems with an immunological basis and is expected to diagnose and manage such patients. The rapid expansion of basic and clinical immunology over the past two decades has resulted in the appearance of increasing numbers of immunology journals and it is impossible for a non-specialist to keep apace with this information overload. The *Immunology and Medicine* series is designed to present individual topics of immunology in a condensed package of information which can be readily assimilated by the busy clinician or pathologist.

K. Whaley, Leicester
May 1994

Preface

The neuromuscular diseases comprise the disorders of peripheral nerve, neuromuscular junction, and muscle (Figure 1). This book addresses the immunologically mediated neuromuscular diseases, including Guillain–Barré syndrome and other autoimmune neuropathies, the Lambert–Eaton myasthenic syndrome, myasthenia gravis, and the autoimmune diseases of muscle. Two chapters are devoted to the vasculitis and human immunodeficiency virus-mediated neuromuscular diseases. The experimental models of neuritis and myasthenia gravis are addressed in separate chapters. An introductory chapter provides a general background to autoimmunity.

I wish to thank my contributing colleagues, all of whom are recognized experts in their respective fields, for their willingness to cooperate in this project. Furthermore, I am grateful to Dr Bill Hoffman of Stanford University who generously assisted in the editing of several chapters during his time spent with us on a sabbatical. I am also indebted to the editor and editorial staff of Kluwer Academic Publishers for their help and advice during preparation of this book.

Munich/Martinsried
March 1994

Reinhard Hohlfeld

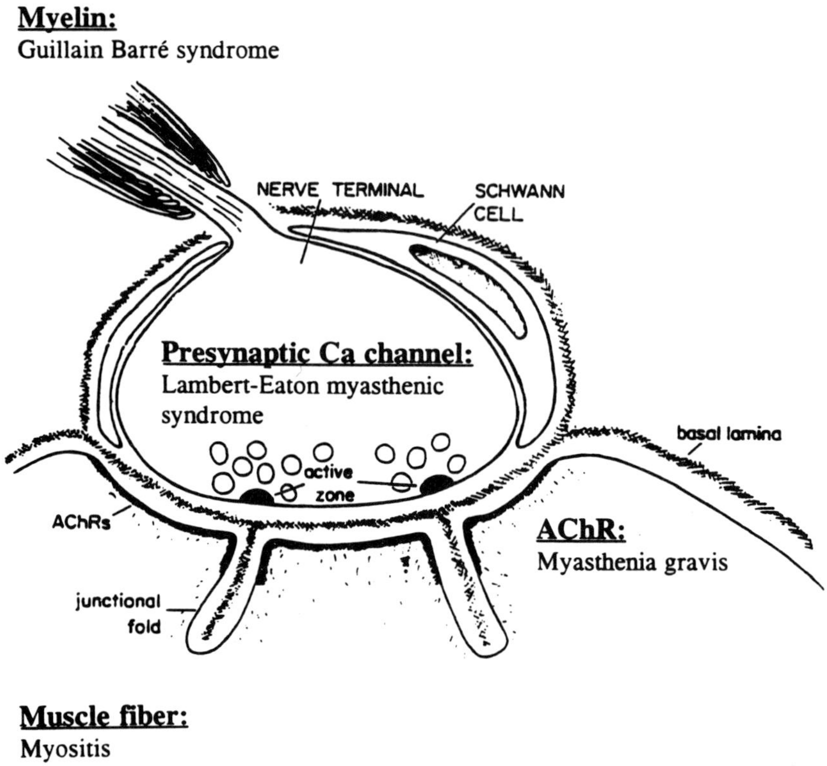

Figure 1 Neuromuscular autoimmune diseases. Schematic drawing of a neuromuscular junction, showing the terminal axon of the nerve ensheathed with myelin, which in the peripheral nervous system is produced by Schwann cells (upper left). Another Schwann cell is shown in close contact with the nerve terminal, which is not myelinated but covered with basal lamina. The basal lamina also fills the synaptic cleft and the junctional folds of the postsynaptic muscle cell membrane, and surrounds the muscle fibre (bottom). The nerve terminal contains synaptic vesicles, which store the transmitter, acetylcholine. When a nerve impulse arrives at the nerve terminal, the presynaptic nerve membrane depolarizes. Presynaptic voltage-gated calcium channels open, allowing influx of calcium into the terminal. This leads to fusion of synaptic vesicles with the presynaptic membrane and release of acetylcholine into the synaptic cleft. The acetylcholine molecules diffuse to the postsynaptic muscle membrane, where they bind to the acetylcholine receptors located on the tips of the postsynaptic folds next to the presynaptic membrane. This leads to depolarization of the postsynaptic membrane above excitation threshold, initiating an action potential that spreads across the entire muscle fibre membrane and eventually triggers the chain of events leading to mechanical contraction of the muscle fibre.

Both pre- and postsynaptic elements of the neuromuscular junction may become targets of autoimmune attack in different diseases. The immunological basis of these neuromuscular autoimmune diseases is the main subject of this book.

List of Contributors

R. J. BAROHN
Department of Medicine (Neurology)
University of Texas Health Science Center
7703 Floyd Curl Drive
San Antonio, TX 78284
USA

D. BURGER
Division of Immunology and Allergy
University Hospital
CH-1211 Geneva 14
Switzerland

M. C. DALAKAS
Neuromuscular Diseases Section
National Institute of Neurological Disorders and Stroke
National Institutes of Health
9000 Rockville Pike
Bethesda, MD 20892
USA

D. B. DRACHMAN
Neuromuscular Unit
Department of Neurology
Johns Hopkins School of Medicine
600 N Wolfe St.
Baltimore, MD 21205
USA

A. G. ENGEL
Department of Neurology and Neuromuscular Laboratory
Guggenheim Building G801
Mayo Clinic
Rochester, MN 55905
USA

H.-P. HARTUNG
Department of Neurology
Julius-Maximilians Universität
Josef-Schneider Str. 11
D-97080 Würzburg
Germany

R. HOHLFELD
Department of Neurology
Klinikum Großhadern
University of Munich
Marchioninistr. 15
D-81366 München
Germany

I. ILLA
Neuromuscular Diseases Section
National Institute of Neurological Disorders and Stroke
National Institutes of Health
9000 Rockville Pike
Bethesda, MD 20892
USA

J. T. KISSEL
Division of Neuromuscular Disease
Department of Neurology
Ohio State University
Columbus, OH 43210
USA

K. A. KROLICK
Department of Microbiology
University of Texas Health Science Center
7703 Floyd Curl Drive
San Antonio, TX 78284
USA

R. W. KUNCL
Department of Neurology
Johns Hopkins School of Medicine
600 N Wolfe St
Baltimore, MD 21205
USA

C. LININGTON
Abteilung für Neuroimmunologie
Max-Planck Institut für Psychiatrie
Am Klopferspitz 18A
D-82152 Martinsried
Germany

J. R. MENDELL
Division of Neuromuscular Disease
Department of Neurology
Ohio State University
Columbus, OH 43210
USA

S. MOHAN
Department of Microbiology
University of Texas Health Science Center
7703 Floyd Curl Drive
San Antonio, TX 78284
USA

M. MONZON
Neuromuscular Diseases Section
National Institute of Neurological Disorders and Stroke
National Institutes of Health
9000 Rockville Pike
Bethesda, MD 20892
USA

J. NEWSOM-DAVIS
Neurosciences Group
Institute of Molecular Medicine
John Radcliffe Hospital
Oxford, OX3 9DU
UK

J. D. POLLARD
Department of Medicine
Division of Neurology
University of Sydney
Sydney, NSW
Australia

K. REINERS
Department of Neurology
Julius-Maximilians Universität
Josef-Schneider Str. 11
D-97080 Würzburg
Germany

A. STECK
Department of Neurology
University Hospital
CH-4031 Basel
Switzerland

P. A. THOMPSON
Department of Microbiology
University of Texas Health Science Center
7703 Floyd Curl Drive
San Antonio, TX 78284
USA

K. V. TOYKA
Department of Neurology
Julius-Maximilians Universität
Josef-Schneider Str. 11
D-97080 Würzburg
Germany

A. VINCENT
Neurosciences Group
Institute of Molecular Medicine
John Radcliffe Hospital
Oxford, OX3 9DU
UK

H. WEKERLE
Abteilung für Neuroimmunologie
Max-Planck Institut für Psychiatrie
Am Klopferspitz 18A
D-82152 Martinsried
Germany

T-M. YEH
Department of Microbiology
University of Texas Health Science Center
7703 Floyd Curl Drive
San Antonio, TX 78284
USA

T. E. ZODA
Department of Microbiology
University of Texas Health Science Center
7703 Floyd Curl Drive
San Antonio, TX 78284
USA

1
Immunological self-tolerance and autoimmunity

H. WEKERLE

The immune system has evolved to distinguish between components of its own organism and foreign molecules. This is of vital importance, since all foreign structures are potentially life-threatening, whether they have invaded the organism from outside (e.g. infectious agents), or have arisen within the tissues (e.g. tumour cells). Distinction between 'self' and 'non-self' is, however, not an easy task. A protective immune cell must be able specifically to recognize a foreign structure and to initiate its destruction and elimination; at the same time, the immune cell has to interact intimately with other cells of the organism during the development of the immune system and even in an ongoing immune response. Obviously, these self tissues must not be destroyed, but tolerated.

For a long time, the notion prevailed that immunological self-tolerance was due to ignorance, i.e. the absence of self-reactive immune cells from the healthy repertoire. This is, however, clearly not the case. Even the healthy immune repertoire contains considerable numbers of T and B lymphocytes bearing receptors that bind self antigens, yet autoimmune diseases are seen only very rarely.

This apparent paradox is well illustrated by naturally occurring humoral autoantibodies. These immunoglobulins, by definition, bind to structures of the own body. Most of these autoantibodies are members of the IgM class, and are produced by $CD5^+$ B lymphocytes. Many, but not all, of these autoantibodies possess a broad spectrum of binding specificity, reacting with determinants on foreign antigens, and also with autoantigens[1,2]. These antibodies are truly 'natural', produced in the absence of an antigenic stimulus, and even without the help of T cells. At least in the mouse, $CD5^+$ B cells often lack somatic mutations in their variable region genes[3], although mutations have been found in human tonsillar populations[4].

Although these IgM 'autoantibodies' do bind to self structures, there is no clear evidence for their pathogenic potential. These immunoglobulins may be indicators of certain immunologically mediated clinical diseases, without being causally involved[5].

There are several criteria for the pathogenic activity of humoral autoantibodies. They include the regular binding to structures showing pathognomonic changes, induction of such changes in tissue culture, and, most convincing, transfer of disease to naïve (animal) recipients.

Remarkably few human or experimental diseases are clearly and exclusively caused by humoral autoantibodies. Perhaps the best known and most thoroughly studied example of a 'humoral' autoimmune disease is myasthenia gravis (MG), and its experimental model, experimental autoimmune myasthenia gravis (EAMG). In both disorders deficits of neuromuscular transmission are caused by autoantibodies binding to the postsynaptic nicotinic acetylcholine receptor (AChR)[6]. It should, however, be noted that the autoantibodies in MG (as in other autoimmune diseases) are polyclonal and heterogeneous. Among the spectrum of anti-AChR autoantibodies, only a minority may be actually pathogenic. It thus may not be surprising to find quite a poor correlation between the total level of anti-AChR autoantibodies and disease severity. This is further emphasized by the fact that only some of the many monoclonal anti-AChR autoantibodies produced by hybridomas are able to transfer passively experimental myasthenia gravis to naïve recipients. Factors such as epitope fine-specificity, and isotype contribute to the pathogenic capacity of an autoantibody[7].

Other diseases caused by humoral autoantibodies include pemphigus vulgaris, bullous pemphigoid, pernicious anaemia, and, possibly, Graves' disease.

The role of the autoreactive immunoglobulins in the pathogenesis of other diseases which have autoantibodies as essential features is much less certain. Most patients with systemic lupus erythematosus (SLE) have autoantibodies against a variety of autoantigens, which are mainly located within the cytoplasm. The most likely effector molecules in the pathogenesis of SLE are the anti-cardiolipin autoantibodies, which bind cardiolipin complexed to the serum apolipoprotein H. These antibodies are closely associated with the human anti-phospholipid syndrome (thrombosis, thrombocytopenia and fetal loss), and their induction in experimental animals causes similar clinical changes[8]. Most of the other autoantibodies found in patients with SLE are directed against nuclear components. Some bind to DNA, others to DNA-binding proteins, and still others react only with DNA/protein complexes[9]. Direct pathogenic activity of these autoantibodies by binding to a defined target structure has not been demonstrated convincingly to date.

The demonstration of autoaggressive T lymphocytes has been much more difficult than the identification of humoral autoantibodies. This is due to the complex manner in which T cells recognize antigen. In contrast to humoral antibodies, which bind to structurally complementary segments on native antigens, T cells recognize antigens only in a specifically processed form, when they are displayed on the surface of an antigen presenting cell (APC). The APC incorporates the antigen and splits the molecule into small peptide fragments. Some of these are bound to products of the major histocompatibility complex (MHC) and transported to the outer membrane of the APC[10]. Accordingly, autoreactive T lymphocytes cannot be identified simply by testing their binding to soluble or particulate autoantigen. Their demonstration requires *in vitro* processing and presentation of these epitopes in cell culture, a technology which has been developed only over the past 10 years[11].

T cells have an undisputed essential role in many, if not most, autoimmune diseases. Autoimmune T cells may be directly involved in the pathogenesis, as effector cells attacking self tissues. Alternatively, autoimmune T cells may act indirectly, either by recruiting and activating inflammatory cells via cytokines, or as helper cells that modulate the production of humoral autoantibodies by B lymphocytes.

Autoaggressive effector T lymphocytes have been identified in most experimentally inducible, organ-specific diseases such as experimental autoimmune encephalomyelitis[12], neuritis[13], uveoretinitis[14], orchitis[15], thyroiditis[16], adjuvant arthritis[17] and autoimmune diabetes mellitus[18,19]. All autoaggressive T lymphocytes express the CD4 membrane phenotype, recognize the autoantigenic epitope in context of MHC class II products, and in most cases, their cytokine pattern follows the Th1 pattern.

In addition, T cells may act as helpers required for the production of high affinity pathogenic IgG autoantibodies, as shown at first in EAMG[20], and MG[21]. In these experiments, AChR specific T cell lines were shown to promote the production of specific autoantibodies by syngeneic AChR-specific B lymphocytes. As is the case for T helper cells in general, the autoimmune T lymphocytes are responsible for inducing in B cells immunoglobulin class switching and somatic mutation in the variable regions, to increase antigen binding affinity. One may assume that T helper cells have a similar role in all other autoantibody-dependent diseases.

There is, however, an additional category of autoimmune diseases, in which the role of T lymphocytes has remained elusive. In SLE and its animal models, for example, there is indirect evidence for a participation of autoimmune T cells. In SLE of humans and mice, anti-DNA autoantibodies often show somatic mutations that should be induced by T helper cells[22]. But, as stressed above, there is no strong evidence for the pathogenic capacity of these autoantibodies. Furthermore, inactivation of T lymphocytes by treatment with T cell-specific monoclonal antibodies has a beneficial effect in SLE-prone mice[23] suggesting a (hitherto undefined) function of T cells in the pathogenesis of lupus-like diseases.

Considering the pivotal role of autoaggressive T lymphocytes in many immunopathological human diseases, determining onset, course and localization of the disorders, these T lymphocytes should be a most attractive target for specific therapeutic strategies[24]. At least in theory, specific neutralization of autoimmune, pathogenic T cells would be the most radical, and at the same time least harmful, therapy for autoimmune disease. A broad spectrum of T cell-targeted therapies has been proposed, with targets ranging from the components of the trimolecular TCR complex, to T cell membrane antigens and cytokines[25].

There is compelling evidence that, at least in the case of certain organ-specific autoantigens, potentially autoaggressive T cells are normal components of the healthy immune system. For example, T cell clones specific for human myelin basic protein or AChR can be readily isolated from the peripheral blood of any healthy volunteer[11], and it appears possible that these cells have an important role in the organization of the immune system[26].

Under physiological conditions, the self-reactive T cell clones never cause 'spontaneous' tissue destruction. How are the autoimmune T cells prevented from causing disease? One way would be to avoid their activation, but this alone does not seem satisfactory. There should be additional, safe control mechanisms, possibly including network-like lymphocytic suppressor circuits. So far, suppressor T cell circuits have not been formally demonstrated in the regulation of immunological self-tolerance, but recent work on CD8 T cell-deprived mice may provide support for such cellular control[27,28].

There may be situations in which the potential autoimmune effector or helper T cells escape from physiological control. In the context of infectious diseases, for example, several interacting factors could trigger autoimmune T cell activation. Structural components of the infectious agent may resemble a self antigen, and may be mistakenly recognized by a truly self-reactive T cell – a mechanism termed molecular mimicry[29]. An ever-increasing number of infectious agents (bacteria and viruses alike) possess structures that act as superantigens, activating large subsets of T cells, often depending on the T cell receptor Vβ gene product used[30]. An exogenous superantigen may activate self-reactive T cell and thus promote disease. Finally, an ongoing infection may create an inflammatory microenvironment that activates by-standing autoimmune T cells, in the absence of direct TCR ligation[31].

Activation of autoreactive T cells may not be sufficient to produce autoimmune disease. Multiple genetic factors seem to influence susceptibility to autoimmunity. This has been particularly well documented for multifactorial autoimmune diseases such as spontaneous insulin-dependent diabetes mellitus (IDDM) in the non-obese diabetic (NOD) mouse. As well as the classical MHC products that influence antigen presentation and generation of the T cell repertoire, polymorphisms of other immunologically relevant genes, such as those coding for the T cell receptor, immunoglobulin, MHC products and cytokines (or their receptors), as well as potentially autoantigenic target structures, have recently been found to co-determine susceptibility to spontaneous autoimmune disease[32].

The principles outlined in this introductory chapter apply to the group of diseases that are the subject of this book. Some of the basic observations mentioned here were initially made in experimental and human myasthenia gravis, the paradigm of the neuromuscular autoimmune disorders.

References

1. Casali P, Notkins A. Probing the human B-cell repertoire with EBV: Polyreactive antibodies and CD5+ B lymphocytes. Annu Rev Immunol. 1989;7:513–35.
2. Kipps TJ. The CD5 B cell. Adv Immunol. 1990;47:117–85.
3. Rajewsky K, Förster I, Cumano A. Evolutionary and somatic selection of the antibody repertoire in the mouse. Science. 1984;238:1088–94.

4. Ebeling SB, Schutte MEM, Logtenberg T. The majority of human tonsillar $CD5^+$ B cells express somatically mutated V_k4 genes. Eur J Immunol. 1993;23:1405–8.
5. Naparstek Y, Plotz PH. The role of autoantibodies in autoimmune disease. Annu Rev Immunol. 1993;11:79–104.
6. Hohlfeld R. Disorders of neuromuscular transmission. Curr Opin Neurol Neurosurg. 1990;3:684–8.
7. Tzartos SJ, Cung MT, Demange P *et al.* The main immunogenic region (MIR) of the nicotinic acetylcholine receptor and the anti-MIR antibodies. Mol Neurobiol. 1992;5:1–29.
8. Gharavi AE, Sammaritano LR, Wen J, Elkon KB. Induction of antiphospholipid autoantibodies by immunization with $\beta 2$ glycoprotein I (apolipoprotein H). J Clin Invest. 1993;90:1105–9.
9. Tan E. Autoantibodies in pathology and cell biology. Cell. 1991;67:841–2.
10. Germain RN, Margulies DH. The biochemistry and cell biology of antigen processing and presentation. Annu Rev Immunol. 1993;11:403–50.
11. Wekerle H. Myelin specific, autoaggressive T cell clones in the normal immune repertoire: Their nature and their regulation. Int Rev Immunol. 1992;9:231–41.
12. Ben-Nun A, Wekerle H, Cohen IR. The rapid isolation of clonable antigen-specific T lymphocytes capable of mediating autoimmune encephalomyelitis. Eur J Immunol. 1981;11:195–9.
13. Linington C, Izumo S, Suzuki M, Uyemura K, Meyermann R, Wekerle H. A permanent rat T cell line that mediates experimental allergic neuritis in the Lewis rat in vivo. J Immunol. 1984;133:1946–50.
14. Caspi RR, Roberge FG, McAllister CG *et al.* T cell lines mediating experimental autoimmune uveoretinitis (EAU) in rats. J Immunol. 1986;136:928–33.
15. Wekerle H, Begemann M. Experimental autoimmune orchitis: *in vitro* induction of an autoimmune disease. J Immunol. 1976;116:159–61.
16. Maron R, Zerubavel R, Friedman A, Cohen IR. T lymphocyte line specific for thyroglobulin produces or vaccinates against autoimmune thyroiditis in mice. J Immunol. 1983;131: 2316–22.
17. Holoshitz J, Naparstek Y, Ben-Nun A, Cohen IR. Lines of T lymphocytes mediate or vaccinate against autoimmune arthritis. Science. 1983;219:56–8
18. Haskins K, MacDuffie M. Acceleration of diabetes in young NOD mice with a $CD4^+$ islet specific T cell clone. Science. 1990;249:1433–6.
19. Elias D, Markowitz D, Reshef T, Van der Zee R, Cohen IR. Induction and therapy of autoimmune diabetes in the non-obese diabetic (NOD/Lt) mouse by a 65-kD heat shock protein. Proc Natl Acad Sci USA. 1990;87:1576–80.
20. Hohlfeld R, Kalies I, Ernst M, Ketelsen U-P, Wekerle H. T lymphocytes in experimental autoimmune myasthenia gravis: isolation of T helper cell lines. J Neurol Sci. 1982;57:265–80.
21. Hohlfeld R, Kalies I, Kohleisen B, Heininger K, Conti-Tronconi BM, Toyka KV. Myasthenia gravis: Stimulation of antireceptor autoantibodies by autoreactive T cell lines. Neurology. 1986;36:618–21.
22. Diamond B, Katz JB, Paul E, Aranow C, Lustgarten D, Scharff MD. The role of somatic mutation in the pathogenic anti-DNA response. Annu Rev Immunol. 1992;10:731–57.
23. Wofsy D, Seaman WE. Reversal of advanced murine lupus in NZB/NZW F1 mice with monoclonal antibody to L3T4. J Immunol. 1987;138:3247–53.
24. Lanzavecchia A. Identifying strategies for immune intervention. Science. 1993;260:937–44.
25. Adorini L, Barnaba V, Bona C *et al.* New perspectives on immunointervention in autoimmune diseases. Immunol Today. 1990;11:383–6.
26. Cohen IR. The cognitive paradigm and the immunological homunculus. Immunol Today. 1992;13:490–4.
27. Koh D-R, Fung-Leung W-P, Ho A, Gray D, Acha-Orbea H, Mak TW. Less mortality but more relapses in experimental allergic encephalomyelitis in $CD8^{-/-}$ mice. Science. 1992;256:1210–13.
28. Jiang H, Zhang S-L, Pernis B. Role of $CD8^+$ T cells in murine experimental allergic encephalomyelitis. Science. 1992;256:1213–15.
29. Oldstone MBA. Molecular mimicry and autoimmune disease. Cell. 1987;50:819–20.
30. Woodland DL, Blackman MA. How do T-cell receptors, MHC molecules and superantigens get together. Immunol Today. 1993;14:208–12.

31. Röcken M, Urban JF, Shevach EM. Infection breaks T-cell tolerance. Nature. 1992;359: 79–82.
32. Ghosh S, Palmer SM, Rodrigues NR, *et al.* Polygenic control of autoimmune diabetes in nonobese diabetic mice. Nature Genet. 1993;4:404–9.

2
Neuropathies associated with anti-myelin antibodies

D. BURGER and A. J. STECK

INTRODUCTION

A number of peripheral neuropathies present with primary demyelination, in which myelin is preferentially damaged or lost and axons remain largely intact. As is the case for other major neurological disorders such as multiple sclerosis and myasthenia gravis, demyelinating neuropathies are likely to be associated with an autoimmune response to structures of the nervous system. Indeed, in these diseases, the pattern of injury to the nervous system is extremely selective, and antibodies and/or pathogenic T cells directed to components of the tissue involved in the disease process can be detected in most patients. Autoimmune diseases result from T or B lymphocytes entering an abnormal state of development in which they escape existing mechanisms that regulate their immunoreactivities and/or other functional activities. However, the mechanisms by which the autoantibodies (produced by pathological B cells) and/or pathogenic T cells cause demyelination remain unknown. In demyelinating lesions of peripheral nerves the final common pathway is invasion of Schwann cell basal lamina by macrophages, penetration of myelin lamellae, phagocytosis of myelin and debris, and stripping of axons. The physiological consequence of this process is the production of conduction blocks. The steps preceding this final damage in autoimmune demyelinating neuropathy are likely to be T cell mediated and/or antibody mediated.

Neuropathies in which humoral autoimmune mechanisms have been implicated include paraproteinaemic polyneuropathies (PPN), acute inflammatory demyelinating polyneuropathy (also called Guillain–Barré syndrome, GBS), and chronic inflammatory demyelinating polyneuropathy (CIDP). With the exception of some PPN, the antigen(s) recognized by autoantibodies in these diseases have not been clearly identified. Furthermore, whether the

Table 2.1 Peripheral nerve myelin lipids

Lipid	*Dry weight* (%)	*Structure*
Total	72	
Phospholipids (total)	55	
Sphingomyelin	19	Phosphorylcholine-Cer
Ethanolamine phosphoglycerides	19	
Cholesterol	23	
Galactolipids (total)	22	
Galactocerebrosides	16	Gal-Cer
Sulphatides	6	SO_4-3Gal-Cer, SO_4-3Galβ1-4Glc-Cer
Gangliosides	0.3–0.7	
LM1		Galβ1-4GlcNAcβ1-3Galβ1-4Glc-Cer 3 | NeuAcα2
GM1		Galβ1-3GalNAcβ1-4Galβ1-4Glc-Cer 3 | NeuAcα2
GD1b		Galβ1-3GalNAcβ1-4Galβ1-4Glc-Cer 3 | NeuAcα2-8NeuAcα2
Minor glycolipids	< 1	
Sulphated glucuronyl paragloboside (SGPG)		Galβ1-4GlcNAcβ1-3Galβ1-4Glc-Cer 3 | SO_4-3GlcUAcβ1
Sulphated glucuronyl lactosaminyl paragloboside (SGLPG)		Galβ1-4(GlcNAcβ1-3Galβ1-4)$_2$Glc-Cer 3 | SO_4-3GlcUAcβ1

autoantibodies found in the blood stream of patients with neuropathy play a role in the pathogenesis of the disease remains to be determined. This chapter summarizes and reviews the recent knowledge on the roles of anti-myelin antibodies in these disorders.

PERIPHERAL MYELIN ANTIGENIC DETERMINANTS

The peripheral nerve myelin sheath is a specialized expansion of the Schwann cell plasma membrane. Myelin is exceptionally rich in lipids (Table 2.1) which accounts for 70–80% of its dry weight, the remaining 20–30% being proteins. The ratio of lipid to protein in myelin is, therefore, the reverse of that found in other plasma membranes. Galactocerebroside, which is found in myelin, oligodendrocytes and Schwann cells, seems to be a myelin-specific constituent, since it is almost absent from other tissues, Sulphatide is present in smaller amounts in myelin, oligodendrocytes, Schwann cells, and perhaps other glial cells. Gangliosides represent less than 1% of PNS myelin lipids, LM_1 being the major ganglioside of human PNS myelin, accounting for more than 50% of the total lipid bound sialic acid[1]. Peripheral human myelin also contains other minor lipid antigens which could play a role in demyelinating diseases, such as the sulphated glucuronyl paragloboside (SGPG) and the sulphated glucuronyl lactosaminyl paragloboside (SGLPG). SGPG and SGLPG are present in myelin and axolemma-enriched fractions in human PNS[1]. Both of these glycolipids are recognized by antibodies of the L2/HNK-1 family.

The protein composition of myelin has long been claimed to be simple: only a few protein bands are visualized by Coomassie blue staining of polyacrylamide gels after electrophoresis. P_0 (M_r approx. 28 000) is the major protein component of PNS myelin, accounting for 50–60% of the myelin proteins[2]. Human P_0 is a glycoprotein containing one unique N-glycosylation site that was found by cDNA sequencing[3]. The N-glycosylation of this site is in agreement with the fact that P_0 possesses only 6–8% carbohydrate by weight[4]. P_0 is one of the smallest members of the immunoglobulin gene superfamily, consisting of 248 amino acids, including 122 residues of a V-like Ig-domain. By homophilic interaction of its extracellular domains, P_0 stabilizes the intraperiod line of compact PNS myelin[5–7]. Two main basic proteins are present in PNS myelin: myelin basic protein (MBP) and P_2. MBP (M_r approx. 18 500) is the major protein of CNS myelin, although it represents only 6% of total proteins in human PNS myelin[2]. Because of its encephalitogenic properties in inducing experimental allergic encephalomyelitis (EAE), MBP has been extensively studied as a potential target antigen in multiple sclerosis. P_2 (M_r approx. 14 500) is the smallest basic protein in PNS myelin, consisting of 131 amino acid residues. The structure and amino acid sequence of P_2 suggest that it is related to a family of cytoplasmic proteins that bind lipid ligands. It has therefore been proposed that P_2 may be involved in transport of fatty acids into Schwann cells[8]. However, its location in compact myelin suggests that P_2 probably fulfils a function in the maintenance of myelin structure. Other minor protein components which are not seen on Coomassie blue staining of gels have been found in PNS myelin. The myelin-associated glycoprotein (MAG, M_r approx. 100 000), which accounts for less than 0.1% of total PNS myelin proteins, is the major glycoprotein of CNS myelin, representing 0.5–1% of the proteins. Like P_0, MAG belongs to the immunoglobulin gene superfamily consisting of one V-like and four C2-like Ig-domains[9]. Human MAG possesses nine potential N-glycosylation sites[10,11], for a calculated peptide molecular weight of 69 100, and contains 30% of carbohydrate by weight[12]. In PNS myelin sheaths, MAG is localized in the periaxonal space, the outer mesaxon, the Schmidt–Lanterman incisures, and the paranodal loops[13]. This localization suggests that MAG is involved in glia–neuron and in glia–glia interactions[12]. The glia–neuron adhesive function of MAG has been recently demonstrated *in vitro*[14]. The expression of MAG occurs early in the myelination process and is regulated by the axon–Schwann cell contact[15]. Experiments carried out by using Schwann cells infected with recombinant retrovirus to introduce either MAG cDNA[16] or MAG antisense RNA[17] have shown that MAG is implicated in the early myelination process by promoting the initial investment of the axon by the myelinating Schwann cell. However, the axonal receptor for MAG remains to be identified. Human MAG bears the L2/HNK-1 carbohydrate epitope, which has been implicated in cell–cell interactions[18,19]. This epitope is also present in other PNS myelin components such as P_0 and the two acidic glycolipids SGPG and SGLPG.

THE BLOOD–NERVE BARRIER

In neuropathies of autoimmune origin, the putative pathogenic antibody or T cell has to reach the target antigen in the nervous parenchyma. As is the case in the CNS with its well known blood–brain barrier, PNS tissues are protected from the external environment. The blood vessels and the perineurium display tight junctions (zonulae occludens) located between endothelial cells of endoneurial blood vessels and between the perineurial cells of the perineurium. Together with the apparent lack of vesicular transport, these observations are highly suggestive of a barrier function, restricting the exchange of large molecules, such as serum proteins, as well as of water-soluble substances between blood and nerves. The PNS microenvironment is thus enclosed by a blood–nerve barrier (BNB), which consists of endoneurial blood vessels and the perineurium[20]. Increased permeability of the BNB may play an important role in the pathogenesis of peripheral neuropathies in which humoral factors such as anti-myelin antibodies are likely to play a causative role.

PARAPROTEINAEMIC POLYNEUROPATHY

Clinical aspects

Among the different polyneuropathies, monoclonal gammopathies are statistically prevalent, particularly in cases with late onset[21]. A monoclonal gammopathy is observed in about 10% of all polyneuropathy patients, representing an incidence 6- to 10-fold higher than that found in a control population. In over 50% of patients the neuropathy is associated with a monoclonal gammopathy of undetermined significance (MGUS), a syndrome displaying benign plasma cell dyscrasia with stable production of M protein over many years[21,22]. The remainder of gammopathies are represented by Waldenström's macroglobulinaemia (a malignant proliferation of a B cell clone) or myeloma. In demyelinating PPN, monoclonal IgM (M-IgM) is much more common than is gammopathy of other immunoglobulin classes, and demyelinating PPN with M-IgM is more frequent in MGUS than in Waldenström's disease[23]. Despite the fact that these two conditions present with quite different prognoses, they seem to damage peripheral nerves in a similar way.

Most patients are males, 40–75 years of age, and neurological signs are usually observed before the gammopathy is detected[24]. Most cases of demyelinating PPN with M-IgM fall into an homogeneous group with well described clinical features[25–29]. Sensory symptoms, consisting of paraesthesias, are usually prominent, accompanied by objective evidence of distal symmetrical sensory loss. About 75% of patients first present with sensory symptoms which, in about half these, are limited to the lower limbs. The neuropathy commonly starts insidiously or subacutely with numbness and paraesthesias in the hands and feet and progresses proximally. Most of the time the disease is painless. Motor signs usually may appear later and are slowly progressive. In about 20% of cases motor function is totally preserved, but when motor deficits do appear, severe muscle wasting may occur in both upper and lower extremities. In some patients, fasciculations have been observed. Footdrop and steppage gait are common, and occasionally motor weakness may proceed to almost total paralysis of limbs. Cranial nerves and autonomic functions usually remain intact, although electrophysiological studies may reveal subclinical involvement. The neurological progression rate in demyelinating PPN with M-IgM directed against myelin is about half that seen in PPN with M-IgM directed against axonal antigen(s)[30]. In PPN with anti-MAG M-IgM, nerve conduction studies show prominent distal slowing: this feature may be useful for selecting patients for specific immunological studies[31].

Some patients with PPN and M-IgM present with distinct diseases, the antibody activity being directed against various gangliosides[32–39]. In such cases, motor symptoms are dominant, mainly as a result of axonal damage. In at least 60% of patients with PPN and IgM gammopathy[33,40,41], the M-IgM reacts with the carbohydrate moiety of MAG[42–44] and P_0[4]. The epitope is also present on two acidic glycolipids occurring in the PNS that have been identified as SGPG and SGLPG[45,46]. Since the first antigen to be identified for these M-IgM was MAG[47], this disease is often referred to as demyelinating polyneuropathy with anti-MAG antibodies.

The annual incidence of PPN with anti-MAG M-IgM has been estimated as 1–5/10 000 of the adult population[48]. The disease is slowly progressive, and remissions with treatment are most unusual. Intringuingly, the clinical condition of patients does not correlate with serum M-IgM concentration or the M-IgM anti-MAG antibody titre[41,49]. There is a similar lack of correlation between the severity of the neuropathy and the affinity of the M-IgM for MAG or SGPG[50]. However, the monoclonal protein (M-protein) appears to play a direct role in the pathogenesis of these neuropathies[26,34,47,51,52].

Pathology of PPN with anti-MAG antibodies

Nerve biopsy usually reveals demyelinating lesions with remyelination and sometimes axonal damage of variable severity[41]. The myelin sheaths are thinner than normal, and segmental demyelination is observed in teased single-fibre preparations. After some years of progression, numerous figures of concentric Schwann cell proliferation, referred to as 'onion bulbs' are observed[26]. Hypermyelinated fibres have been sometimes observed[53]. Two additional features characteristic of PPN with anti-MAG M-IgM are deposits of M-IgM on the myelinated sheaths, and an ultrastructural alteration,

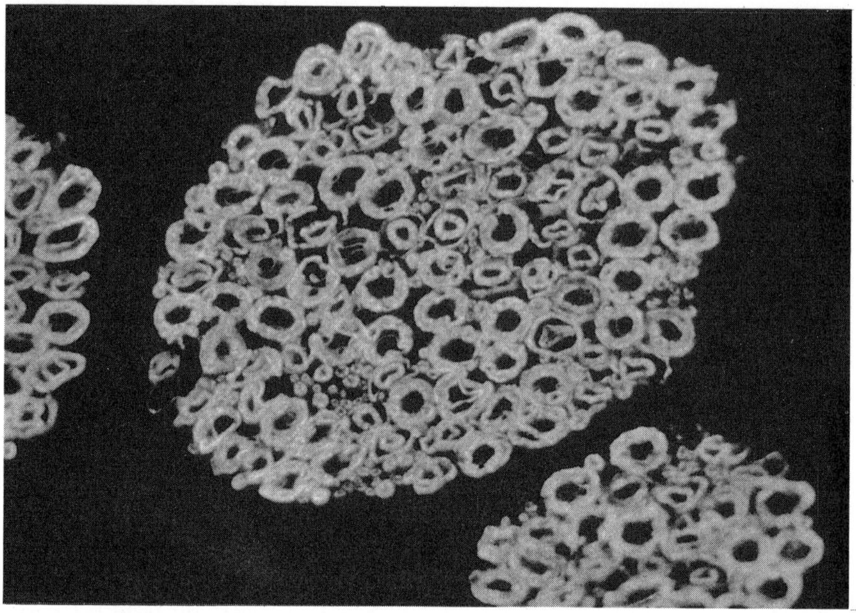

Figure 2.1 Indirect immunofluorescence staining of normal human peripheral nerve section by anti-myelin-associated glycoprotein M-IgM from a patient with paraproteinaemic polyneuropathy. Antibodies bind specifically to myelin sheaths and not to axons

consisting of a widening of myelin lamellae in peripheral nerves with a 23 nm spacing between the separated leaflets of the intermediate line.

M-IgM deposits on the affected nerve were first observed in biopsy material by direct immunofluorescence, using fluorescent anti-immunoglobulin[25,54], or immunohistochemically, using peroxidase–anti-peroxidase staining of paraffin-embedded sections[55]. More recently, M-IgM deposits were demonstrated within the compact myelin using direct electron microscopic immunocytochemical techniques[56]. Indirect immunofluorescence or immunoperoxidase techniques demonstrate fixation of M-IgM on myelin sheaths of normal peripheral nerves and lumbar roots[30,57,58]. Figure 2.1 shows immunofluorescence-labelled M-IgM strongly attached to the normal compact myelin sheaths. No labelling is observed in the axons. Direct immunofluorescence examination shows specific binding of μ, κ or λ chains on a variable number of myelinated fibres in nerve biopsies from afflicted patients. In most cases the M-IgM light chain is of the κ type.

Ultrastructurally, normal myelin appears as an ordered structure of stacked membrane leaflets with alternating dense lines, representing the cytoplasmic part (major dense line), and intermediate lines, representing the extracellular part (minor dense line). Patients with PPN and anti-MAG antibodies show a widening of myelin lamellae (Figure 2.2): the intermediate lines disappear and the major dense lines which remain intact are separated by abnormally large spaces of 23 nm, that may contain some granular materials[41,59] or orderly criss-crossed organization[60]. The widening of myelin lamellae is often

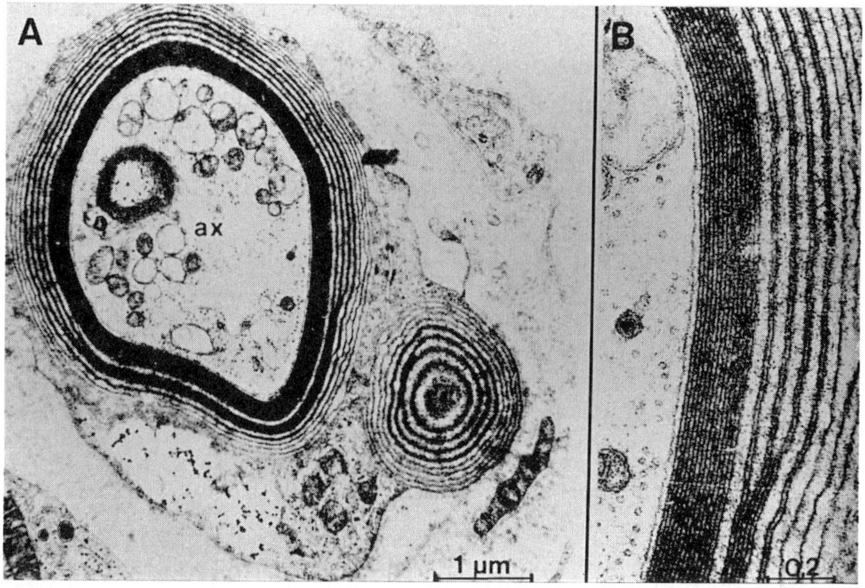

Figure 2.2 Electron micrograph of a sural nerve biopsy from a patient with paraproteinaemic polyneuropathy and anti-myelin-associated glycoprotein M-IgM. (A) Pathologically myelinated axon; (B) larger magnification showing the widening of the external myelin lamellae at the level of the intraperiod line (ax = axon). Reproduced by permission from *Neurology*[24] (Journal copyright 1983)

observed in remyelinating fibres[53], and is usually observed in the external leaflets, where only the outermost lamella can be dilated. However, widening in the middle or both internal and external parts of myelin sheaths has also been observed[41,59]. Generally, high magnification electron microscopy is required to detect only few abnormalities[59]. Widening of the myelin lamellae is reported to occur in 50% of patients with PPN and M-IgM, and in more than 90% of those with PPN and anti-MAG M-IgM[41]. The widening of myelin lamellae has been attributed to the incorporation of M-IgM into the myelin sheaths[54] and/or to myelin overhydration[59].

Patient management

Plasmapheresis and chemotherapy are usually used to treat patients with PPN. Individually, these treatments seem to be inefficient in most cases[27,58,61]. When applied intensively, plasma exchanges alone can result in patient improvement: Mussini *et al.*[62] obtained improvement in six of seven patients, and Haas *et al.*[63] in one patient. For maximum effectiveness, plasmapheresis and immunosuppressive treatment are often combined, although no consensus has been obtained concerning the efficiency of this treatment programme. Responses showed intraindividual variation: some patients show no change, others experience rapid improvement of clinical and electrophysiological signs, although these relapse when treatment is stopped[64]. A combination of corticosteroids and chlorambucil treatment, with or without plasmapheresis[58,65,66] may produce improvement after some months of treatment. A correlation between the reduction in circulating M-IgM concentration and clinical condition has been described in two patients[66].

Role of M-IgM in the pathogenesis

Although plasmapheresis may not produce a systematic improvement in PPN patients, a causative role for anti-MAG M-IgM in the disorder is strongly suggested by the finding of deposits of the corresponding class of heavy and light chain within the myelin of the affected nerve[67]. Deposits of the terminal complement complex (C1q, C3d, and C5), corresponding to the sites of myelin lamellae widening, have been demonstrated by direct and indirect immunofluorescence and immunoperoxidase assays[68,69]. Despite the above observations, some authors suggest that the secretion of circulating M-IgM is a secondary response to a primary damage of the nerve[28,67]. In this case, the chronic stimulation by nerve (myelin) antigens is suggested to be the origin of IgM[70], which would cross the BNB passively, accumulating on the damaged nerve[71].

More frequently, the pathogenesis of PPN with anti-MAG M-IgM is attributed to an autoimmune mechanism in which the M-IgM is the primary factor inducing myelin (nerve) damage[65,72,73]. Current evidence obtained in animal models strongly argues in favour of this hypothesis. First, the systemic transfusion of patients' M-IgM into chickens produces the characteristic widening of the myelin lamellae[74]. Second, M-IgM deposits are observed in close contact with myelin sheaths following a short period of passive transfer of human anti-MAG M-IgM into the marmoset, although clinical signs are not observed[75]. Third, intraneural injection of purified anti-MAG M-IgM and complement into feline sciatic nerve causes focal demyelination[76] and induces progressive conduction blocks[77]. In the latter case it should be noted that patient serum causes extensive inflammatory, macrophage-mediated demyelination of the feline peripheral nerve, a pathological change that bears little resemblance to that seen in human PPN[78]. Therefore, it is generally accepted that, in demyelinating PPN with anti-MAG M-IgM, following an unidentified stimulation, naturally occurring B cells secreting IgM directed against myelin proliferate and secrete large amounts of anti-myelin M-IgM[79,80]. The secreted M-IgM may reach the nerve tissue by crossing the damaged BNB[67]. The nervous lesion could be produced directly by the M-IgM[29] or by secondary complex deposits[65]. Anti-myelin IgM could also interfere with the turnover of myelin and induce secondary demyelination[72]. The autoimmune hypothesis outlined above raises three main questions (Figure 2.3):

(1) Which factors or conditions are responsible for the proliferation of anti-MAG M-IgM secreting B cell clones?

(2) How does the M-IgM cross the blood–nerve barrier (BNB) to reach their PNS targets?

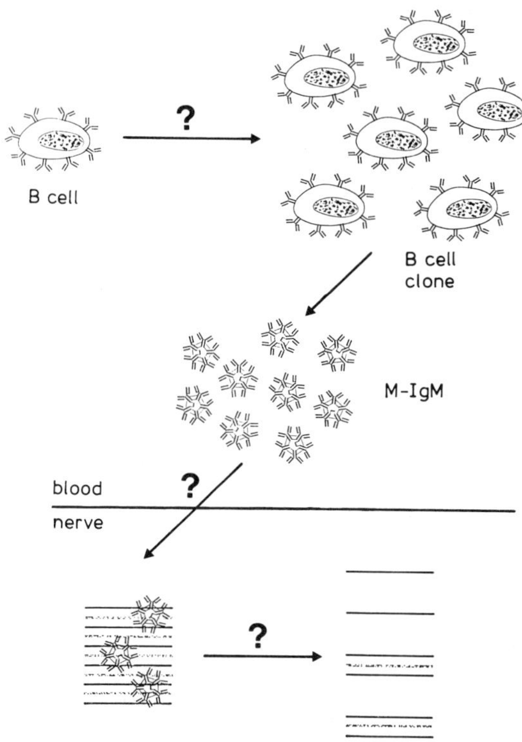

Figure 2.3 Scheme of the pathogenesis of paraproteinaemic neuropathy with anti-myelin-associated glycoprotein (MAG) M-IgM. Unidentified factors are responsible for the proliferation of a B cell clone which secretes anti-MAG M-IgM. The M-IgM cross the blood–nerve barrier by an unknown mechanism to reach their targets within the myelin sheath where they produce the 23 nm widening of the lamellae at the intermediate line

(3) How do these particular immunoglobulins produce such singular abnormalities of myelin structure as the 23 nm spacing of the lamellae at the intermediate line?

As part of our investigations on demyelinating PPN, we have focused our attention on the second question; namely, the mechanism by which anti-MAG M-IgM crosses the BNB. Despite the high concentrations of circulating anti-MAG M-IgM in demyelinating PPN (5–20 mg/ml in MGUS), only a small fraction of the total M-IgM seems to penetrate the BNB. This fact argues against physical damage to or rupture of the BNB, which would be expected to produce a drastic infiltration of the nerve by the antibody. On the other hand, there is no correlation between the circulating level and/or the titre of the antibody and the clinical condition in most patients, suggesting that myelin is not accessible to the whole pool of anti-MAG M-IgM, but that the antibody that is able to cross the BNB is pathogenic. However, the anti-MAG IgM are monoclonal antibodies, i.e., structurally and chemically homogeneous molecules, and the only molecular diversity to be found is in

Table 2.2 Relative occurrence of IgM [^{14}C]glycopeptide fractions

Type of oligosaccharide structure	*Relative occurrence (% of total)* IgM normal	M-IgM paraproteinaemic polyneuropathies	M-IgM Waldenström
Tri- and/or tetra-antennary (total)	34.3	38.0	24.1
Fully sialylated	1.5	0.0	0.3
With core fucose	25.8	33.8	21.8
With α(2-3)sialic acid	1.0	0.8	0.0
Biantennary (total)	28.4	22.0	36.2
With core fucose	16.4	11.4	30.8
With α(2-3)sialic acid	0.0	0.0	0.0
High mannose and/or hybrid (total)	37.3	40.0	39.7
With core fucose	3.3	3.3	8.4
With α(2-3)sialic acid	1.8	0.0	0.4

the heterogeneity and microheterogeneity of their oligosaccharide structures. IgM possesses five N-glycosylation sites on each heavy chain[81], and one on the J chain[82]. Interactions between carbohydrates and carbohydrate receptors have recently been shown to be important for the interaction and extravasation of a number of inflammatory cells through vascular endothelium. One can hypothesize that carbohydrate–selectin interaction(s) may play a role in the crossing of the BNB by the neuropathogenic M-IgM. This transvascular shift may, for example, be mediated by endothelial cell expression of cell surface carbohydrate receptors[83]. M-IgM bearing a particular carbohydrate structure may be able to interact with an endothelial cell selectin, which may facilitate crossing of the BNB to reach and damage nerve tissues. In agreement with this hypothesis, in a preliminary analysis of IgM [^{14}C]glycopeptides (D. Burger, unpublished data), we have observed some structural differences between oligosaccharides of M-IgM from a patient with PPN, from a patient with Waldenström's macroglobulinaemia without neurological signs, and normal IgM (from a pool of 15 normal sera). As shown in Table 2.2 the proportion of tri- and/or tetra-antennary oligosaccharides is enhanced in the M-IgM of the PPN patient. Sialylated structures are slightly diminished in PPN patient M-IgM and some differences are also observed in the proportion of core fucosylated structures. Interestingly, enhancement of branching (increased tri- and/or tetra-antennary compared to biantennary oligosaccharides) is often observed in neoplastic cells of both murine and human origin, and seems to be associated with metastatic potential[84,85], which requires the tumour cell to cross the vascular endothelial cell layer to invade target tissue. However, whether these structural differences account for the pathogenicity of a particular anti-MAG M-IgM pool in patients with PPN remains to be determined.

Structure of the carbohydrate epitope

The epitope recognized by patient M-IgM on MAG, P_0 and glycolipids is also recognized by the mouse monoclonal IgM HNK-1[86,87] raised against human natural killer cells[88]. However, it seems probable that the anti-MAG M-IgM does not recognize natural killer cells, since it displays a lower affinity for these cells than does mouse M-IgM[89]. The results obtained by Chou *et al.*[45], together with the fact that human M-IgM binds other glycoproteins that are not recognized by HNK-1[90], suggest that the epitopes recognized by HNK-1 and human M-IgM are closely related but may be different. Other monoclonal antibodies from rat have also been raised against the same epitope, which is now referred to as L2/HNK-1[18]. Structural characterization and chemical modifications of the carbohydrate moiety of SGPG allowed the identification of the sulphated glucuronic acid as an important determinant for the binding of the antibodies belonging to the L2/HNK-1 family[45,46,91]. Although the presence of sulphate groups in the carbohydrate moiety of both MAG and P_0 was demonstrated earlier[92,93], the presence of glucuronic acid residues in the oligosaccharide structures of glycoproteins bearing the L2/HNK-1 epitope has only been clearly demonstrated in the ependymins of fish brain[94]. The presence of sulphate on these glucuronic acid residues has not been directly demonstrated. Other attempts have also failed to demonstrate the presence of a sulphated glucuronic acid residue in N-linked oligosaccharides of bovine P_0[95], human P_0[96] or whole murine brains[97]. The removal of sialic acids and sulphate groups by neuraminidase and methanolysis neutralizes > 95% of oligosaccharide structures of L2/HNK-1-positive human P_0, suggesting that glucuronic acid is absent from these structures[96]. It seems, therefore, that the L2/HNK-1 epitope in glycoproteins is definitely different from that in glycolipids, since it may lack the glucuronic acid residue. Recently, our attention has been focused on the oligosaccharide structures that bear the L2/HNK-1 epitope in human MAG and P_0. In one study[98] we found that the epitope for HNK-1 and M-IgM is borne by complex and hybrid types of N-linked oligosaccharide structures on MAG and P_0. The N-linked oligosaccharides possess a common pentasaccharide core with the structure Manα1-3(Manα1-6)Manβ1-4GlcNacβ1-4GlcNAcβ1-N-Asn. As a function of the sugar residues added to this core structure three different types of oligosaccharides can occur: high mannose type structures that contain exclusively additional mannose residues; complex structures containing additional residues such as N-acetylglucosamine, galactose, fucose and sialic acid; and hybrid types of these two structures. Taking advantage of the fact that N-linked oligosaccharide structures display different affinities for lectins, we have used serial lectin affinity chromatography to characterize the N-linked oligosaccharide structures of human MAG and P_0[99] and to identify the structures bearing the epitope for human M-IgM and HNK-1[100]. Both these studies have shown that the L2/HNK-1 epitope is mainly, or exclusively, borne by oligosaccharide structures with an α(1-6)fucose residue in the core in MAG and in P_0. This result has been confirmed by Field *et al.*[96], who showed a high degree of fucosylation in L2/HNK-1-positive N-oligosaccharides of human P_0. The L2/HNK-1 epitope is not present, however, on all the fucosylated structures of MAG and P_0. Considering that sulphation occurs after fucosylation of P_0 oligosaccharides[101], the α(1-6)fucose residue may affect the processing of the sulphated antigenic residue(s), perhaps by acting as a 'no-go, go' signal[102] for a glycosyltransferase responsible for epitope synthesis. Nevertheless, the fact that all fucosylated structures do not bear the epitope suggests that other control mechanisms or signals may affect epitope synthesis. Comparison of oligosaccharide structures of human MAG and P_0[99] showed that, in spite of wide structural heterogeneity, the oligosaccharide content of the glycoproteins is homologous to an extent that may reflect similarities in their functions in the myelination process and the maintenance of myelin structure. However, in these analyses, we assigned oligosaccharide structures to glycopeptide fractions as a function of their behaviour on lectin affinity columns[103]. Since then, a comparative analysis of bovine and human P_0 has shown that both glycoproteins bear very similar oligosaccharide structures (D. Burger and K. Uyemura, unpublished results); mainly hybrid type structures, as demonstrated by mass spectrometry[95]. These results, together with those recently published by Field *et al.*[96], indicate that the major oligosaccharide structures present on P_0 are of the hybrid type and that these structures may be multiply sulphated. Therefore, we now suggest that the major human P_0 oligosaccharide structures (P_0 fraction A′, in reference 99) are probably of the multisulphated hybrid type. By analogy, we hypothesize that MAG glycopeptides interacting with lectins in a similar manner to P_0 glycopeptide fraction A′ (dMAG fractions A′ in reference 99) probably bear multisulphated hybrid type oligosaccharides rather than the bisected biantennary structures that we previously suggested[99]. In MAG and P_0, the L2/HNK-1 epitope seems to be present on multisulphated structures with an α(1-6)fucose residue in the core and lacking the glucuronic acid residue. Whether the α(1-6)fucose residue and/or the sulphate groups are involved in the antibody binding site remains to be determined.

In the nervous system, a number of glycoproteins involved in cellular recognition and/or adhesion share common carbohydrate structures, including the L2/HNK-1 epitope[18]. These carbohydrate epitopes are well conserved during evolution[104], suggesting that they play an important functional role in the development and maintenance of the nervous system. The L2/HNK-1 carbohydrate epitope is present mainly, if not exclusively, in molecules such as MAG, P_0, L1, NILE, Ng-CAM, N-CAM, J1, hexabrachion, tenascin, cytotactin, F11, cytotactin receptor, and integrin, which are involved in adhesion[18]. Recent evidence supports the idea that the L2/HNK-1 epitope acts as a ligand in cell adhesion[105,106]. However, whether the carbohydrate moiety is implicated in the recognition and/or adhesion function of MAG, P_0, and other neural cell adhesion molecules remains to be determined.

Diversity of the fine specificity of anti-MAG M-IgM

Although most, if not all, anti-MAG M-IgM recognize the same carbohydrate epitope(s) related to the L2/HNK-1 epitope, some heterogeneity has been observed in their specificity and affinity. Studies carried out with chemically modified SGPG have shown that M-IgM display subtle distinct specificities[45,91,107]. The diversity of anti-MAG antibodies is also indicated by their differential immunostaining patterns on avian embryonic tissues[108] and by the fact that they display various affinities for glycoprotein and glycolipid antigens[50,109]. The search for a 'public' idiotype has been proven particularly difficult, since both polyclonal and monoclonal anti-idiotypic antibodies to anti-MAG M-IgM rarely share idiotypic determinants[110–114]. However, it seems that M-IgM do express a public idiotype, as demonstrated with polyclonal antiserum generated in primates[115]. This type of public idiotype would be very helpful in the application of specific immunotherapy. Since evidence suggests that the primary pathological factor in demyelinating PPN is the anti-MAG M-IgM, current therapies are designed to decrease the serum titre of this immunoglobulin. This is generally accomplished by plasmapheresis or by killing autoreactive B cells with immunosuppressive drugs, as described above. This kind of treatment is usually inefficient in PPN[116], and problems with drug resistance and toxic side-effects due to interaction with normal tissue also limit the clinical effectiveness of chemotherapy. The development of more selective immunosuppressive therapy is therefore important. Since B cell malignancies are usually monoclonal, the idiotype of the surface immunoglobulin of each clone is unique to the individual and can be viewed as a tumour-specific antigen. Hence anti-idiotypic antibodies represent ideal targeting vehicles for guiding toxic agents to B cells[117]. Highly toxic proteins, generally derived from plant, fungi, or bacteria, can be bound covalently to monoclonal anti-idiotypic antibodies, to produce immunotoxins that combine the extreme potency of the toxin with the selectivity of the ligand. Current experiments carried out in our laboratory are designed to investigate the efficiency and specificity of such an immunotoxin against immortalized patient B cells (S. Bourdenet-Picasso, D. Burger and A. J. Steck, unpublished results).

Main target antigen

Since different antigenic targets have been identified, the question arises of the identity of the major target, or the target which is first recognized by the pathogenic M-IgM. The localization of the different targets within the peripheral myelin sheath is well established. MAG is mainly present in 'semi-compact' myelin membranes that have a gap of 12–14 nm between extracellular leaflets and a spacing of 5 nm or more between cytoplasmic leaflets (Schmidt–Lanterman incisures, the periaxonal space, the outer mesaxon, and the paranodal myelin loops)[13]. P_0 is present in compact multilamellar myelin[118]. The two glycolipids, SGPG and SGLPG, are present in myelinated fibres in myelin and axolemma[1]. However, their precise localization within the myelin sheath by immunocytochemical methods is hampered by the cross-reaction of anti-SGPG/SGLPG antibodies with MAG and P_0. In addition to the localization of the antigen, the affinity of M-IgM for the antigen may play a role in the pathogenesis of PPN. It has been shown that M-IgM display affinities for MAG that are 10- to 100-fold higher than those for P_0[119].

Different experimental approaches have been used to identify the main antigen target in demyelinating PPN. Mouse monoclonal antibody to MAG produces widening of myelin lamellae and vesiculation when injected into guinea pig optic nerve[120], a central nervous system site that contains neither P_0 nor SGPG. This study demonstrates that MAG is an effective target for inducing demyelinating features comparable to those observed in PPN. Another study has shown that when SGPG and SGLPG are the only available target, for example, in rat peripheral nerve, anti-SGPG antiserum is able to produce demyelination, along with mild to moderate clinical symptoms[121]. However, in this latter study, although myelin vesiculation was observed, the typical widening of myelin lamellae was not induced, and, as with intraneural injection of human M-IgM into feline sciatic nerve, after a few days, extensive inflammatory and macrophage-mediated demyelination was observed. This type of pathology bears little resemblance to that seen in human PPN.

These two studies seem to exclude P_0 as a major target antigen in PPN with anti-MAG M-IgM. However, the fact that deposits of M-IgM occur within compact myelin *in vivo*[56] may be indicative for a role of P_0 as a potential important target antigen. Indeed, P_0, by interacting with itself, is probably responsible for myelin compaction at the level of the intermediate line in PNS[5–7]. One can therefore hypothesize that the pathogenic M-IgM, by interacting with the L2/HNK-1 epitope on P_0, could account for the maintenance of the 23 nm spacing between myelin leaflets in patients, and that the criss-crossed structures observed in the abnormally wide intermediate line could represent the 'adhesive' M-IgM. In fact, the diameter of an IgM molecule is about 20 nm – a range that fits well with the 23 nm widening observed in PPN. Taken together, these studies indicate that MAG, P_0 and the glycolipids SGPG and SGLPG could play a role in the pathogenesis of PPN with anti-MAG M-IgM.

ACUTE AND CHRONIC INFLAMMATORY DEMYELINATING POLYNEUROPATHIES

Since GBS and CIDP are the subjects of another chapter in this book, here we will merely point out the studies concerned with anti-myelin antibodies in these inflammatory demyelinating diseases of the PNS.

Anti-myelin antibodies in GBS

As has been proposed in the case of multiple sclerosis, it is generally accepted that Guillain–Barré syndrome (GBS) is also an autoimmune disease mediated by T cells reactive against myelin antigens. Because of its neuritogenic properties in experimental allergic neuritis, P_2 is considered to be the major T cell antigen in GBS. In addition to cellular autoimmunity, humoral demyelinating factors have also been demonstrated in GBS by various techniques, but their role as primary pathogenic agents remains uncertain. However, several lines of evidence indicate that anti-myelin antibodies may play a subsidiary immunopathogenic role in GBS. First, antibodies against

Table 2.3 Antibodies against myelin or myelin containing tissues in Guillain–Barré syndrome (GBS)

		Positive (%)		
Antigen	*Method*	*GBS*	*Controls and other neurological diseases*	*Reference*
Human spinal cord	Complement fixation	50.0	4.3	122
Dorsal root ganglion	Tissue culture	83.9	31.5	123
Myelin, spinal cord, peripheral nervous system	Immunofluorescence	66.7	2.2	124
Peripheral nervous system	Antiglobulin consumption	50.0	10.0	125
Peripheral nervous system	Complement fixation	27.3	6.5	126
Human myelin	Complement fixation	11.8	0.2	127
Rabbit myelin	Complement fixation	29.4	0.0	127
Human optic nerve	Complement fixation	11.0	2.0	128
Human sciatic nerve	Complement fixation	7.0	1.0	128
Rabbit sciatic nerve	Complement fixation	7.0	0.0	128
Lumbar nerve root	Complement fixation, mixed haemagglutination	83.3	0.0	129
Sciatic nerve	Mixed haemagglutination, immunofluorescence	68.8	4.4	130
Human peripheral nerve myelin	C1 fixation	91.7	27.3	131
Human peripheral nerve myelin	C1 fixation	100.0	0.0	132
Human peripheral nerve myelin	Enzyme-linked immunosorbent assay	59.0	7.9	133

myelin or myelin-containing tissues are found more frequently in patients with GBS than in normal subjects or in patients with other neurological diseases (Table 2.3). Second, antibody titre is maximal at the onset of the disease[131] and decreases in parallel with clinical improvement in untreated patients[134]. Third, beneficial responses to plasma exchange are often observed in the first few weeks of the disease[135,136]. Fourth, endoneurial injection of acute-phase patient serum into rat sciatic nerve produces focal demyelination[137–139] and conduction block[140]. Finally, acute phase GBS serum induces *in vitro* complement-dependent demyelination, the degree of which is a function of the anti-peripheral myelin antibody titre[141].

Numerous studies have attempted to identify the putative target antigen in GBS: those concerned with anti-myelin antibodies are summarized in Table 2.4. Various results have been obtained using the different antigens. In a study using galactocerebroside as an antigen, antibodies were detected in 17 GBS patients in one study[127], but in none of 100 patients in another study[128]. Inconsistent results have also been found with antibodies directed against P_2, which have been reported in 0.6–100% of GBS patients[127,142–144]. Some discrepancies are also observed in the proportion of GBS patients with anti-ganglioside antibodies or anti-sulphatide antibodies (Table 2.4). Such variations may be due to the technique used to detect the antibody, the origin of the antigen (for example, the response to

Table 2.4 Antibodies against myelin antigens in Guillain–Barré syndrome (GBS)

Antigen	*Method*	*Positive (%)* GBS	*Positive (%)* Controls and other neurological diseases	*Reference*
Galactocerebroside	Complement fixation	11.8	0.2	127
Galactocerebroside	Complement fixation	0.0	0.0	128
P_2 (bovine)	$[^{125}I]P_2$ binding	0.6	0.0	126
P_2 (bovine)	Enzyme-linked immunosorbent assay	5.3	0.0	142
P_2 (bovine)	Enzyme-linked immunosorbent assay	54.5	9.4	143
P_2 (human)	Direct plaque-forming cell assay	100.0	0.0	144
Gangliosides	Enzyme-linked immunosorbent assay	19.2	0.0	36
GM1	Enzyme-linked immunosorbent assay, thin layer chromatography immunostaining	28.3	1.8	145
Neutral myelin glycolipid, Forssman-like antigen	C1 fixation, thin layer chromatography immunostaining	100.0	33.3	146
SGPG	Enzyme-linked immunosorbent assay	25.0	9.0	147
Sulphatide	Enzyme-linked immunosorbent assay	21.0	6.5	147
LM1	Thin layer chromatography–enzyme-linked immunosorbent assay	43.0	20.0	148
Sulphatide	Thin layer chromatography–enzyme-linked immunosorbent assay	65.0	15.0	148

human P_2 is greater than that to bovine P_2 (Table 2.4)), the phase of the disease when the serum was taken (sera of patients obtained during the acute phase display greater demyelinating activity than those obtained during the recovery phase), and the choice of the antigen. The studies to date have produced a wide spectrum of results and have not clarified the nature of the main target antigen (if there is but one) for antibodies in GBS.

Anti-myelin antibodies in CIDP

CIDP is a demyelinating disease which is distinguishable from GBS by clinical criteria[149] and by the fact that it presents with less prominent inflammation[150]. As is the case for multiple sclerosis, CIDP may be subacute, chronic progressive, or remitting[151]. Since plasmapheresis, with or without immunosuppression, is the current treatment of choice, and produces

Table 2.5 Antibodies against myelin antigens or myelin containing tissues in chronic inflammatory demyelinating polyneuropathy (CIDP)

		Positive (%)		
Antigen	*Method*	*GBS*	*Controls and other neurological diseases*	*Reference*
Human peripheral nerve myelin	C1 fixation	75.0	27.3	131
Human peripheral nerve myelin	Enzyme-linked immunosorbent assay	51.0	7.9	132
P_2	$[^{125}I]$-P_2 binding	0.9	0.0	127
Galactocerebroside	Complement fixation	0.9	0.9	127
LM1	Thin layer chromatography–enzyme-linked immunosorbent assay	67.0	20.0	133
Sulphatide	Thin layer chromatography–enzyme-linked immunosorbent assay	87.0	15.0	133
SGPG	Enzyme-linked immunosorbent assay and thin layer chromatography	0.1	9.0	147
Sulphatide	Enzyme-linked immunosorbent assay and thin layer chromatography	0.1	6.5	147
GM1	Thin layer chromatography–enzyme-linked immunosorbent assay	67.0	68.0	153

improvement in 30–60% of patients[152], humoral factors seem to be implicated. The search for a humoral pathogenic factor has focused on myelin tissues and myelin antigens (Table 2.5). In the relatively few studies that have attempted to identify the target antigen in CIDP, the incidence of anti-myelin antibody was 3- to 6-fold higher than in controls, suggesting a role for these antibodies in the pathogenesis of the disease. However, as is the case for GBS, the main target antigen(s) for autoantibodies in CIDP remains to be determined.

CONCLUSION

Most of the antibodies implicated in the pathogenesis of demyelinating neuropathies of autoimmune origin are directed against carbohydrate epitopes, with the exception of those directed against the basic protein P_2, which are detected in some GBS and CIDP patients. Usually, the immune system displays distinct reactivities against carbohydrates or proteins. The carbohydrates are mostly recognized by B cells, whereas proteins are usually recognized by both T and B cells. However, T cell responses may be observed against glycoconjugates, although activation of T cells by the carbohydrate carrier (i.e. the protein) is required. The antibody response to a carbohydrate epitope is therefore dependent upon its carrier and upon the presence of B and/or T cells able to recognize the glycoconjugate. T cells do not seem to be implicated in the pathogenesis of PPN, and inflammatory features are therefore mild or absent. In GBS and CIDP, however, inflammation is the main pathological finding, but this does not preclude convergence of both humoral and cellular autoimmune response, as recently pointed out by Hartung and Toyka[154].

ACKNOWLEDGEMENTS

The experiments reported here were carried out with the support of the Swiss National Science Foundation, the Swiss Multiple Sclerosis Society and the Roche Research Foundation.

References

1. Ariga T, Kusunoki S, Asano K *et al.* Localization of sulfated glucuronyl glycolipids in human dorsal root and sympathetic ganglia. Brain Res. 1990;519:57–64.
2. Greenfield S, Brostoff S, Eylar EH, Morell P. Protein composition of myelin of the peripheral nervous system. J Neurochem. 1973;20:1207–16.
3. Hayasaka K, Nanao K, Tahara M *et al.* Isolation and sequence determination of cDNA encoding the major structural protein of human peripheral myelin. Biochem Biophys Res Commun. 1991;180:515–18
4. Bollensen E, Steck AJ, Schachner M. Reactivity with the peripheral myelin glycoprotein P_0 in sera from patients with IgM monoclonal gammopathy and polyneuropathy. Neurology. 1988;38:1266–70.
5. Filbin MT, Walsh FS, Trapp BD, Pizzey JA, Tennekoon GI. Role of myelin P_O protein as a homophilic adhesion molecule. Nature. 1990;344:871–2.
6. D'Urso D, Brophy PJ, Staugaitis SM *et al.* Protein zero of peripheral nerve myelin: biosynthesis, membrane insertion, and evidence for homotypic interaction. Neuron. 1990;2:e449–60.
7. Schneider-Schaulies J, von Brunn A, Schachner M. Recombinant peripheral myelin protein P_0 confers both adhesion and neurite outgrowth-promoting properties. J Neurosci Res. 1990;27:286–97.
8. Jones TA, Bergfors T, Sedzik U, Unge T. The three dimensional structures of P_2 myelin protein. EMBO J. 1988;7:1597–604.
9. Pedraza L, Owens GC, Green LAD, Salzer JL. The myelin-associated glycoprotein: membrane disposition, evidence of a novel disulfide linkage between immunoglobulin-like domains, and posttranslational palmitylation. J Cell Biol. 1990;111:2651–61.
10. Sato S, Fujita N, Kurihara T, Kuwano R, Sakimura K, Takahashi Y, Miyatake T. cDNA cloning and amino acid sequence for human myelin-associated glycoprotein. Biochem Biophys Res Commun. 1989;163:1473–80.
11. Spagnol G, Williams M, Srinivasan J, Golier J, Bauer D, Lebo RV, Latov N. Molecular cloning of human myelin-associated glycoprotein. J Neurosci Res. 1989;24:137–42.
12. Brady RO, Quarles RH. Developmental and pathophysiological aspects of the myelin-associated glycoprotein. Cell Mol Neurobiol. 1988;8:139–48.
13. Trapp BD, Quarles RH. Presence of the myelin-associated glycoprotein correlates with alterations in the periodicity of peripheral myelin. J Cell Biol. 1982;92:877–82.
14. Sadoul R, Fahrig T, Bartsch U, Schachner M. Binding properties of liposomes containing

the myelin-associated glycoprotein MAG to neural cell cultures. J Neurosci Res. 1990;25: 1–13.
15. Owens GC, Bunge RP. Evidence for an early role for myelin-associated glycoprotein in the process of myelination. Glia. 1989;2:119–28.
16. Owens GC, Boyd CJ, Bunge RP, Salzer JL. Expression of recombinant myelin-associated glycoprotein in primary Schwann cells promotes the initial investment of axons by myelinating Schwann cells. J Cell Biol. 1990;111:1171–82.
17. Owens GC, Bunge RP. Schwann cells infected with a recombinant retrovirus expressing myelin-associated glycoprotein antisense RNA do not form myelin. Neuron. 1991;7: 565–75.
18. Schachner M. Families of neural adhesion molecules. In: Carbohydrate recognition in cellular function. Ciba Foundation Symposium 145. Chichester: John Wiley & Son, 1989: 156–68.
19. Margolis RK, Ripellino JA, Goosen B, Steinbrich R, Margolis RV. Occurrence of the HNK-1 epitope (3-sulfoglucuronic acid) in PC 12 pheochromocytoma cells, chromaffin granule membranes, and chondroitin sulfate proteoglycans. Biochem Biophys Res Commun. 1987;145:1142–8.
20. Olsson Y. Microenvironment of the peripheral nervous system under normal and pathological conditions. Crit Rev Neurobiol. 1990;5:265–311.
21. Kelly JJ, Kyle RA, Miles JM, O'Brien PC, Dyck PJ. The spectrum of peripheral neuropathy in myeloma. Neurology. 1981;31:24–31.
22. Kyle RA. Monoclonal gammopathy of undetermined significance: Natural history of 241 cases. Am J Med. 1978;64:814–26.
23. Kelly JJ, Kyle RA, O'Brien PC, Dyck PJ. Prevalence of monoclonal protein in peripheral neuropathy. Neurology. 1981;31:1480–3.
24. Steck AJ, Murray N, Meier C, Page N, Perruisseau G. Demyelinating neuropathy and monoclonal IgM antibody to myelin-associated glycoprotein. Neurology. 1983;33:19–23.
25. Julien J, Vital C, Vallat JM, Lagueny A, Deminiere C, Darriet D. Polyneuropathy in Waldenström's macroglobulinemia. Deposition of M component on myelin sheaths. Arch Neurol. 1978;35:423–5.
26. Latov N, Sherman WH, Nemni R, Galassi G, Shyong J, Penn AS, Chess L, Olarte M, Rowland LP, Osserman EP. Plasma cell dyscrasia and peripheral neuropathy with a monoclonal antibody to peripheral nerve myelin. N Engl J Med. 1980;303:618–21.
27. Melmed C, Frail D, Duncan I, Braun P, Danoff D, Finlayson M, Stewart J. Peripheral neuropathy with IgM kappa monoclonal immunoglobulin directed against myelin associated glycoprotein. Neurology. 1983;33:1397–405.
28. Smith IS, Kahn SN, Lacey BW, King RHM, Eames RA, Whybrew DJ, Thomas PK. Chronic demyelinating neuropathy associated with benign IgM paraproteinaemia. Brain. 1983;106:169–95.
29. Steck AJ, Meier C, Vandavelde M, Regli F. Polyneuropathies et gammapathies: une forme avec anti-glycoproteine MAG. Rev Neurol (Paris). 1984;140:28–36.
30. Dellagi K, Dupouey P, Brouet JC, Billecocq A, Gomez D, Clauvel JP, Seligman M. Waldenström's macroglobulinemia and peripheral neuropathy: a clinical and immunologic study of 25 patients. Blood. 1983;62:280–5.
31. Kaku DA, Sumner AJ. Characteristic electrophysiological findings in anti-MAG polyneuropathy. Neurology. 1992;42(suppl.3):408.
32. Ilyas AA, Quarles RH, Dalakas MC, Fishman PH, Brady RO. Monoclonal IgM in a patient with paraproteinemic neuropathy binds to gangliosides containing disialolsyl groups. Ann Neurol. 1985;18:655–9.
33. Quarles RH, Ilyas AA, Willison HJ. Antibodies to glycolipids in demyelinating diseases of the human peripheral nervous system. Chem Phys Lipids. 1986;42:235–48.
34. Freddo L, Yu RK, Latov N, Donofrio P, Hays AP, Greenberg HS, Albers JW, Allessi AG, Leavitt A, Davar G, Keren D. Gangliosides GM_1 and GD_{1b} are antigens for IgM M-protein in a patient with motor neuron disease. Neurology. 1986;36:454–8.
35. Miyatani N, Baba H, Sato S, Nakamura K, Yuasa T, Miyatake T. Antibody to sialosylactosaminylparagloboside in a patient with IgM paraproteinemia and polyradiculoneuropathy. J Neuroimmunol. 1987;14:189–96.
36. Ilyas AA, Willison HJ. Dalakas MC, Whitaker JN, Quarles RH. Identification and

characterization of gangliosides reacting with IgM paraproteins in three patients with neuropathy associated with biclonal gammopathy. J Neurochem. 1988;51:851–8.
37. Nardelli E, Steck AJ, Barkas T, Schluep M, Jerusalem F. Motor neuron syndrome and monoclonal IgM with antibody activity against gangliosides GM_1 and GD_{1b}. Ann Neurol. 1988;23:524–8.
38. Kusunoki S, Shimizu T, Matsumura K, Maemura K, Mannen T. Motor dominant neuropathy and IgM paraproteinemia: the IgM M-protein binds to specific gangliosides. J Neuroimmunol. 1989;21:177–81.
39. Yuki N, Miyatani N, Sato S, Hirabayashi Y, Yamazaki M, Yoshimura N, Hayashi Y, Miyatake T. Acute relapsing neuropathy associated with IgM antibody against B-series gangliosides containing a GalNAcβ1-4(Gal3-2αNeuAc8-2αNeuAc)β1 configuration. Neurology. 1992;42:686–9.
40. Nobile-Orazio E, Francomano E, Daverio R, Barbieri S, Marmiroli P, Manfredini E, Carpo M, Moggio M, Legname G, Baldini L, Scarlato G. Anti-myelin-associated glycoprotein IgM antibody titers in neuropathy associated with macroglobulinemia. Ann Neurol. 1989;26:543–50.
41. Vital A, Vital C, Julien J, Baquey A, Steck AJ. Polyneuropathy associated with IgM monoclonal gammopathy. Immunological and pathological study in 31 patients. Acta Neuropathol. 1989;79:160–7.
42. Frail DE, Edwards AM, Braum PE. Molecular characteristics of the epitope in myelin-associated glycoprotein that is recognized by a monoclonal IgM in human neuropathy patients. Mol Immunol. 1984;21:721–5.
43. Ilyas AA, Quarles RH, McIntosh TD, Dobersen RJ, Trapp BD, Dalakas MC, Brady RO. IgM in a human neuropathy related to paraproteinemia binds to a carbohydrate determinant in the myelin-associated glycoprotein and to ganglioside. Proc Natl Acad Sci USA. 1984;81:1225–9.
44. Nobile-Orazio E, Hays AP, Latov N, Perman G, Golier J, Shy M, Freddo L. Reactivity of mouse and human monoclonal anti-MAG antibodies: antigenic specificity and immunofluorescence studies. Neurology. 1984;34:1336–42.
45. Chou DKH, Ilyas AA, Evans JE, Quarles RH, Jungalwala FB. Structure of a glycolipid reacting with monoclonal IgM in neuropathy and with HNK-1. Biochem Biophys Res Commun. 1985;128:383–8.
46. Ariga T, Kohriyama T, Freddo L, Latov N, Saito M, Kon K, Ando S, Suzuki M, Hemling ME, Rinehart KL, Kusunoki S, Yu RK. Characterization of sulfated glucuronic acid containing glycolipids reacting with IgM M-proteins in patients with neuropathy. J Biol Chem. 1987;262:846–53.
47. Braun PE, Frail E, Latov N. Myelin-associated glycoprotein is the antigen for a monoclonal IgM in polyneuropathy. J Neurochem. 1982;39:1261–5.
48. Latov N, Hays AP, Sherman WH. Peripheral neuropathy and anti-MAG antibodies. CRC Crit Rev Neurobiol. 1988;3:301–32.
49. Jauberteau MO, Henin D, Bouche P, Vallat JM, Dumas M, Dellagi S, Leger JM, Harpin ML, Ratinahirana H, Chaunu MP, Quarles R, Baumann N. Study of antiglycolipid antibodies in patients with IgM monoclonal dysglobulinemias and peripheral neuropathy. Rev Neurol (Paris). 1988;144:474–80.
50. Brouet JC, Mariette X, Chevalier A, Hauttecoeur B. Determination of the affinity of monoclonal human IgM for myelin-associated glycoprotein and sulfated glucuronic paragloboside. J Neuroimmunol. 1992;36:209–15.
51. Sherman WJ, Latov N, Hays AP, Takatsu M, Nemni R, Galassi G, Osserman EF. Monoclonal IgMk antibody precipitation with chondroitin sulfate C from patients with axonal polyneuropathy and epidermolysis. Neurology. 1983;33:192–201.
52. Ilyas AA, Quarles RH, Dalakas MC, Brady RO. Polyneuropathy with monoclonal gammopathy: glycolipids are frequently antigens for IgM paraprotein. Proc Natl Acad Sci USA. 1985;82:6697–700.
53. Vital C, Pautrizel B, Lagueny Z, Vital A, Bergouignan FX, David B, Loisaue P. Hypermyélinisation dans un cas de neuropathie périphérique avec gammapathie monoclonale benigne à IgM. Rev Neurol (Paris). 1985;141:729–34.
54. Propp RP, Means E, Deibel R, Sherer G, Barron K. Waldenström's macroglobulinemia and neuropathy. Deposition of M-component on myelin sheaths. Neurology. 1975;25:980–8.

55. Nardelli E, Pizzighella S, Tridente G, Rizzuto N. Peripheral neuropathy associated with immunoglobulin disorders. An immunological and ultrastructural study. Acta Neuropathol. 1981;suppl.VII:258–61.
56. Mata M, Kahn SN, Fink DJ. A direct electron microscopic immunocytochemical study of IgM paraproteinemic neuropathy. Arch Neurol. 1988;45:693–7.
57. Abrams GM, Latov N, Hays AP, Sherman W, Zimmerman EA. Immunocytochemical studies of human peripheral nerve with serum from patients with polyneuropathy and paraproteinemia. Neurology. 1982;32:821–6.
58. Meier C, Roberts K, Steck AJ, Hess A, Miloni E, Tschopp L. Polyneuropathy in Waldenström's macroglobulinemia: reduction of endoneurial IgM-deposits after treatment with chlorambucil and plasmapheresis. Acta Neuropathol. 1984;64:297–307.
59. King RHM, Thomas PK. The occurrence and significance of myelin with unusually large periodicity. Acta Neuropathol. 1984;63:318–29.
60. Jacobs JM, Scadding JW. Morphological changes in IgM paraproteinaemic neuropathy. Acta Neuropathol. 1990;80:77–84.
61. Dyck PJ, Low PA, Windebank AJ, Jaradeh SS, Gosselin S, Bourque P, Smith BE, Kratz KM, Karnes JL, Evans BA, Pineda AA, O'Brien PC, Kyle RA. Plasma exchange in polyneuropathy associated with monoclonal gammopathy of undetermined significance. N Engl J Med. 1991;325:1482–6.
62. Mussini JM, Planchon B, Barrier J, Guimbretiere J. Plasma exchange in polyneuropathies accompanying IgM monoclonal gammopathy. Plasma Ther Transfus Technol. 1985;6: 443–7.
63. Haas DC, Tatum AH. Plasmapheresis alleviates neuropathy accompanying IgM anti-myelin-associated glycoprotein paraproteinemia. Ann Neurol. 1988;23:394–6.
64. Lassoued K, Dellagi K, Brouet JC, Clauvel JM, Bussel A, Seligmann M. Effects of plasma exchange in nine patients with peripheral neuropathy and monoclonal IgM directed to myelin-associated glycoprotein. Plasma Ther Transfus Technol. 1985;6:449–52.
65. Dalakas MC, Flaum MA, Rick M, Engel WK, Gralnick HR. Treatment of polyneuropathy in Waldenström's macroglobulinemia and immunologic studies. Neurology. 1983;33: 1406–10.
66. Nobile-Orazio E, Baldini L, Barbieri S, Marmiroli P, Spagnol G, Francomano E, Scarlato G. Treatment of patients with neuropathy and anti-MAG IgM M-proteins. Ann Neurol. 1988;24:93–7.
67. Mendell JR, Sahenk Z, Whitaker JN, Trapp BD, Yates AJ, Griggs RC, Quarles RH. Polyneuropathy and IgM monoclonal gammopathy: studies on the pathogenic role of anti-myelin-associated glycoprotein antibody. Ann Neurol. 1985;17:243–54.
68. Hays AP, Lee SSL, Latov N. Immune reactive C3d on the surface of myelin sheaths in neuropathy. J Neuroimmunol. 1988;18:231–44.
69. Monaco S, Bonetti B, Ferrari S, Moretto G, Nardelli E, Tedesco F, Mollnes TE, Nobile-Orazio E, Manfredini E, Bonazzi L, Rizzuto N. Complement-mediated demyelination in patients with IgM monoclonal gammopathy and polyneuropathy. N Engl J Med. 1990; 322:649–52.
70. Hafler DA, Johnson D, Kelly JJ, Panitch H, Kyle R, Weiner HL. Monoclonal gammopathy and neuropathy: myelin-associated glycoprotein reactivity and clinical characteristics. Neurology. 1986;36:75–8.
71. Swash M, Perrin J, Schwartz MS. Significance of immunoglobulin deposition in peripheral nerve in neuropathies associated with paraproteinemia. J Neurol Neurosurg Psychiatry. 1979;42:179–83.
72. Takatsu M, Hays AP, Latov N, Abrams GM, Nemni R, Sherman WH, Nobile-Orazio E, Saito T, Freddo L. Immunofluorescence study of patients with neuropathy and M-IgM proteins. Ann Neurol. 1985;18:173–81.
73. Steck AJ, Murray N, Dellagi K, Brouet J-C, Seligmann M. Peripheral neuropathy associated with monoclonal IgM antibody. Ann Neurol. 1987;22:764–7.
74. Tatum AH. Experimental IgM anti-myelin paraprotein demyelinating neuropathy: ultrastructural characterization. Ann Neurol. 1989;26:298.
75. Dancea S, Dellagi K, Renaud F, Mahouy G, Hauw JJ, Brouet JC. Effect of passive transfer of human anti-myelin-associated glycoprotein IgM in marmoset. Autoimmunity. 1989;3: 29–37.

76. Hays AP, Latov N, Takatsu M, Sherman WH. Experimental demyelination of nerve induced by serum of patients with neuropathy and anti-MAG IgM M-protein. Neurology. 1987;37:242–56.
77. Trojaborg W, Galassi G, Hays AP, Lovelace RE, Alkaitis M, Latov N. Electrophysiologic study of experimental demyelination induced by serum of patients with IgM M-proteins and neuropathy. Neurology. 1989;39:1581–6.
78. Willison HJ, Trapp BD, Bacher JD, Dalakas MC, Griffin JW, Quarles RH. Demyelination induced by intraneural injection of human antimyelin-associated glycoprotein antibodies. Muscle Nerve. 1988;11:1169–76.
79. Guilbert B, Dighiero G, Avrameas S. Naturally occurring antibodies against nine common antigens in human sera. I. Detection, isolation and characterization. J Immunol. 1982;128:2779–87.
80. Freddo L, Ariga T, Saito M, Macala LC, Yu RK, Latov N. The neuropathy of plasma cell dyscrasia: binding of IgM M-proteins to peripheral nerve glycolipids. Neurology. 1985;35:1420–4.
81. Anderson DR, Grimes WJ. Heterogeneity of asparagine-linked oligosaccharides of five glycosylation sites on immunoglobulin M heavy chain from mineral oil plasmaycytome 104E. J Biol Chem. 1982;257:14858–64.
82. Baenziger JU. Structure of the oligosaccharides of human J chain. J Biol Chem. 1979;254:4063–71.
83. Springer TA, Lasky LA. Sticky sugars for selectins. Nature. 1991;349:196–7.
84. Collard JG, van Beek WP, Janssen JW, Schijven JF. Transfection by human oncogenes: concomitant induction of tumorigenicity and tumor-associated membrane alterations. Int J Cancer. 1985;35:207–13.
85. Dennis JW, Laferte S, Waghorne C, Breitman ML, Kerbel RS. Beta 1-6 branching of Asn-linked oligosaccharides is directly associated with metastasis. Science. 1987;236:582–5.
86. McGarry RC, Helfand SL, Quarles RH, Roder JC. Recognition of myelin-associated glycoprotein by the monoclonal antibody HNK-1. Nature. 1983;306:376–8.
87. Sato S, Baba H, Tanaka M, Yanagisawa K, Miyatake T. Antigenic determinant shared between myelin-associated glycoprotein from human brain and natural killer cells. Biomed Res. 1983;4:489–94.
88. Abo T, Blach CM. A differentiation antigen of human NK and K cells identified by a monoclonal antibody (HNK-1). J Immunol. 1981;127:1024–9.
89. Miller SL, Kahn SN, Perussia B, Trinchieri G. Comparative binding of murine and human monoclonal antibodies reacting with myelin-associated glycoprotein to myelin and human lymphocytes. J Neuroimmunol. 1987;15:229–42.
90. Dennis RD, Antonicek H, Wiegandt H, Schachner M. Detection of the L2/HNK-1 carbohydrate epitope on glycoproteins and acidic glycolipids of the insect *Calliphora vicina.* J Neurochem. 1988;51:1490–6.
91. Ilyas AA, Chou DKH, Jungalwala FB, Costello C, Quarles RH. Variability in the structural requirements for binding of human monoclonal anti-myelin-associated glycoprotein immunoglobulin M antibodies and HNK-1 to sphingolipid antigens. J Neurochem. 1990;55: 594–601.
92. Matthieu JM, Quarles RH, Poduslo JF, Brady RO. [^{35}S]sulfate incorporation into myelin glycoproteins. I. Central nervous system. Biochim Biophys Acta. 1975;392:159–66.
93. Matthieu JM, Everly JL, Brady RO, Quarles RH. [^{35}S]sulfate incorporation into myelin glycoproteins. II. Peripheral nervous system. Biochim Biophys Acta. 1975;392:167–74.
94. Shashoua VE, Daniel PF, Moore ME, Jungalwala FB. Demonstration of glucuronic acid on brain glycoproteins which react with HNK-1 antibody. Biochem Biophys Res Commun. 1986;183:902–9.
95. Uyemura K, Kitamura K. Comparative studies on myelin proteins in mammalian peripheral nerve. Comp Biochem Physiol. 1991;98C:63–72.
96. Field MC, Wing DR, Dwek RA, Rademacher TW, Schmitz B, Bollensen E, Schachner M. Detection of multisulphated N-linked glycans in the L2/HNK-1 carbohydrate epitope expressing neural adhesion molecule P_0. J Neurochem. 1992;58:993–1000.
97. Wing DR, Field MC, Schmitz B, Schachner M, Dweck RA, Rademacher TW. Use of whole brain oligosaccharides as probe for a functional neural epitope. Proceedings of the Xth International Symposium on Glycoconjugates, Jerusalem, Israel. 1989, pp. 374–5.

98. Burger D, Simon M, Perruisseau G, Steck AJ. The epitope(s) recognized by HNK-1 antibody and IgM paraprotein in neuropathy is present on several N-linked oligosaccharide structures on human P_0 and myelin-associated glycoprotein. J Neurochem. 1990;54:1569–75.
99. Burger D, Perruisseau G, Simon M, Steck AJ. Comparison of the N-linked oligosaccharide structures of the two major human myelin glycoproteins MAG and P_0: Assessment and relative occurrence of oligosaccharide structures by serial lectin affinity chromatography of [^{14}C]-glycopeptides. J Neurochem. 1992;58:845–53.
100. Burger D, Perruisseau G, Simon M, Steck AJ. Comparison of the N-linked oligosaccharide structures of the two major human myelin glycoproteins MAG and P_0: Assessment of the structures bearing the epitope for HNK-1 and human monoclonal immunoglobulin M found in demyelinating neuropathy. J Neurochem. 1992;58:854–61.
101. Poduslo JF. Golgi sulfation of the oligosaccharide chain of P_0 occurs in the presence of myelin assembly but not in its absence. J Biol Chem. 1990;265:3719–25.
102. Schachter H. Biosynthetic controls that determine the branching and microheterogeneity of protein-bound oligosaccharides. Biochem Cell Biol. 1986;64:163–81.
103. Cummings D, Merkle RK, Stults NI. Separation analysis of glycoprotein oligosaccharides. Methods Cell Biol. 1989;32:141–83.
104. Bajt ML, Schmitz M, Schachner M, Zipser B. Carbohydrate epitopes involved in neural cell recognition are conserved between vertebrates and leech. J Neurosci Res. 1990;27: 276–85.
105. Keilhauer G, Faissner A, Schachner M. Differential inhibition of neurone-neurone, neurone-astrocyte, and astrocyte-astrocyte adhesion by L1, L2, and N-CAM antibodies. Nature. 1985;316:728–30.
106. Künemund V, Jungalwala FB, Fischer G, Chou DKH, Keilhauer G, Schachner M. The L2/HNK-1 carbohydrate of neural cell adhesion molecules is involved in cell interactions. J Cell Biol. 1988;106:213–23.
107. Ilyas AA, Dalakas MC, Brady RO, Quarles RH. Sulfated glucuronyl glycolipids reacting with anti-myelin-associated glycoprotein monoclonal antibodies including IgM paraproteins in neuropathy: species distribution and partial characterization of epitopes. Brain Res. 1986;385:1–9.
108. Tucker GC, Dellagi K, Schmitt C, Brouet JC, Thiery JP. Heterogeneity of human anti-MAG IgM as revealed by their activity on avian embryonic tissues. Clin Exp Immunol. 1987;67:352–61.
109. Lieberman F, Marton LS, Stefansson K. Pattern of reactivity of IgM from sera of eight patients with IgM monoclonal gammopathy and neuropathy with components of neural tissue: evidence for interaction with more than one epitope. Acta Neuropathol. 1985;68: 196–200.
110. Saito T, Sherman WH, Latov N. Specificity of idiotypes of M-proteins that react with MAG in patients with neuropathy. J Immunol. 1983;2496–8.
111. Page N, Murray N, Perruisseau G, Steck AJ. A monoclonal anti-idiotypic antibodies against a human monoclonal IgM with specificity for myelin-associated glycoprotein. J Immunol. 1985;134:3094–9.
112. Kahn SN. Human IgM monoclonal antibodies with restricted antigenic specificity for myelin express unrelated idiotype. J Neurol Sci. 1985;67:161–70.
113. Schmitt C, Dellagi K, Mihaesco E, Brouet JC. Detection of cross-reactive determinants shared by human monoclonal IgM reacting with myelin-associated glycoprotein. J Immunol. 1987;138:1442–6.
114. Steck AJ, Page N. Analysis of the human anti-myelin associated glycoprotein IgM system with anti-idiotypic antibodies. NATO-ASI series. 1987;129:95–102.
115. Brouet JC, Dellagi K, Gendron MC, Chevalier A, Schmitt C, Mihaesco E. Expression of a public idiotype by human monoclonal IgM directed to myelin-associated glycoprotein and characterization of the variability subgroup of their heavy and light chains. J Exp Med. 1989;170:1551–8.
116. Brouet JC, Danon F, Mihaesco E, Bussel A, Oskenhendler E. Peripheral polyneuropathies associated with monoclonal IgM. Antibody activity of monoclonal IgM and therapeutic implications. Nouv Rev Fr Hematol. 1990;32:307–10.
117. Krolick KA. Selective elimination of autoreactive lymphocytes with immunotoxins. Clin Immunol Immunopathol. 1989;50:273–82.

118. Quarles RH. Human monoclonal antibodies associated with neuropathy. Methods Enzymol. 1989;179:291–9.
119. Van den Berg LH, Sadiq SA, Thomas FP, Latov N. Characterization of HNK-1 bearing glycoproteins in human peripheral nerve myelin. J Neurosci Res. 1990;25:295–9.
120. Sergott RC, Brown MJ, Lisak RP, Miller SL. Antibody to myelin-associated glycoprotein produces central nervous system demyelination. Neurology. 1988;38:422–6.
121. Maeda Y, Bigbee JW, Maeda R, Miyatani N, Kalb RG, Yu RK. Induction of demyelination by intraneural injection of antibodies against sulfoglucuronyl paragloboside. Exp Neurol. 1991;113:221–5.
122. Melnick SC. Thirty-eight cases of the Guillain–Barré syndrome: an immunological study. Br Med J. 1963;1:368–73.
123. Cook DS, Dowling PC, Murray MR, Whittaker JN. Circulating demyelinating factors in acute idiopathic polyneuropathy. Arch Neurol. 1971;24:136–44.
124. Tse KS, Arbesman CE, Tomast TB, Tourville D. Demonstration of antimyelin antibodies by immunofluorescence in Guillain–Barré syndrome. Clin Exp Immunol. 1971;8:881–7.
125. Nyland H, Aarli JA. Guillain–Barré syndrome: demonstration of antibodies to peripheral nerve tissue. Acta Neurol Scand. 1978;58:35–43.
126. Latov N, Gross RB, Kastelman J, Flanagan T, Lamme S, Alkaitis DA, Olarte MR, Sherman WH, Chess L, Penn AS. Complement fixing antiperipheral nerve myelin antibodies in patients with inflammatory polyneuritis and with polyneuropathy and paraproteinemia. Neurology. 1981;31:1530–4.
127. Hughes RCA, Gray IA, Gregson NA, Kadlubowski M, Kennedy M, Leibowitz S, Thompson H. Immune responses to myelin antigens in Guillain–Barré syndrome. J Neuroimmunol. 1984;6:303–12.
128. Winer JB, Gray IA, Gregson NA, Hughes RCA, Leibowitz S, Shepherd P, Taylor WA, Yewdall V. A prospective study of acute idiopathic neuropathy. III. Immunological studies. J Neurol Neurosurg Psychiatry. 1988;51:619–25.
129. Osterman PO, Vedeler CA, Ryberg B, Fagius J, Nyland H. Serum antibodies to peripheral nerve tissue in acute Guillain–Barré syndrome in relation to outcome of plasma exchange. J Neurol. 1988;235:285–9.
130. Van Doorn PA, Brand A, Vermeulen M. Clinical significance of antibodies against peripheral nerve tissue in inflammatory polyneuropathy. Neurology. 1987;37:1798–802.
131. Koski CL, Humphrey R, Shin ML. Anti-peripheral myelin antibody in patients with demyelinating neuropathy: Quantitative and kinetic determination of serum antibody by complement component 1 fixation. Proc Natl Acad Sci USA. 1985;82:905–9.
132. Koski CL. Complement-fixing anti-peripheral myelin antibodies and C9 neoantigen in serum from patients with Guillain–Barré syndrome: quantitation, kinetics, and clinical correlation. Ann NY Acad Sci. 1988;540:319–25.
133. Vedeler CA, Matre R, Nyland H. Class and IgG subclass distribution of antibodies against peripheral nerve myelin in sera from patients with inflammatory demyelinating polyradiculoneuropathy. Acta Neurol Scand. 1988;78:401–7.
134. Koski CL, Gratz E, Sutherland J, Mayer RF. Clinical correlation with anti-peripheral-nerve myelin antibodies in the Guillain–Barré syndrome. Ann Neurol. 1986;19:573–7.
135. Guillain–Barré syndrome study group. Plasmapheresis and acute Guillain–Barré syndrome. Neurology. 1985;35:1096–104.
136. Osterman PO, Lundemo G, Pirskanen R, Fagius J, Pihlstedt P, Siden A, Safwenberg J. Beneficial effect of plasma exchange in acute inflammatory polyradiculoneuropathy. Lancet. 1984;2:1296–312.
137. Feasby TE, Hahn AF, Gilbert JJ. Passive transfer studies in Guillain–Barré polyneuropathy. Neurology. 1982;32:1159–67.
138. Saida T, Saida K, Lisak RP, Brown MJ, Silberberg DH, Asbury AK. In vivo demyelinating activity of sera from patients with Guillain–Barré syndrome. Ann Neurol. 1982;11:69–75.
139. Brown MJ, Rosen JL, Lisak RP. Demyelination in vivo by Guillain–Barré syndrome and other human serum. Muscle Nerve. 1987;10:263–71.
140. Harrison BM, Hansen LA, Pollard JD, McLeod JG. Demyelination induced by serum from patients with Guillain–Barré syndrome. Ann Neurol. 1984;15:163–70.
141. Sawant-Mane S, Clarck MB, Koski CL. *In vitro* demyelination by serum antibody from patients with Guillain–Barré syndrome requires terminal complement complexes. Ann

Neurol. 1991;29:397–404.
142. Zweiman B, Rostami A, Lisak RP, Moskovitz AR, Pleasure DE. Immune reactions to P_2 protein in human inflammatory demyelinative neuropathies. Neurology. 1983;33:234–7.
143. Negishi T, Yamashita T, Nomura K, Hosokawa T, Ohno R, Hamaguchi K, Uyemura K. Serum antibodies to peripheral nerve antigens in Guillain–Barré syndrome. Ann NY Acad Sci. 1988;540:376–7.
144. Luijten JAFM, De Jong WAC, Demel RA, Heijnen CJ, Ballieux RE. Peripheral nerve P_2 basic protein and the Guillain–Barré syndrome. J Neurol Sci. 1984;66:209–16.
145. Ilyas AA, Mithen FA, Chen ZW, Cood SD. Anti-GM_1 antibodies in Guillain–Barré syndrome. J Neuroimmunol. 1992;36:69–76.
146. Koski CL, Chou DKH, Jungalwala FB. Anti-peripheral nerve myelin antibodies in Guillain–Barré syndrome bind a neutral glycolipid of peripheral myelin and cross-react with Forssman antigen. J Clin Invest. 1989;84:280–7.
147. Ilyas AA, Mithen FA, Dalakas MC, Wargo M, Chen ZW, Bielory L, Cook SD. Antibodies to sulfated glycolipids in Guillain–Barré syndrome. J Neurol Sci. 1991;105:108–17.
148. Fredman P, Vedeler CA, Nyland H, Aarli JA, Svennerholm L. Antibodies in sera from patients with inflammatory demyelinating polyradiculoneuropathy react with ganglioside LM_1 and sulfatide of peripheral nerve myelin. J Neurol. 1991;238:75–9.
149. Report from an Ad Hoc Subcommittee of the American Academy of Neurology AIDS Task Force. Research criteria for diagnosis of chronic inflammatory demyelinating polyneuropathy (CIDP). Neurology. 1991;41:617–18.
150. Haymaker W, Kernohan JW. The Landry–Guillain–Barré syndrome: a clinicopathologic report of fifty fatal cases and critique of the literature. Medicine (Baltimore). 1949;28: 59–141.
151. McCombe PA, Pollard JD, McLeod JG. Chronic inflammatory demyelinating polyneuropathy. Brain. 1987;110:1617–30.
152. Heininger K, Gibbels E, Besinger UA, Borberg H, Hartung HP, Grabensee B, Toyka KV. Role of therapeutic plasmapheresis in chronic inflammatory demyelinating polyneuropathy. Prog Clin Biol Res. 1990;337:275–81.
153. Lamb NL, Patten BM. Clinical correlation of anti-GM_1 antibodies in amyotrophic lateral sclerosis and neuropathies. Muscle Nerve. 1991;14:1021–7.
154. Hartung HP, Toyka KV. T-cell and macrophage activation in experimental autoimmune neuritis and Guillain–Barré syndrome. Ann Neurol. 1990;27(suppl.):S57–S63.

3
Guillain–Barré syndrome and CIDP

H.-P. HARTUNG, K. REINERS, K. V. TOYKA and J. D. POLLARD

GUILLAIN–BARRÉ SYNDROME (GBS)

Since poliomyelitis has been almost completely eradicated, Guillain–Barré syndrome (GBS), described in 1916[1], has become the most common cause of acute paralysis in Western countries. It occurs with an annual incidence of 1–2 cases/100 000 and affects all ages, men slightly more frequently than women. There is no seasonal preponderance. A viral or bacterial infection precedes GBS by 1–4 weeks in more than two-thirds of cases[2–4].

Clinical features

While patients often report distal paraesthesiae as the initial complaint, weakness is the predominant symptom. This most often takes the form of distally accentuated, relatively symmetrical paresis that, in the course of the disease, may involve more proximal muscle groups. Arms and legs are affected by flaccid paralysis to a similar degree at the nadir of disease in the majority of cases. Bilateral facial palsy is present in 30–50% of patients. Deep tendon reflexes are absent or greatly diminished. The diaphragm and ancillary respiratory muscles are involved in 25–30% of patients, who require artificial ventilation. Oropharyngeal muscles are affected in 25–50% and some degree of oculomotor palsy is observed in up to 15% of patients (Table 3.1). Sensory loss is rarely severe, but mild impairment of sensation in a glove and stocking distribution is usual. Paraesthesiae and pain are not uncommon features[4–17].

Motor weakness can progress rapidly in a matter of hours or more, but commonly progresses over a period of several days to 4 weeks. Four weeks is the arbitrary cut off in the differentiation of GBS from chronic polyneuritis, according to recently redefined criteria (Table 3.2)[18].

Table 3.1 Frequency of clinical features in Guillain–Barré syndrome

	% of patients
Weakness	
Upper extremities	20–90
Lower extremities	60–95
Facial	50
Oropharyngeal	20–50
Oculomotor paresis	10
Areflexia/hyporeflexia	95
Sensory abnormalities	
Paraesthesiae	70–80
Mild sensory loss	50
Pain	20–30
Respiratory failure	25
Autonomic	
Sphincter disturbance	10–20
Arterial hypotension	15
Arterial hypertension	30
Sinus tachycardia	30–40
Arrhythmia	10–20

Figures given first denote frequency at the onset of the disease, second at nadir

Autonomic symptoms in Guillain–Barré syndrome

Symptoms of autonomic dysfunction, affecting both sympathetic and parasympathetic systems, often develop acutely and early in patients with GBS[19–21]. Autonomic dysfunction may decrease or increase a given response; thus, parasympathetic denervation may lead to either tachycardia or bradycardia, and sympathetic dysregulation may produce hyperhidrosis as well as hypohidrosis. While the decrease of specific activity is usually attributable to the loss of transmission to the receptors, hyperfunction of autonomic receptors is thought to result from denervation hypersensitivity. In the case of the cardiovascular system, derangement of baroreceptor function is probably the most important factor, but up- or down-regulation of afferent baroreceptor and efferent receptor sensitivity, as well as alterations in circulating compounds such as catecholamines, atrial natriuretic factor[22,23] and other vasoactive substances may also play a role.

Acute neurophysiological and histological alterations in the preganglionic parasympathetic (vagus) and sympathetic (greater splanchnic) nerve were demonstrated in the guinea pig model of GBS, experimental allergic neuritis (EAN)[24]. Only 17 days after inoculation with myelin, marked slowing of nerve conduction in myelinated fibres, temporal dispersion of the compound action potential, and histological evidence of demyelination and axonal damage were shown in teased fibres. As in earlier studies, small myelinated fibres showed the greatest damage but unmyelinated fibres also showed axonal degeneration. All pathological alterations were more pronounced in the sympathetic than in the parasympathetic nerve.

The reported frequency of autonomic dysfunction in GBS depends on the battery of tests applied to screen for such symptoms. In larger series,

Table 3.2 Criteria for diagnosis of Guillain–Barré syndrome

Features required for diagnosis

Progressive motor weakness of more than one limb. The degree ranges from minimal weakness of the legs, with or without mild ataxia, to total paralysis of the muscles of all four extremities and the trunk, bulbar and facial paralysis, and external ophthalmoplegia

Areflexia or distal areflexia with definite hyporeflexia of biceps and knee jerks

Features supporting the diagnosis

Clinical features (ranked in order of importance)

- Progression. Symptoms and signs of motor weakness develop rapidly but cease to progress by 4 weeks into the illness. Approximately 50% reach the nadir by 2 weeks, 80% by 3 weeks, and 90% by 4 weeks
- Relative symmetry of weakness
- Only mild sensory symptoms or signs
- Cranial nerve involvement, most commonly bilateral facial palsy
- Recovery within 2–4 weeks after progression stops
- Autonomic dysfunction: tachycardia, arrhythmia, postural hypotension, arterial hypertension may be present and fluctuate
- Absence of fever at onset of neuropathic symptoms

Cerebrospinal fluid (CSF) features strongly supportive of the diagnosis

- CSF protein. After the first week of symptoms, CSF protein is elevated or has been shown to rise on serial lumbar punctures
- CSF cells: $\leq$ 10 mononuclear leukocytes/mm^3

Electrodiagnostic features: nerve conduction slowing or block

Features casting doubt on the diagnosis

Marked, persistent asymmetry of weakness

Persistent bladder or bowel dysfunction

Bladder or bowel dysfunction at onset

$>$ 50 mononuclear leukocytes/mm^3 in CSF

Presence of polymorphonuclear leukocytes in CSF

Sharp sensory level

Features excluding the diagnosis

Hexacarbon abuse (paint lacquer vapours or glue-sniffing)

Acute intermittent porphyria

Diphtheria

Lead neuropathy

Purely sensory syndrome

Poliomyelitis, botulism, toxic neuropathy (nitrofurantoin, organophosphorus compounds, dapsone)

Modified from reference 18

autonomic dysfunction has been found in more than 50% of patients[19,20,25–27]. Valuable tests for assessing autonomic function in GBS patients include investigations of parasympathetic function such as analysis of spontaneous heart rate variability[28] (Figure 3.1), heart rate response to deep inspiration and tilting and heart rate variation during Valsava manoeuvre, as well as those of sympathetic regulation, including the thermal sweat test, sympathetic skin response, blood pressure response to tilting and during Valsava manoeuvre and plasma noradrenalin response to tilting (for an overview see references 29, 30).

There have been numerous reports of patients with GBS showing hypersensitivity to drugs acting on the autonomic system, in particular those with a cardiovascular target (e.g., phentolamine, nitroglycerin, phenylephrine,

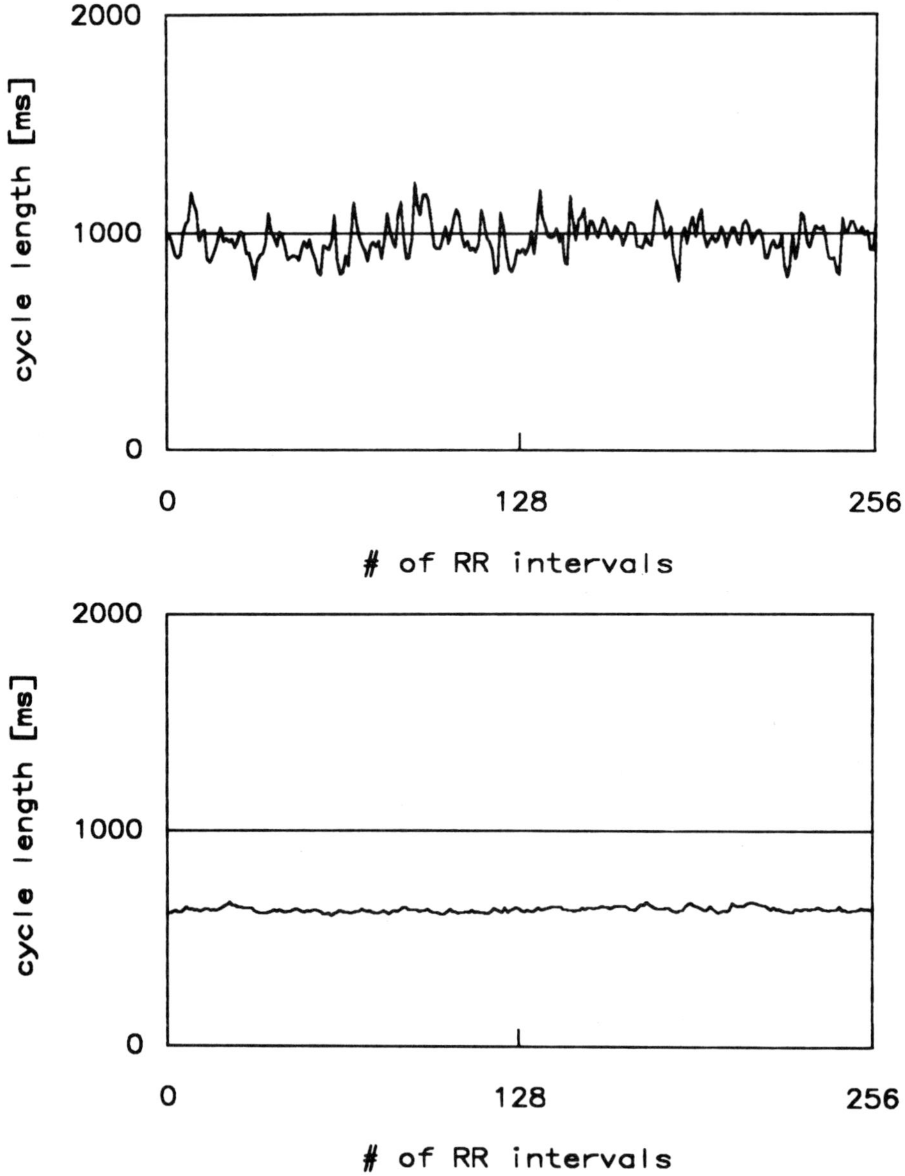

Figure 3.1 Autonomic failure in acute Guillain–Barré syndrome: Lack of spontaneous heart rate variation. Spontaneous heart rate (expressed as RR intervals; ordinate) recorded over 256 consecutive heart beats (abscissa) in a healthy control (male, aged 20 years; upper panel) and in patients with acute Guillain–Barré syndrome, 8 days after onset of symptoms (lower panel). At the time of recording, the patient required artificial ventilation. Note two characteristic alterations in GBS-induced autonomic (parasympathetic) dysfunction: (1) tachycardia (mean rate, 96/min); (2) lack of physiological sinus arrhythmia. This situation is comparable to the denervated heart after heart transplantation surgery. (Recording courtesy of Dr P. Flachenecker)

ephedrine, isoproteronol, various anaesthetics and narcotics, muscle relaxants; for an overview see reference 31).

As a consequence of autonomic denervation, altered receptor sensitivity and erratic responses, the regulation of autonomic function is less tight in GBS patients than in healthy individuals, and swings in autonomic tone become more pronounced. It is not clear whether tachycardia or bradycardia, which are both found in GBS, is more likely to lead to asystole. Sinus tachycardia is usually accompanied by paroxysmal hypertension and excessive sweating, and bradycardia and atrioventricular block rhythms may be seen in the context of 'vagal spells'[19] with flushing, bronchorrhoea and hypotension. Hypotensive episodes are not invariably the consequence of bradycardia but may also be due to vasodilatation with normal heart rate. Manipulations that lead to vagal stimulation in healthy individuals (e.g. voiding, urinary catheter manipulation, suctioning) may give rise to dramatic cardiac depression in GBS patients. Careful observation of patients in an intensive care unit is therefore strongly advised during such manoeuvres[32]. However, many acute exacerbations of autonomic function resolve spontaneously. While no clear-cut correlation between the severity of motor or sensory symptoms or nerve conduction velocities and the frequency and severity of autonomic disturbance has been found, patients with pronounced axonal damage and those requiring artificial ventilation more often develop severe autonomic dysregulation.

Autonomic disturbance other than cardiovascular presents as pupillary, gastrointestinal (gastroparesis, rectal incontinence, diarrhoea, constipation, ileus), and urogenital (urinary retention or incontinence, impairment of sexual function) dysfunction[19].

Patients with subgroups of GBS-like disorders may exhibit more pronounced autonomic symptoms than are usually encountered in typical GBS. Autonomic dysfunction is particularly impressive in some cases of inflammatory neuropathy that start with a rapid onset of autonomic symptoms and later develop additional sensorimotor symptoms. Pathology in these cases reveals mainly axonal degeneration. Patients with acute pandysautonomia, which may represent the purely autonomic end of a spectrum of GBS-like neuropathies, show severe autonomic symptoms and variable sensorimotor deficits at the onset[33–35] or developing later[36].

Course and prognosis

The different speed with which paralysis may develop has already been mentioned. In one large series of 100 patients from Southern England, 34% reached their nadir within 7 days, 70% within 14 days, 84% within 21 days, and 92% within 1 month, 1 month being the arbitrary cut off which distinguishes acute and chronic inflammatory polyradiculoneuropathy[17]. Hughes *et al.*[37] observed several patients who reached maximum disease severity after 4 weeks, but no later than 8 weeks, and thought this to constitute a separate entity, for which they suggested the term 'subacute idiopathic demyelinating polyradiculoneuropathy'. These patients made a

Table 3.3 Prognostic factors suggesting poor outcome

Older age
Need for artificial ventilation
Very low distal motor amplitudes (probably reflecting axonal damage)
Rapid progression (time < 1 week)
Presence of GM1 antibodies (controversial)
Preceding *Campylobacter jejuni* infection (controversial)

faster and more complete recovery. Mildly affected patients with GBS recover within weeks, but about half of the patients become bed-bound or chair-bound through the course of their disease and up to one-third require artificial ventilation. Mortality figures range from 3 to 13%[6,8,17,38–46]. Typically, recovery starts 1–4 weeks after the nadir and proceeds to the extent that patients regain their ability to walk unaided within 2–3 months of onset; 10–20% are left with some degree of disability after 12 months.

Recurrences of GBS have been recorded. One or more relapses of acute paralysis are seen in 1–5% of patients, who are asymptomatic or only mildly affected between attacks. Episodes may be months or years apart, but otherwise show the typical features of monophasic GBS[47–49].

Complications that may determine the fate of the patient are due to autonomic disturbances, respiratory failure, and thromboembolism from immobilization and intercurrent infections, particularly pneumonia. A number of prognostic factors have been identified in multicentre therapeutic trials (Table 3.3)[46,50].

Variant forms of GBS

In 1956, Fisher described the triad of ophthalmoplegia, limb ataxia and areflexia[51]. There is still debate about the nature of the neuropathy in Fisher syndrome but most would agree that there is no indication of central nervous system involvement[52–57].

More recently, sveral authors have proposed the existence of a separate subgroup of GBS characterized by prominent axonal degeneration on electrodiagnostic and pathological examination. Some autopsy studies on single cases have shown a conspicuous paucity or complete absence of inflammatory demyelination, suggesting the possibility that this clinically indistinguishable neuropathy has a different pathogenesis. However, it is also conceivable that this simply represents the extreme end of a disease spectrum and that early massive inflammation causes severe axonal changes. These patients have a poor prognosis[58–61].

Epidemics of acute flaccid paralysis have occurred in Mexico, South America, China and India[62–64]. The clinical presentation is similar but electrophysiological features and pathology, characterized by Wallerian-like degeneration of motor fibres in the absence of inflammatory changes, distinguish this condition from classical demyelinating GBS. For the Chinese cases, the term 'acute motor axonal neuropathy' was recently suggested[64].

Table 3.4 Differential diagnosis of Guillain–Barré syndrome

Locked-in syndrome
Brainstem infarction
Brainstem encephalomyelitis
Spinal cord compression
Transverse myelitis
Acute necrotic myelopathy
Vasculitic neuropathy
Acute motor neuron diseases
poliomyelitis, rabies/enterovirus anterior myelopathies, Chinese paralytic syndrome (acute motor axonal neuropathy), cytoplasmic and nuclear neuronopathy
Biological toxins
botulism, tick paralysis, diphtheria, ciguatera, buckthorn, snake bite
Environmental toxins
heavy metals, arsenic, lead, thallium, gold
Hexacarbons
industrial solvents, glue-sniffing
Organophosphates
Alcohol
Porphyric neuropathy
Borreliosis
Critical illness polyneuropathy
Acute pandysautonomia
CIDP with acute onset
Hysteria
Hypokalaemia
Hyperkalaemia

Differential diagnosis

The history and clinical features are sufficiently characteristic to establish the diagnosis in most cases, but several disorders may be confused with GBS (Table 3.4)[3,15,41].

Antecedent events

Approximately 70% of patients give a history of acute infectious illness antedating neuropathic symptoms by 1–3 weeks. Influenza-like symptoms, upper respiratory infection or diarrhoea have usually cleared before onset of the neurological disorder. A plethora of viral, bacterial, and mycoplasma agents have been associated with GBS, but good evidence for a more than chance link with a virus is available only for cytomegalovirus, Epstein–Barr virus, vaccinia, variola, and human immunodeficiency virus[65–69]. Varicella zoster and measles may also possibly be added to this list (summarized by Arnason and Soliven[3]) (Table 3.5). More recently, the bacterial diarrhoeal agent *Campylobacter jejuni* has been identified as a common infectious trigger[70–76]. *C. jejuni* infection is the most common diarrhoeal illness in the western world, and depending on the serological methodology used and the geographic background, a preceding *C. jejuni* infection can be proven in 10–60% of all patients. It is of particular note that specific serotypes of the organism have been identified that are associated with GBS but uncommon

Table 3.5 Infections associated with GBS

Viral	
	Cytomegalovirus
	Epstein–Barr virus (EBV)
	Human immunodeficiency virus (HIV)
	Possible: varicella zoster, vaccinia, variola
Bacterial	
	Campylobacter jejuni
	Mycoplasma pneumoniae

in enteritis not associated with neuropathy (e.g. Penner type 19 in Japan; Lior 11 in Germany)[70,73,77]. The implications of these findings are discussed below.

There have also been numerous reports that GBS may follow certain types of vaccination. The most publicized outbreak was that occurring during the swine influenza vaccination programme in the USA in 1976. A small increase in the number of cases relative to that expected in non-vaccinated individuals was reported; however, this occurred only with some lots of vaccine[78–81]. Cases of an acute motor neuropathy following rabies vaccination have been reported from South America, where the vaccine is prepared from rabies virus-infected suckling mouse or rat brain[82–84]. More recently, a report from Finland claimed an increased incidence of GBS after vaccination with live-attenuated poliovirus, but the numbers are too small to draw definite conclusions[85].

Anecdotal reports are available which linked GBS with therapeutic or illicit use of drugs, including gold, amitryptiline, zimeldine, danazol, captopril, streptokinase, and heroin (reviewed by Arnason and Soliven[3]).

Electrophysiological features in Guillain–Barré syndrome

Electrophysiological testing of the peripheral nervous system has helped to elucidate the functional consequences of demyelination and axonal damage and has proved useful in the early diagnosis of GBS before abnormalities in the cerebrospinal fluid can be found, i.e. within the first days of the disease[86,86a]. The mechanisms of the conduction deficit and its clinical implications will now be reviewed, and a strategy for approaching the patient is proposed.

Pathophysiology of nerve conduction in demyelinating neuropathies

Segmental demyelination combined with a variable degree of axonal degeneration is the characteristic pathological feature of GBS. Patients in later stages of GBS, like those suffering from chronic inflammatory demyelinating neuropathy (CIDP), also show remyelination of nerve fibres. The effects of demyelination alone have rarely been properly separated from those of the simultaneous remyelination, largely because motor nerve or even sequential nerve biopsies cannot usually be obtained. The electrophysiological characteristics will therefore be discussed primarily on the basis of experimental animal data.

Slowing of nerve conduction

Mechanisms underlying the slowing of conduction have been elucidated in a series of studies on single nerve fibres in mammalian diphtheric neuropathy[87,88]. From these and other experiments it is clear that slowing of nerve conduction velocity can be evoked by focal (segmental) increases in internodal conduction time owing to continuous rather than saltatory conduction along an internode. The same phenomenon was seen in regenerating tips of crushed dorsal root fibres in the rat[89], demonstrating that demeylinating and remyelinating segments may be present simultaneously in an individual fibre, and share common electrophysiological properties. Conduction slowing is even more likely to occur in remyelination than in demyelination[90]. Physiologically, continuous conduction requires a redistribution of sodium channels from nodal to internodal segments of the nerve fibre; this has not yet been demonstrated in demyelination. Paranodal demylination, which may sometimes precede segmental demyelination, is more effective in slowing conduction[91]. This may explain why conduction slowing can occasionally be noted early in the course of GBS, before segmental demyelination has occurred.

Conduction block

Conduction block describes the complete failure of transmission along a nerve fibre segment: a stimulus applied proximal to the lesion fails to produce a response distally, while the same stimulus applied distal to the lesion elicits a normal response. After transection of a nerve fibre, conduction in the distal segment is maintained transiently, while Wallerian degeneration develops. Depending on the length of the distal stump and the site of stimulation, such conduction may last for some days. In contrast, conduction block in axonal neuropathies develops in the degenerating distal segment. However, in demyelinating neuropathies, conduction block occurs in the absence of axonal damage[92]. McDonald[93] was the first to directly demonstrate conduction block evoked by administration of diphtheria toxin in the region of the dorsal root ganglion in the cat. Demyelinative processes occurring in experimental allergic neuritis[94], and in mechanical derangement[95,96] were later also shown to cause conduction block.

Observations in the demyelinating and remyelinating stage of the disease suggest that intermittent (frequency-dependent) conduction block may be a transient stage between normal transmission and total conduction block. Intermittent conduction block can best be assessed by examining the refractory period of transmission, that is, the longest interval during which the second of two impulses does not traverse a region of demyelination[97–99]. In the clinical situation it is difficult to assess the failure of a nerve to transmit a series of impulses. First, intermittent block of single fibres cannot be detected by the common recording of compound muscle or nerve action potentials; and second, repetitive appropriate stimulation (20–100 Hz) is not tolerated by most patients. This technique has not, therefore, gained wide acceptance.

The effect of temperature on nerve conduction

Another physiological feature of demyelination is the detrimental effect of increased temperature on transmission[100]. Differential effects of temperature on sodium and potassium channels, together with a reduced safety factor of transmission in demyelination, result in conduction failure at higher temperatures. While patients with central demyelination may experience more severe symptoms at raised temperatures (Uhthoff's phenomenon in multiple sclerosis) similar observations are rarely reported in patients with GBS. However, the accentuation of unpleasant or painful paraesthesia with increasing temperature (e.g. while resting in bed at night) experienced by some patients may have an analogous physiological basis.

Ectopic nerve excitation

Symptoms may also be due to the fact that demyelination gives rise to spontaneous (ectopic) impulse generation within the nerve[101]. This is the physiological basis for twitching and fasciculations of motor nerves, experienced by both the patient and the electromyographer. In more severe cases, even cramps may be generated by such spontaneous excitation of nerve fibres. Myokymia affecting the extremities and facial muscles are occasionally seen in patients with GBS or CIDP[102–106].

Important indications of the type of abnormality that can be expected in demyelinating neuropathies have come from computer simulations[106]. Such modelling demonstrates that the interpretation of electrophysiological data is much easier if repetitive examinations have been performed during the course of the disease.

Problems in interpreting electrophysiological findings in GBS

The electrodiagnostic correlates of demyelination

Major pitfalls in the interpretation of electrophysiological data in demyelinating neuropathies arise from the common misconception that demyelination means conduction slowing, and vice versa. In interpreting nerve conduction studies, however, slowing of conduction velocity only indicates demyelination along the nerve if there is no axonal loss, i.e. if compound muscle action potential (CMAP) amplitudes are near normal. It is important to realize that, in the absence of demyelination, preferential loss of axons of the fastest conducting fibres alone may slow conduction velocity by as much as 40% relative to that in the fibres that normally determine the velocity obtained in nerve conduction studies[107]. In patients with the acute axonal form of GBS, inexcitability of axons develops within 3 days of onset of symptoms[59,108]; by preferentially affecting fastest conducting fibres, this can also delay the earliest CMAP components, imitating early demyelination.

Distal conduction block

Another major pitfall arises from disregarding the possibility of a very distal conduction block, and thus considering an unobtainable CMAP as evidence of axonal degeneration. While conduction block in a more proximal segment of the nerve can easily be detected by comparing CMAP waveform and amplitude obtained at two or more stimulation sites along the nerve, conduction block distal to the most distal stimulation site possible remains undetected by neurographic investigation alone. Needle examination of the paretic muscle must be added to the spectrum of tests. If performed after time has been allowed for spontaneous activity to develop in the muscle (about 3–5 days in proximal muscles or 5–8 days in distal muscles) needle electromyography (EMG) will unequivocally distinguish between distal conduction block and denervation due to axonal degeneration.

'Partial' conduction block

Other difficulties relate to the concept of 'partial' conduction block described in demyelinating neuropathies[5]. This term is meant to indicate failure of conduction in a proportion of fibres within a nerve. As discussed above, for an individual nerve fibre, there is nothing between orderly transmission on one hand and conduction failure, or conduction block, on the other. 'Partial' conduction block in an individual nerve fibre can, therefore, only mean something which is more precisely described as 'intermittent' conduction block (see above). There is good reason to avoid the ambiguous term 'partial' conduction block, although it has been included in the current criteria for diagnosing demyelination[18] (see Table 3.2).

The electromyographer must be warned against diagnosing ('partial') conduction block simply from differences in CMAP amplitudes between distal and proximal stimulation sites. First, the examiner must ensure truly supramaximal stimulation at the proximal stimulation site[109] to avoid producing partial conduction block as a technical artefact. Second, the effect of interphase cancellation is often underestimated. In the normal arm nerve, an amplitude difference of up to 15% is found between proximal stimulation at the elbow and distal stimulation at the wrist. In patients with neuropathies, temporal dispersion with inherent interphase cancellation[110] is sufficient to account for a greater decrease in amplitude with no conduction block. While under these circumstances comparisons based on amplitudes alone require a decrease of > 15–40%[90,111–112] comparisons of areas under the curve may be more consistent in establishing the existence of a real conduction block. However, computer simulations even suggest that amplitude or area decreases of up to 50% can be produced by interphase cancellation alone, without conduction block. Identifying conduction block properly is thus difficult in many cases, and the electromyographer should interpret his data cautiously[113]. In general, conduction block can be identified more reliably as the length of the segment over which the alteration in waveform occurs decreases, and when alteration can be demonstrated to occur abruptly while the stimulating electrode travels stepwise along the nerve. Thus, short segment stimulation is an important ancillary technique to help define focal

Table 3.6 Electrodiagnostic criteria for peripheral nerve demyelination[18]

Patient must have three of the following four features:

1. Reduction in conduction velocity in two or more motor nerves
   a. < 80% of lower limit of normal (LLN) if amplitude > 80% of LLN
   b. < 70% of LLN if amplitude < 80% of LLN
2. Conduction block or abnormal temporal dispersion in one or more motor nerves: either peroneal nerve between ankle and below fibular head, median nerve between wrist and elbow, or ulnar nerve between wrist and below elbow.

   Criteria for conduction block:
   a. < 15% change in duration between proximal and distal sites and > 20% drop in negative-peak area of peak-to-peak amplitude between proximal and distal sites.

   Criteria for abnormal temporal dispersion and possible conduction block:
   a. > 15% change in duration between proximal and distal sites and > 20% drop in negative-peak area or peak-to-peak amplitude between proximal and distal sites.
3. Prolonged distal latencies in two or more nerves.
   a. > 125% of upper limit of normal (ULN) if amplitude > 80% of LLN
   b. > 150% of ULN if amplitude < 80% of LLN
4. Absent F-waves or prolonged minimum F-wave latencies (10–15 trials) in two or more motor nerves.
   a. > 120% of ULN if amplitude > 80% of LLN
   b. > 150% of ULN if amplitude < 80% of LLN.

conduction block[114]. Electrodiagnostic criteria for demyelination are summarized in Table 3.6 (after ref. 18).

Large versus small fibre involvement

Larger nerve fibres carry more myelin than do small fibres and have therefore been assumed to be more resistant to demyelination in GBS. In experimentally induced demyelination in the rat, earlier and more severe damage was found in small than in thick fibres[115]. This may explain the symptoms of a small fibre neuropathy in terms of pain and the high proportion of GBS patients with autonomic dysfunction (see above).

Electrophysiological findings

On the background of time-dependent alterations of physiological nerve properties in GBS, it is clear that electrodiagnostic findings in the individual patient strongly depend on the stage of the disease, i.e. its severity, as well as the point in time when investigations are performed (Table 3.7). The following account describes the typical sequence of events in the course of the disease.

Electrophysiology in early GBS

Nerve conduction studies (Figure 3.2)

Demyelination first reduces the safety factor of transmission[97-99]. At this stage, intermittent conduction block can be detected. Distal latencies may

Table 3.7 Sequential electrophysiological features of demyelination/remyelination

Intermittent conduction block (prolonged refractory period; reduction of safety factor of neural transmission; increased temperature sensitivity)
Conduction block in a proportion of fibres within a nerve ('partial' conduction block)
F-wave impersistence
Slowed conduction
Conduction block in whole nerve
Abnormal (spontaneous) impulse generation
Abnormal irritability of the nerve fibre to mechanical stimuli (Tinel's sign)
Repetitive discharges/neuromyotonia
'Late' components in CMAP

become prolonged while conduction in the forearm segment of the median or ulnar nerve is still within normal limits. As the conduction block affects more and more fibres, CMAPs decrease. Only later does conduction slow measurably[86]; this occurs in the roots and proximal parts of the nerves earlier than in distal segments, corresponding to the clinical notion that paresis of proximal muscles heralds weakness in more distal muscles.

Neurophysiological data in the preclinical stage of acute demyelination rely on investigations in experimental animals. In these studies, the first abnormalities were found in proximal nerve conduction, i.e. in F-waves or in somatosensory evoked potentials (SEP) recorded from the scalp or the spinal cord[116]. Ropper and Chiappa[117] found similar changes in proximal conduction in patients with early GBS. As expected from a radicular site of damage, sensory conduction time between Erb's point potential and N13 (spinal) is prolonged the most.

F-wave studies are particularly useful in electrodiagnosis of early GBS because impulses travel the whole length of motor nerve fibres, including the motor roots. F-waves represent the recurrent discharge of antidromically activated α-motoneurones[118] and can be elicited in about 2–5% of motoneurones[119]. F-wave studies have long been used to identify proximal conduction abnormalities in GBS[120]. In contrast to the results of earlier studies[121] a more recent study[122] places the sensitivity of peripheral nerve conduction and F-wave studies above that of SEP, which were found to be helpful only if peripheral conduction and F-waves were normal. Since F-wave latencies alone may be prolonged irrespective of the site of damage along the nerve[123] they must be compared to more distal nerve conduction to be useful diagnostically.

Recently, F-waves have attracted more attention as an indicator of incipient GBS[86]; delayed F-waves and F-wave impersistence (< 6 responses obtained from 10 stimuli) are the earliest indicators of beginning demyelination in neuropathies. The value of F-wave minimum latency determination, chronodispersion and persistence was recently confirmed for GBS and CIDP[124]. Pathological F-wave parameters with normal CMAP were found to be highly specific for the presence of demyelination in the peripheral nerve.

In order to demonstrate early demyelination, serial studies including

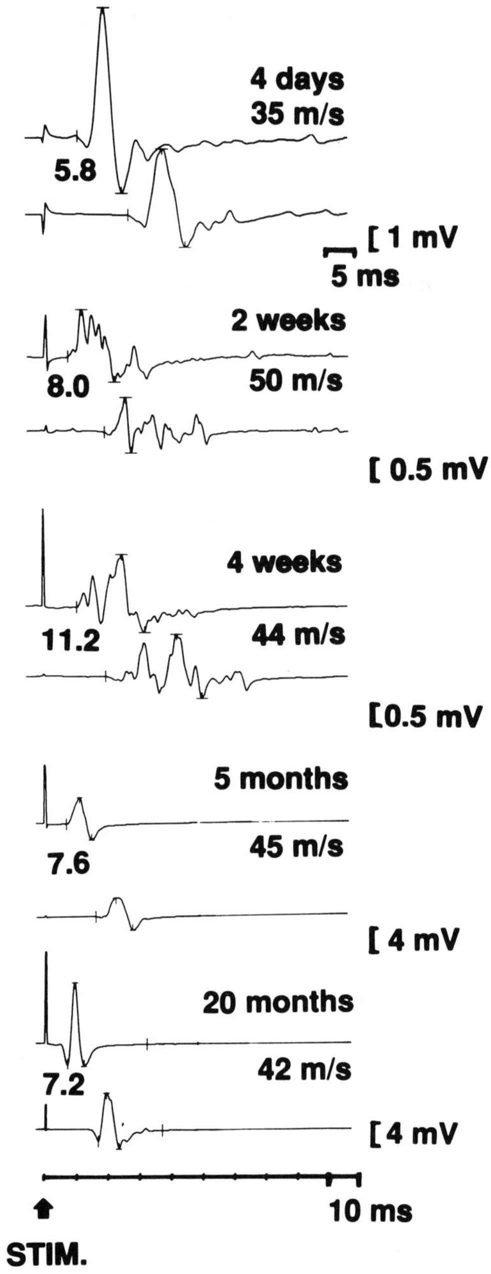

Figure 3.2 Electrophysiological findings in Guillain–Barré syndrome: sequential nerve conduction studies. All recordings were taken from the right tibial nerve in a 34-year-old woman. Skin temperature was kept at 34°C during all recordings. The upper trace of each recording represents

continued

proximal nerve segments are useful, and distal latencies and CMAPs should be followed. Investigations should include at least three different nerves: the diagnostic yield is then more than 90%, whereas abnormalities are found in only 50% of patients in whom only one nerve is tested[125].

Conduction in nerves innervating proximal muscles is difficult to assess because only one point for stimulation is accessible. To avoid this problem one may determine motor latencies from Erb's point to proximal muscles of the upper extremities. If early neurophysiological assessment is possible, a prolongation of the axillary nerve latency to the deltoid muscle may be detected while other conduction studies are still normal. More pronounced slowing in proximal segments of longer nerves compared to more distal segments, is of similar importance[86].

Recording of magnetically evoked motor potentials offers a new means to investigate proximal motor pathways. In GBS, abnormalities suggesting proximal conduction block in a proportion of fibres have been found in patients at a stage when conventional nerve conduction studies were still normal[126].

Figure 3.2 *continued* the compound muscle action potential (CMAP) recorded from the abductor hallucis muscle after stimulation of the tibial nerve at the ankle. The figure under the curve indicates the distal motor latency (DML, ms). The lower trace shows the CMAP recorded following stimulation of the tibial nerve at the knee level. The time after first symptoms is indicated together with the motor conduction velocity (MCV, m/s) as calculated for the calf segment of the tibial nerve. First symptoms of GBS (tingling in both hands, followed by minor weakness of handgrip, grade 4, MRC) occurred 4 days after a late abortion induced in the 18th week of pregnancy because of organic heart defect. There was no overt infection preceding the GBS. Four days after onset (note that time scale is different from later recordings): the CMAP amplitude on distal stimulation was relatively small but still within the normal range. The CMAP waveform, however, was abnormally dispersed owing to subnormal conduction velocities in a proportion of nerve fibres. CMAP dispersion was even more pronounced on proximal stimulation. The comparison of CMAP amplitudes on proximal vs. distal stimulation revealed a decrease of 47%, strongly suggesting (but not proving) conduction block in a proportion of fibres. DML was marginal, MCV was slightly reduced. F wave persistence was reduced to 40% (4/10). Sensory nerve conduction studies on the sural nerves were normal, median nerve DML at this stage was moderately prolonged, and the median nerve sensory action potential was small with a slightly reduced conduction velocity. At 2 and 4 weeks after onset the disease progressed, and the patient became wheel-chair bound. Five plasma exchanges were administered up to day 12. The nadir of the disease was reached at day 10, with a pleateau phase until week 3. Clinical deterioration was paralleled by gross reduction in CMAP amplitude with major dispersion. Note that distal motor latencies became progressively prolonged while MCV in the calf segment had actually recovered to low normal values. By week 4, F wave persistence returned to 80%. Despite severe paresis, needle EMG of the intrinsic foot muscles showed only minor spontaneous activity, even after 4 weeks. This confirmed that the rapid decrease of CMAP amplitudes was largely due to conduction block rather than the consequence axonal degeneration thereby indicating a more favourable prognosis. At 5 months after onset (note change in amplitude calibration), despite a steady and subjectively full clinical recovery from week 3 onward, deep tendon reflexes were still missing. CMAP amplitudes increased and became more compact, and distal latencies slowly decreased. At 20 months after onset motor and sensory function had been fully restored, knee jerks had returned, but ankle jerks were still missing. CMAP amplitudes increased to normal. MCV stayed in the lower normal range but DML remained slightly prolonged. F wave studies were all normal

Electromyography

The reduction in the number of recruitable motor units due to conduction block prompts those units already active to discharge at a higher rate than normal to reach a given force. An experienced electromyographer will often be able to detect this relatively high discharge frequency of smaller motor units without additional equipment. Modern EMG machines provide routines to quantify motor unit discharge rate and to detect disturbed recruitment of motor units. However, for more precise comparison it is necessary to measure the force output of the muscle while sampling single motor unit discharges. Such analysis has been shown to provide additional information in chronic neuropathies, enabling a distinction between axonal and demyelinating neuropathies[127].

At present, EMG examination in GBS patients focuses on the identification of:

(1) Altered recruitment of motor units, in that only a reduced number of units is recruitable, each discharging at higher rates than normal; identification requires an experienced examiner and/or computer support.

(2) Spontaneous activity which may appear in proximal muscles as early as 2 days after onset. If present, it can often be tracked further distally, usually arriving in distal muscles after 2–3 weeks.

(3) Motor units that can be stimulated electrically but cannot be recruited voluntarily, thus suggesting conduction block in single fibres.

(4) Reinnervation potentials in later stages of the disease indicating incipient recovery while there is still no voluntary movement of limbs.

Electrodiagnostic criteria of GBS

The electrodiagnostic section of the current criteria for diagnosing GBS[18] is designed for use in the first 3 weeks of illness only and therefore focuses on nerve conduction studies to identify demyelination.

In more severe cases, however, early EMG also has an important role in identifying patients with early axonal damage who usually have a poorer prognosis (see Table 3.3). According to the proposed criteria, the diagnosis of GBS can be made if, in addition to the appropriate clinical picture and cerebrospinal findings (see Table 3.2), three of the criteria listed in Table 3.6 are fulfilled.

With respect to the identification of conduction block, these criteria were rather permissive. The flood of reports claiming identification of conduction block has prompted a reappraisal of the electrophysiological criteria of conduction block[113]. The recommended term is now ‘suggestive of conduction block in individual fibres’ for data fulfilling the old criteria only, while additional evidence is required for the diagnosis of definite conduction block. The investigations recommended to corroborate the presence of conduction block are listed in Table 3.8.

For routine nerve conduction studies, most of the additional criteria are

Table 3.8 Investigations corroborating the presence of conduction block[130]

Procedure	*Criteria*
Short-segment stimulation	Abrupt change in area and/or amplitude over 2–4 cm
Recording of single motor units (MU)	MU can be activated on distal but not on proximal stimulation, or MU can be activated electrically but not voluntarily
Computer-reconstruction of CMAP from single MU	Reconstruction incomplete

Table 3.9 Screening criteria for conduction block in routine electrophysiology (modified from reference 128)

Most important: ensure supramaximal stimulation!
Decrease in CMAP negative phase area and/or amplitude of > 50% on proximal as compared to distal stimulation

technically difficult to meet. Therefore, based mainly on the experimental data reported by Rhee *et al.*[110], Lange *et al.*[128] have proposed the following screening method (Table 3.9). Conduction block can be assumed if the area and/or amplitude of the negative phase of the CMAP on proximal stimulation is 50% or less than that on distal stimulation. An area decrease of less than 50% together with an increase of the duration of the negative phase by more than 30% merely suggests temporal dispersion of the potential without real conduction block, while the reduction of the area by more than 50% together with an increase of the duration by less than 30% would indicate the combination of conduction block and temporal dispersion (Figure 3.2). Variants of innervation must be excluded when testing for conduction block (e.g. the median nerve in patients with Martin–Gruber anastomosis).

Electrophysiology in advanced GBS

In advanced GBS, i.e. at the time of the clinical nadir (usually about 1–3 weeks after onset of symptoms) the electrophysiological situation is best described as cumulative demyelination with superimposed axonal lesions[111]. About 50% of patients show segmental demyelination within 2 weeks of onset, increasing to 85% in the third week of the disease. Less than 10% of patients never exhibit clear-cut electrophysiological signs of demyelination because of the rapid onset of axonal degeneration[106,111].

Nerve conduction studies

Maximal nerve conduction abnormalities are found at the time of the clinical nadir in both adults[111,129] and in children[130]. While clinical deterioration usually ceases within 4 weeks, some patients with only prolonged distal latencies after 3 weeks may continue to develop conduction block in a portion of nerve fibres, and slowing of conduction velocities in the following weeks[131]. Conduction velocity in distal nerve segments, for example, may further diminish while there is already clinical improvement at more proximal sites[111].

Motor nerve conduction abnormalities are generally predominant in GBS and are much more common than sensory abnormalities during the first weeks of illness[5]. With time, sensory abnormalities tend to become more obvious, so that after 3 weeks sensory nerve conduction is abnormal in 80% of patients. Sensory abnormalities are more common in the median than in the sural nerve[132]. This seemingly odd finding may have a methodological and not a biological basis: while sensory median nerve conduction is measured over the distal segment of the nerve, conduction studies examine more proximal parts of the sural nerve, thereby preventing the distally pronounced abnormalities of nerve conduction from influencing the test result.

Electromyography

Although in patients with the acute axonal form of the disease axonal degeneration may be seen as early as a few days after first signs of muscle weakness, needle EMG studies usually become informative only later in the disease. Spontaneous activity (fibrillation and fasciculation potentials and positive sharp waves) is rare in the first 2 weeks, except for patients with the axonal form of GBS. Spontaneous activity may persist for longer in distal muscles[111], tested at 2–4 months after the onset. A continuing decrease in CMAP amplitude on distal stimulation indicates either axonal degeneration with conduction failure or (more favourably) distal conduction block. Preservation of distal conduction in the early stage of the disease does not, however, ensure a favourable outcome, because axonal degeneration may follow very soon[46]. Close EMG monitoring within the following days can make a clear distinction between the two possibilities.

Electrodiagnosis in variants of GBS

The electrophysiological findings in the Fisher variant of GBS[51] resemble those of classical GBS[133,134] but in 60% of patients show slowed conduction in the facial nerve and equivalently prolonged latencies in the blink reflex[135]. Isolated facial nerve conduction slowing may also be seen in classical GBS. Conduction slowing has been found to be more pronounced in children with GBS than in adult patients, particularly in the patient group under 10 years of age; the outcome in children, however, is generally much more favourable[42,135a].

It is still doubtful whether the 'Chinese paralytic syndrome' (CPS; acute motor axonal neuropathy[63,64]) and similar cases reported in Mexican children[62] represent a variant of the acute axonal form of GBS. Electrophysiological findings in these syndromes differ considerably from those of typical GBS and, like the nerve pathology, suggest an underlying axonopathy[64].

Table 3.10 Correlation between nerve pathology and neurophysiological deficit

Pathology	*Neurophysiology*
Segmental demyelination	
Early, moderate degree	Conduction block, CMAP (↓)
Severe, wide-spread	Conduction failure, very low and dispersed or no CMAP recordable
Late, with remyelination	Conduction slowing (< 60% of normal CV possible), CMAP low and dispersed
Severe distal demyelination, even if early	Proximal conduction preserved but cannot be assessed in routine investigation because CMAP is lost; no spontaneous activity in EMG
Axonal (Wallerian) degeneration	
Early, if only part of nerve fibres affected	Conduction slowing (no less than 60% of normal CV), CMAP ↓
Late, if all fibres affected	Conduction failure, no CMAP recordable; spontaneous activity in EMG

CMAP = compound motor action potential; CV = nerve conduction velocity; EMG = needle electromyography

Correlation of clinical features with electrophysiology and prognostic significance

Prognostic factors other than those derived from electrophysiological data have been discussed above (Table 3.3). It is not the degree of conduction slowing but the amount of conduction block and failure that correlates best with clinical impairment[5] (Table 3.10): rapid reversal of proximal conduction block was seen to underlie early clinical recovery in three GBS patients[136]. The marked slowing sometimes observed in GBS is mostly indicative of remyelination, that is known to take place even while further demyelination occurs along other segments of the same nerve fibre.

Patients in whom the CMAP amplitude on distal stimulation is reduced by more than 80% in the initial nerve conduction study generally have a poor prognosis[137]. However, as discussed above, low CMAP amplitudes on distal stimulation are ambiguous with respect to pathogenesis. Needle EMG clarifies the physiological basis of this phenomenon, and thereby gives an important prognostic clue. While distal conduction block may resolve within a few weeks, axonal regeneration proceeds over weeks to months, is ineffective over longer nerve segments, and is rarely complete. The degree of axonal damage therefore appears to be the limiting factor in prognosis.

Long-term follow-up studies generally show improved and mostly normal nerve conduction after about 1 year, almost in parallel with the recurrence of tendon reflexes[129]. About 30% of clinically recovered patients retain some abnormality in nerve conduction[125]. The fact that the internodal length in remyelinated segments of peripheral nerves is only about half that found in unaffected nerve segments is not a sufficient explanation for this: in conditions such as diphtheric neuropathy conduction velocity finally recovers to normal, despite shorter internodes in the remyelinated nerve fibre[138].

Pathology

Asbury and colleagues[1a] were the first to report in an autopsy series of 19 cases the features that are now considered the pathological hallmarks of the disease: mononuclear cellular infiltration and demyelination, with lymphocytes infiltrating the peripheral nervous system from the most proximal root levels down to the intramuscular arborization of motor nerves. Lymphocytes were seen both in the endoneurium and the epineurium in a perivenular distribution (Figure 3.3). Demyelination occurred in those areas which were heavily infiltrated by lymphocytes. Subsequent studies of sural nerve biopsies revealed different degrees of pathology and various frequencies of mononuclear cell infiltration[138a,139,140] (Figure 3.4). Obviously, timing of biopsy in a disease that evolves at different rates and is characterized by multifocal lesions could explain these divergent observations. Prineas[141] was the first to stress the second cardinal feature of the pathology in GBS: macrophage-mediated demyelination (Figures 3.5 and 3.6). Ultrastructurally, he showed vesicular disintegration and splitting of myelin lamellae and penetration by macrophages of the basal lamina of the Schwann cell[142]. Macrophages insinuate processes between myelin lamellae, which they then phagocytose. Macrophage processes have also been observed within meylinated axons; this may explain some of the associated axonal degeneration. Almost invariably, some degree of associated axonal degeneration is observed in this primarily demyelinating neuropathy. In single cases, an extraordinary degree of axonal degeneration was noted early in the course of the disease[60]. Feasby *et al.*[59] and Ropper[143] called attention to a primary axonal form of the disease that was clinically indistinguishable from typical GBS but had characteristic electrophysiological features suggestive of primary axonal degeneration. Two autopsy studies have been reported[59,144]. The pathogenesis of these cases is elusive and it has been argued that they constitute a separate entity.

The pathological findings obtained in biopsy and autopsy studies support the existence of both cellular and humoral mechanisms in the pathogenesis of the disease[1,139,140,144–146].

Immunopathogenesis

There have been two schools of thought with regard to the pathogenesis of GBS. Despite the early pathological descriptions of significant cellular infiltration of the peripheral nervous system, for almost two decades most investigators favoured the view that a humoral immune reaction underlies nerve damage in GBS[3,145,147,148]. Several lines of evidence serve to support this notion (Table 3.11). Particularly important evidence was provided by experiments in which varying degrees of inflammatory demyelination could be produced in rodent nerves following intraneural injection of GBS sera although such effects were later shown to be relatively non-specific[145,149,150].

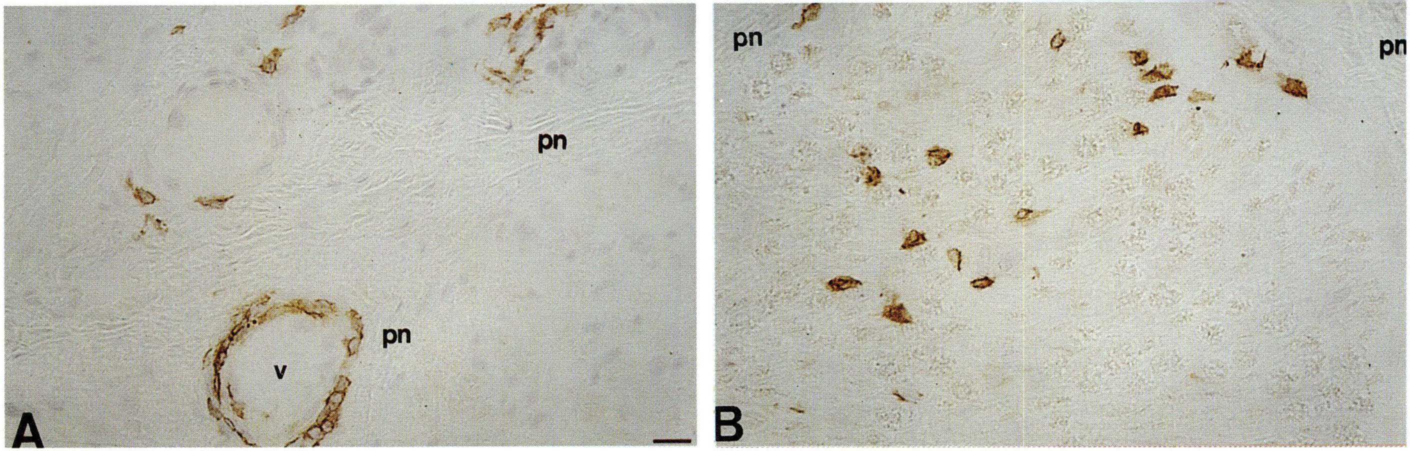

Figure 3.3 T lymphocyte infiltration of nerves in GBS. Perivascular epineurial (**A**) and diffuse endoneurial (**B**) infiltration of $CD3^+$ T lymphocytes in a sural nerve biopsy from patients with GBS. Immunohistological identification of T cells with the Leu4 monoclonal antibody in a frozen section counterstained with hematoxylin. V = venule, pn = perineurium, scale bar = 20 μm

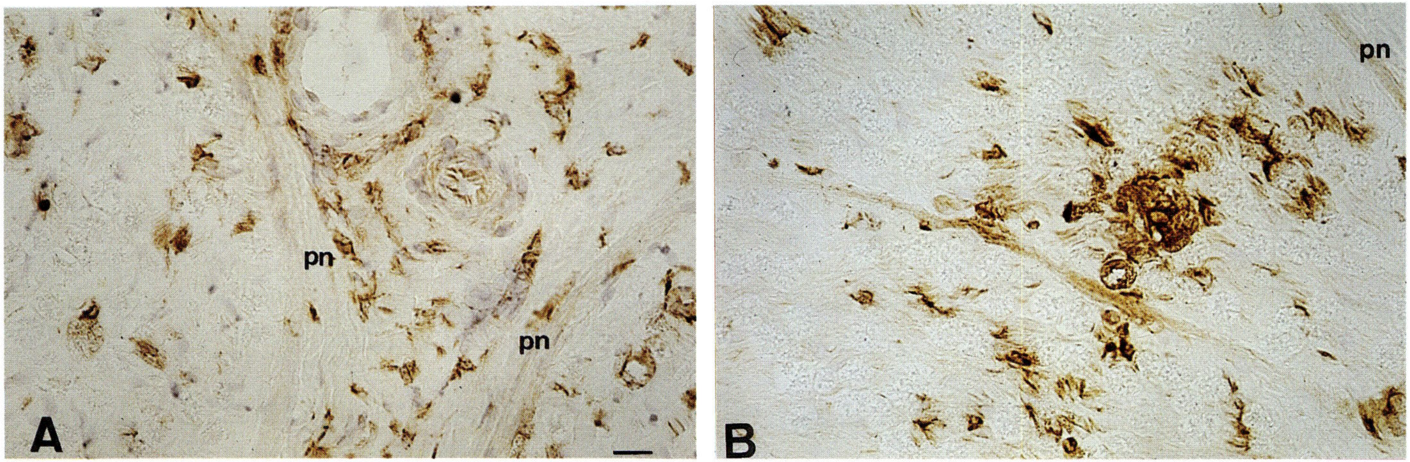

Figure 3.4 Macrophage invasion of nerve in GBS. Increased numbers of $CD68^+$ macrophages are present in the epineurium (**A**) and in the endoneurium (**B**). Frozen section (8 μm) of a sural nerve biopsy from a patient with GBS immunostained with a marker for macrophages and counterstained with hematoxylin. pn = perineurium, scale bar = 20 μm

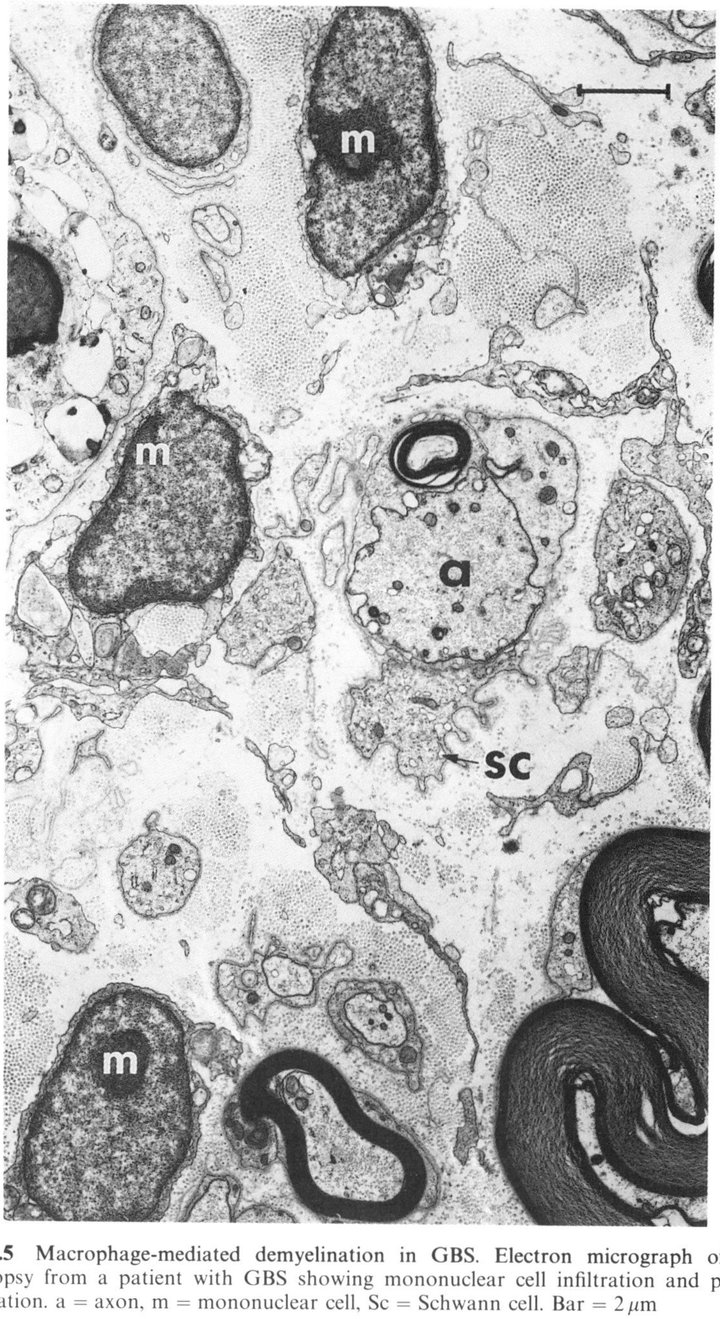

Figure 3.5 Macrophage-mediated demyelination in GBS. Electron micrograph of sural nerve biopsy from a patient with GBS showing mononuclear cell infiltration and primary demyelination. a = axon, m = mononuclear cell, Sc = Schwann cell. Bar = 2 μm

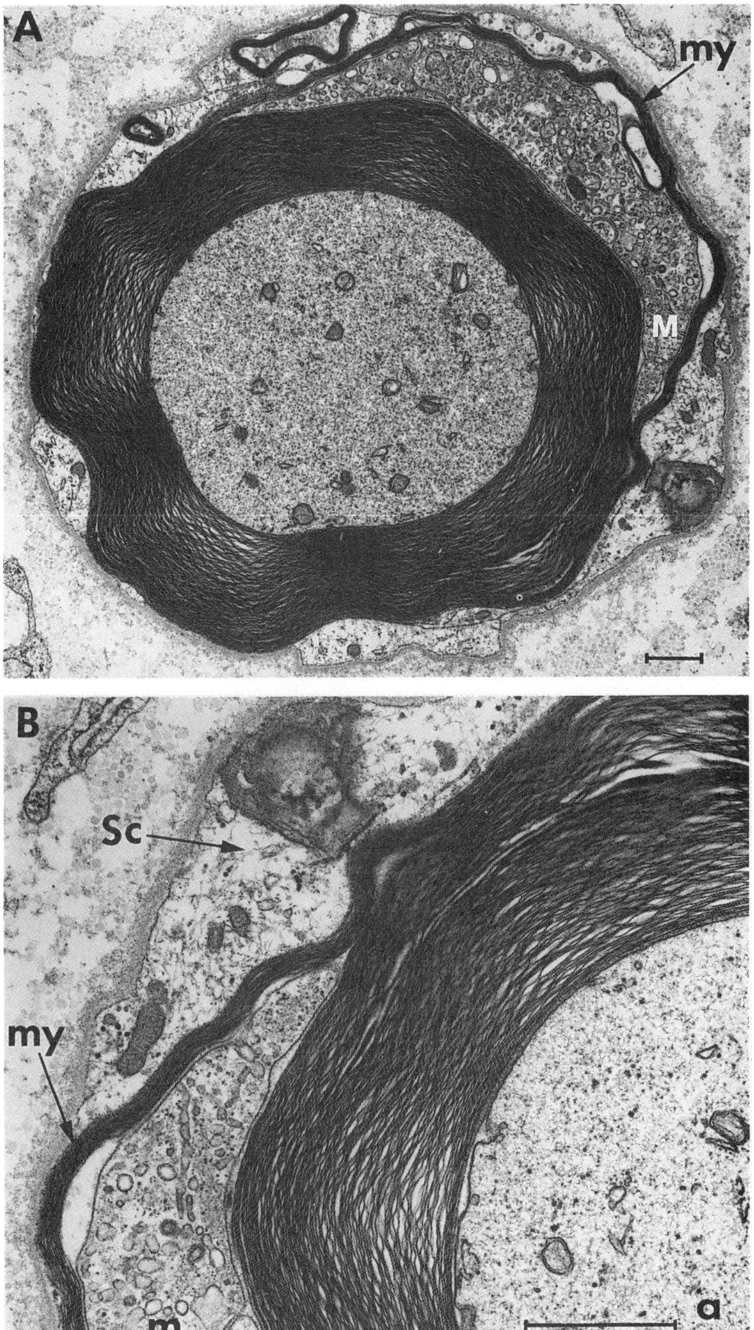

Figure 3.6 **Macrophage-mediated demyelination in GBS. Electron micrograph of sural nerve** biopsy from a GBS patient showing macrophage stripping of the myelin sheath. (**A**) A macrophage process (m) is separating several outer myelin lamellae (my) from the main sheath. Bar = 1 μm. (**B**) High power showing macrophage process (m) insinuating between myelin lamellae (my). Note Schwann cell cytoplasm (sc) is markedly oedematous. Bar = 1 μm

Table 3.11 Evidence for a humoral pathogenesis of Guillain–Barré syndrome (GBS)

Transfer studies
Demyelination of organotypic nerve cultures by GBS sera
Macrophage-associated demyelination of rat sciatic nerve following intraneural transfer of GBS sera
Production of conduction block after intraneural injection of GBS sera into rat sciatic nerve
Immunofluorescent studies on IgG, IgM, complement deposition on nerve fibres
Circulating antibodies to peripheral nerve/peripheral nerve myelin
Circulating antibodies to glycolipids
Detection of circulating cytokines in GBS sera
Activated complement components (C3a, C5a, C5b-9) detected in plasma, cerebrospinal fluid and *in situ*
Therapeutic efficacy of plasma exchange
Therapeutic efficacy of high-dose intravenous immunoglobulin

Humoral pathogenesis

Numerous studies attempted to identify disease specific circulating antibodies binding to peripheral nerve or purified myelin components utilizing different techniques. Many groups found antibodies to peripheral nerve myelin with varying frequency in GBS but also in other neurological disorders or healthy individuals[145,148,151]. Occasionally antibodies have been detected with specificity for two of the major proteins of peripheral myelin, the 29 kDa 219 amino acid transmembrane glycoprotein P0 and the 14 kDa 131 amino acid protein P2[152], but this has not been disease-specific. Recently, Connolly and co-workers[153] reported high titres of IgM and IgG antibodies to the cytoskeletal protein β-tubulin in 20% of GBS patients, 57% of those with CIDP, and only 2% of controls. However, the significance of these findings is at present unclear.

More recently, attention has focused on lipid antigens as targets for B cell immune responses in GBS. Lipids make up about 75% of the total nerve dry weight. Major myelin lipids are cholesterol, galactosylceramide (cerebroside) and galactosylceramide-3-O-sulphate (sulphatide); smaller amounts of several different gangliosides and complex neutral glycolipids (GD1a, GD1b, GT1b, GM1, GM2, GM3, GD2, GD3, LM1) are also present[154,155]. 3′-LM1 has been identified as the major monosialoganglioside, accounting for approximately 30% of total ganglioside sialic acid (Table 3.12).

Using the C1 fixation and transfer assay, complement fixing antibodies to human myelin were originally identified in 90% of GBS patients and were reported to belong mostly to the IgM class[156–158]. Serial determinations disclosed the absence of immunoglobulin isotype switching to IgG which would be compatible with the (auto)antigen being a thymus-independent antigen (i.e. carbohydrate/glycoconjugate rather than protein)[157]. These IgM antibodies were found to bind to carbohydrate residues similar to those of the Forssman antigen, a ceramide containing five carbohydrate residues which is present in many mammalian species and infectious agents. The Forssman antigen gives rise to a heterophilic antibody response, which can be determined in low titre in about one-third of normal individuals. However,

Table 3.12 Structures of glycolipids

	Carbohydrate sequence
GM1	Galβ1-3GalNAcβ1-4Galβ1-4Glcβ1-1Cer 3 | NeuAcα2
GT1b	NeuAcα2-3Galβ1-3GalNAcβ1-4Galβ1-4Glcβ-1Cer 3 | NeuAcα2-8NeuAcα2
GD1a	NeuAcα2-3Galβ1-3GalNAcβ1-4Galβ1-4Glcβ11Cer 3 | NeuAcα2
GD1b	Galβ1-3GalNAcβ1-4Galβ1-4Glcβ1-1Cer 3 | NeuAcα2-8NeuAcα2
GM3	NeuAcα2-3Galβ1-4Glcβ1-1Cer
GM2	GalNAcβ-4Galβ1-4Glcβ1-1Cer 3 | NeuAcα2
LM1	NeuAcα2-3Galβ1-4GlcNAcβ1-3Galβ1-4Glcβ1-1Cer
HexLM1	NeuAcα2-3Galβ1-4GlcNAcβ1-3Galβ1-4GlcNAcβ1-3Galβ1-4Glcβ1-1
Sulphatide	SO_4-3Galβ1-1Cer
SGPG	SO_4-3GlcAβ1-3Galβ1-4GlcNAcβ1-3Galβ1-1Cer

Cer, ceramide (N-acylsphingosine); LM1, sialosyl paragloboside; HexLM1, sialosyl lactosaminyl paragloboside; SGPG, sulphoglucuronyl paragloboside

recently Ilyas and co-workers[158a] were unable, using a different assay, to detect increased serum titres of antibodies to neutral glycolipids, particularly the Forssman antigen, in a series of 54 GBS patients when compared to individuals with other diseases or healthy controls.

Several groups have now provided evidence for a humoral immune response to acidic glycoconjugates in 5–6% of GBS patients. Antibodies were directed to one or more of the gangliosides GM1, GD1a, GD1b, GT1b, asialo-GM1, and LM1[70,75,76,152,155,158,158a,159–173] (Table 3.13). A number of investigators found a convincing association of GM1 antibodies with a more severe and predominantly axonal type of GBS. These antibodies could also be detected more frequently in patients who had a preceding *Campylobacter jejuni* infection than in those without[76,171–174]. However, others[70,75] found no association with preceding infection. Yuki *et al.*[172,173] reported on the association of anti-GD1a antibodies with severity of GBS. The reported discrepancies in the frequency of these antibody responses may reflect differences in the detecting system applied and in patient selection[175]. Immunogenetic background may also play a role: most Japanese patients with severe GBS, anti-ganglioside antibodies and evidence of a preceding

Table 3.13 Ganglioside antibodies in Guillain–Barré syndrome (GBS) and Miller-Fisher syndrome (MFS)

Reference	*Syndrome*	*Frequency*	*Isotype*	*Glycolipid antigens*
163	GBS	1/26	IgG	LM1, hexose
		2/26	IgG	GD1b
		2/26	IgM	GD1a, GT1b
155	GBS	29/50	IgG/IgM	LM1
	GBS	1/50	IgG/IgM	GM1
	GBS	1/50	IgG/IgM	GD1b, GT1b
171	GBS	2/2	IgG	GM1
76	GBS	14/95	IgG/IgM	GM1, GD1b
46	GBS	34/100	IgG/IgM	GM1
170	GBS	4/22	IgG/IgM/IgA	GM1, GD1b, asialo-GM1
174	GBS	5/16	IgG/IgM	GM1, GD1b
166	GBS	36/53	IgG/IgM	Acid glycolipids
158a	GBS	11/53	IgG	LM1
	GBS	12/53	IgG/IgM	GD1a and/or GD1b
	GBS	16/53	IgG/IgM	GM1 and/or GD1b
	GBS	18/53	IgG	GM1
172	GBS	2/10	IgG	GD1a
173	GBS	7/37	IgG/IgM	GM1, GD1a
161	GBS	1/1	IgG	GM1, GD1b, asialo-GM1
183	GBS	2/20	IgG	GM1
162	GBS	12/42	IgG/IgM	GM1, GD1b, asialo-GM1
169	GBS	13/24	IgG/IgM	GM1, GD1b
70	GBS	7/31	IgG/IgM/IgA	GM1, GD1a, GD1b
75	GBS	6/58	IgG/IgM	GM1, GD1b
180	MFS	6/6	IgG	GQ1b
181	MFS	4/4	IgG	GQ1b
178	MFS	13/16	IgG/IgM	GQ1b

C. jejuni infection were found to have the HLA-B35 haplotype[176,177]. Interestingly, in a study of 19 Japanese patients with the Fisher variant, a statistically significant association with a different haplotype, HLA-B39, was noted[188]. In Caucasians no particular association between MHC class I or II gene haplotypes and GBS has been found[179]. Fredman *et al.*[160] found antibody activity predominantly to LM1 in 43% of GBS patients and also in 67% of CIDP patients, as well as in 20% of blood donors who served as controls. Anti-sulphatide antibodies were detected with even higher frequency (65% of GBS and 87% of CIDP cases)[164]. In view of the higher incidence of these antibodies in patients with chronic polyneuritis, the authors surmised that these antibodies may result secondarily from repeated shedding of myelin antigens following the initial insult to the nerve. This seems attractive because, in contrast to earlier reports, Fredman *et al.*[160] found that most of these antibodies belong to the IgG class, that is, they are part of a secondary immune response. IgM and IgA class antibodies have also been observed[158,160,163–166]. Anti-SGPG antibodies of IgM or IgG class were detected in 13 of 53 (25%) GBS sera[164].

It is noteworthy that in a high proportion of patients with the Fisher variant of GBS, antibodies were detected that reacted with the ganglioside GQ1b[178,180,181]. In a recent series of 31 consecutive patients with GBS we have been unable to find a significant correlation between the presence of GM1 antibodies and any clinical features of the disease[70].

The common structural denominator of the glycolipid antigens is the terminal Gal(β1-3)GalNac carbohydrate moiety. It has been proposed that at least part of this antibody reactivity results from natural immunity, and that the level of such antibodies is increased following polyclonal stimulation of immunoglobulin production[155]. Interestingly, studying the effects of GBS sera on rat Schwann cell cultures, Mithen *et al.*[182] observed cytotoxic damage in 31% of 52 samples but found no correlation between cytotoxic activity and the presence of antibodies directed to glycolipids.

A key question is to what extent gangliosides and other glycoconjugates are immunogenic[183]. Ganglioside antibodies can be detected in many autoimmune diseases and in normal individuals[155]. Intramuscular administration of gangliosides to healthy individuals apparently does not yield significant serum levels of anti-ganglioside antibodies[184] and no changes in serum cytokine levels or local production of cytokines by peripheral blood monocytes are observed. One study found no significant formation of serum antibody to GM1 following therapeutic administration of gangliosides to a population of patients with Alzheimer's disease[155]. The situation may, however, be different if gangliosides are administered to patients with ongoing nerve inflammation. There are single cases on record of patients presenting with GBS in temporal association with parenteral administration of a ganglioside mixture; in some instances this was associated with high titres of anti-GM1 antibodies[174,185,186]. In another study from Italy, no increase in serum titres of GM1 antibodies was noted in GBS patients who had previously received gangliosides for therapeutic purpose[169]. An epidemiological survey in the Ferrara region of Italy showed that the incidence of GBS was not related to the widespread use of a ganglioside mixture for therapeutic purposes; this argues against a disease-precipitating role of gangliosides[187].

Addition of gangliosides to the inoculum used to produce EAN did not increase disease severity[188,189]. Administration of gangliosides to animals with active EAN neither improved nor worsened the neuropathy[190]. Anti-GM1 antibodies generated in Lewis rats by immunization with a ganglioside preparation containing GM1 showed cross-reactivity with other glycolipids but did not bind the Galβ(1-3)GalNac glycoprotein, although this epitope is commonly recognized by anti-GM1 antibodies found in patients with lower motor neuron syndromes[167,191]. This has been taken to indicate that anti-ganglioside antibodies in patients with lower motor neuron disease, and by extrapolation in those with GBS, probably do not result from autoreactivity to gangliosides released after nervous tissue damage. Collectively, these data point out the immunological relevance of carbohydrate structures as target epitopes that are shared extensively with glycolipids and glycoproteins.

The ganglioside GM1, while being a minor glycolipid of peripheral nerves, is of particular interest as a potential autoantigen since it is localized at and around the nodes of Ranvier. Antibodies to GM1 binding to this region could conceivably interfere with regular impulse propagation but experimental evidence for this is still incomplete[192].

It should be noted that the mechanisms by which immune responses are initiated against carbohydrate antigens differ from those mounted against proteins. Carbohydrates contain repetitive sugar sequences that can directly activate B cells by cross-linkage of the surface immunoglobulin receptors in an antigen-specific manner, obviating the need for helper T cells. Alternatively, as has been mentioned, these repetitive structures can induce polyclonal activation of B cells with ensuing generation of long-lived IgM responses. Hence, without isotype class switch of the immunoglobulins produced, no immunological memory is generated[193]. It is, however, conceivable that bystander T cell-derived cytokines could modulate this response and induce class switching from IgM to IgG or to affinity maturation[194,195]. Humoral immune responses to peptide antigens require helper T cells. This in turn implies the trimolecular interaction of the autoantigen(s), T cell receptors and MHC class II antigens to initiate clonal proliferation for all antigen specific T helper cells. As a consequence, affinity maturation, class switching from IgM to IgG and instruction of memory B cells occur[196]. Gangliosides themselves, however, cannot be intracellularly processed and presented in the context of MHC class II molecules[197]. It follows that in order to be rendered immunogenic, gangliosides must be bound to a protein or be part of a cross-reactive glycoprotein. In this instance, a pre-existing CD5 population-derived anti-carbohydrate antibody-positive B cell could act as antigen presenting cell to process and present a peptide fragment from the carrier protein to the T cell. The T cell could then provide cognate help to B cells, with resulting IgG antibody production. Gangliosides have been reported to exert immunosuppressive actions[190,198], and their neutralization might release immunostimulatory mechanisms. However, at present, the pathogenic significance of antibodies to glycolipids remains elusive.

Circulating antibodies to nerve antigens must pass the blood–nerve barrier to gain access to the myelin sheath. Blood–nerve barrier disruption is an early event in inflammatory demyelination. Several lines of evidence indicate that antibodies act by initiating the complement cascade with subsequent generation of the proinflammatory peptides C3a and C5a[199] and the assembly of the membrane attack complex C5b-9[157,200–203]. These activated complement components have been detected in plasma and cerebrospinal fluid of GBS patients, as has been mentioned earlier, and in situ deposition at the sural nerve has been observed[157,204]. In EAN the terminal complement complex could be localized by immunocytochemistry on Schwann cells and along myelin sheaths prior to demyelination[205].

An alternative role of antibodies pertinent to the mechanisms of demyelination could be their engagement in antibody-dependent cellular cytotoxicity (ADCC)[206]. Antibodies bind to macrophage via their Fc portion and guide them to the potential autoantigen(s).

Cellular immune reactions

The landmark paper of Asbury *et al.*[1a] first emphasized the role of mononuclear cells in GBS. Results in the animal model of experimental autoimmune

Table 3.14 Evidence for the involvement of T cells in Guillain–Barré syndrome

Pathological findings: multifocal infiltration of nerve roots and nerves in perivascular distribution
Induction of experimental autoimmune neuritis by myelin specific T cells
Presence of activated T cells in peripheral blood (increased HLA-DR expression, up-regulation of transferrin receptor; increased soluble interleukin-2 receptor; increased interleukin-2 concentrations)
Proliferative responses of T cells in peripheral blood to P0, P2, and peptides

neuritis clearly documented a pivotal role of T cells in initiating inflammatory demyelination[145,147,207]. Lewis rats that were T cell depleted or thymectomized did not develop EAN upon active immunization with myelin. Transfer of lymph node cells recovered from animals with actively induced EAN could produce the disease. Most tellingly, EAN could be induced by adoptive transfer of autoreactive P2- and P0-specific T cell lines[208–210], while ablation of T cell function suppressed EAN[211].

Attempts to demonstrate disease-specific T cell sensitization in GBS patients yielded inconsistent results[207,212–214]. Most recently, Taylor *et al.*[215] and Khalili-Shirazi *et al.*[216] reported an early transient proliferative response of blood mononuclear cells to the myelin protein P0 and synthetic peptides thereof in GBS and some CIDP patients, and a continued response to P2 and P2 peptides in up to 60% of GBS patients. Responses to at least one of these antigens were also found in 36% of CIDP patients and 25% of normal controls. It has been possible to isolate P2-specific T cell lines from one GBS patient and three normal individuals[217]. Evidence for systemic T cell activation has been furnished (Table 3.14). GBS patients have a higher number of circulating T cells carrying on their surface the activation markers HLA-DR, the transferrin receptor, and the interleukin-2 (IL-2) receptor[218]. Furthermore, concentrations of the soluble interleukin-2 receptor as well as of IL-2 itself are increased in patients with GBS; titres paralleled disease activity[219–222].

At present we do not know whether T cells specific for P2 or P0 play any pathogenic role. Clearly, further investigations are required to explore in more detail the T cell repertoire to myelin antigens in GBS patients and in controls. Autoreactive T cells in order to gain access to peripheral nerve have to be activated and migrate across the blood–nerve barrier. Adhesion molecules expressed on T cells, monocytes, and endothelial cells govern cellular trafficking: recent work in animals with EAN suggests that intercellular adhesion molecule 1 (ICAM-1) may be of particular importance[223–225]. T lymphocytes could be instrumental in several ways[145,207] including providing cognate help to B cells such that these are instructed to synthesize myelin antigen-specific antibodies, and recruiting macrophages in a delayed hypersensitivity reaction and stimulating them to enhanced phagocytic activity and elaboration of inflammatory mediators[200]. Most of the data obtained in experimental autoimmune neuritis would be compatible with such a function. T cells could exert direct cytotoxic damage to the myelin sheath or the Schwann cell[226]. There is little *in vivo* evidence to support this notion. It is, of course, also conceivable that T cells may suppress the ongoing immune response and terminate the acute monophasic disease. One study reported that the $CD8^+$ cytotoxic/suppressive subset of T lymphocytes in blood was diminished compared with hospital controls early in the course of the disease[227].

As has been mentioned above, macrophages feature prominently in the cellular infiltrate of the nerve lesion in GBS. They may be derived from blood-borne monocytes that have crossed the blood–nerve barrier or from endoneurial macrophages. These are numerous in normal nerves, where they are situated outside the basal lamina of the blood vessels[228,229]. This perivascular distribution renders them uniquely suited to act as antigen presenting cells in the peripheral nervous system. One prerequisite for a cell to function as professional antigen presenter is the display on its surface of MHC class II gene products. Biopsy studies in GBS patients documented the presence of MHC class II molecules both on Schwann cells and macrophages (Figures 3.7–3.9)[240]. Further studies have shown that MHC class II antigens are expressed on Schwann cells not only in GBS but also in a variety of non-inflammatory neuropathies[230–233]. Work carried out in experimental autoimmune neuritis would suggest that macrophages act as chief professional antigen presenters in peripheral nerves[234]. Recently, Atkinson *et al.*[235] presented immunoelectron microscopic evidence that MHC class II antigens were expressed exclusively on endothelial and perivascular mononuclear cells.

Beyond their role in the induction phase of an immune response, macrophages have been shown to be of pivotal importance in the amplification and effector phase of immune-mediated demyelination[200,207,236]. Mechanisms by which macrophages can damage peripheral nerves include phagocytosis of myelin, the generation of proinflammatory cytokines such as IL-1, IL-6 and tumour necrosis factor-α (TNF-α), and the release of potent inflammatory mediators acting at short range such as proteases, oxygen radicals, eicosanoids, complement components and possibly nitric oxide metabolites[36,200,205,215,237–239,241,244,248,249]. Macrophages are known to be rendered activated by T cells through the T cell-derived cytokines, interferon (IFN)-γ, and TNF-α. Their role in the pathogenesis of immune-mediated demyelination has been clarified again in the animal model EAN. An immunocytochemical study demonstrated the presence of cells positive for IFN-γ in nerve roots; this correlated with the number of MHC class II antigen-positive macrophages during the course of EAN[243]. The functional role of IFN-γ was established by *in vivo* manipulation. Administration of recombinant rat IFN-γ greatly worsened myelin-induced and T cell line-mediated EAN. Conversely, *in vivo* administration of a monoclonal antibody to IFN-γ, neutralizing the endogenously produced cytokine, abrogated EAN[245,246]. TNF-α was also identified in EAN lesions, where it appeared around the time of first clinical symptoms. Intraperitoneal administration of antibody to TNF-α reduced the severity of the disease[247]. Finally 20–50% of GBS patients have raised serum levels of TNF-α[249a]. Both IFN-γ and TFN-α stimulate the release of inflammatory mediators from macrophages and, in addition, TNF-α apparently possesses toxic properties towards myelin[224,250]. It is also possible that cytokines also modulate nerve impulse propagation and channel properties of Schwann cells.

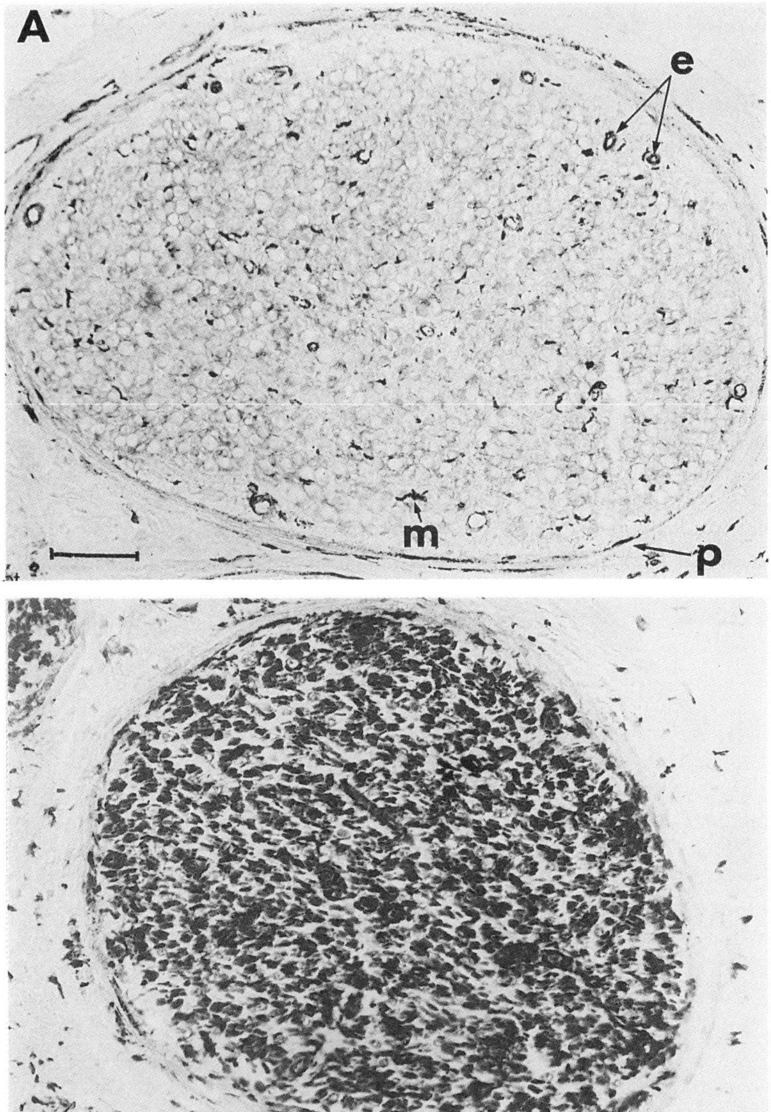

Figure 3.7 MHC class II molecules in GBS. Transverse section of sural nerve immunostained with mouse monoclonal antibody to MHC class II molecules and peroxidase-conjugated goat antimouse IgG. (**A**) normal human nerve reaction product (black stain) is seen on occasional resident mononuclear cells (m), endothelial cell (e) and perineurial cells (p). In **B**, from a patient with GBS, dense reaction product is present throughout the endoneurium. Bar = 10 μm

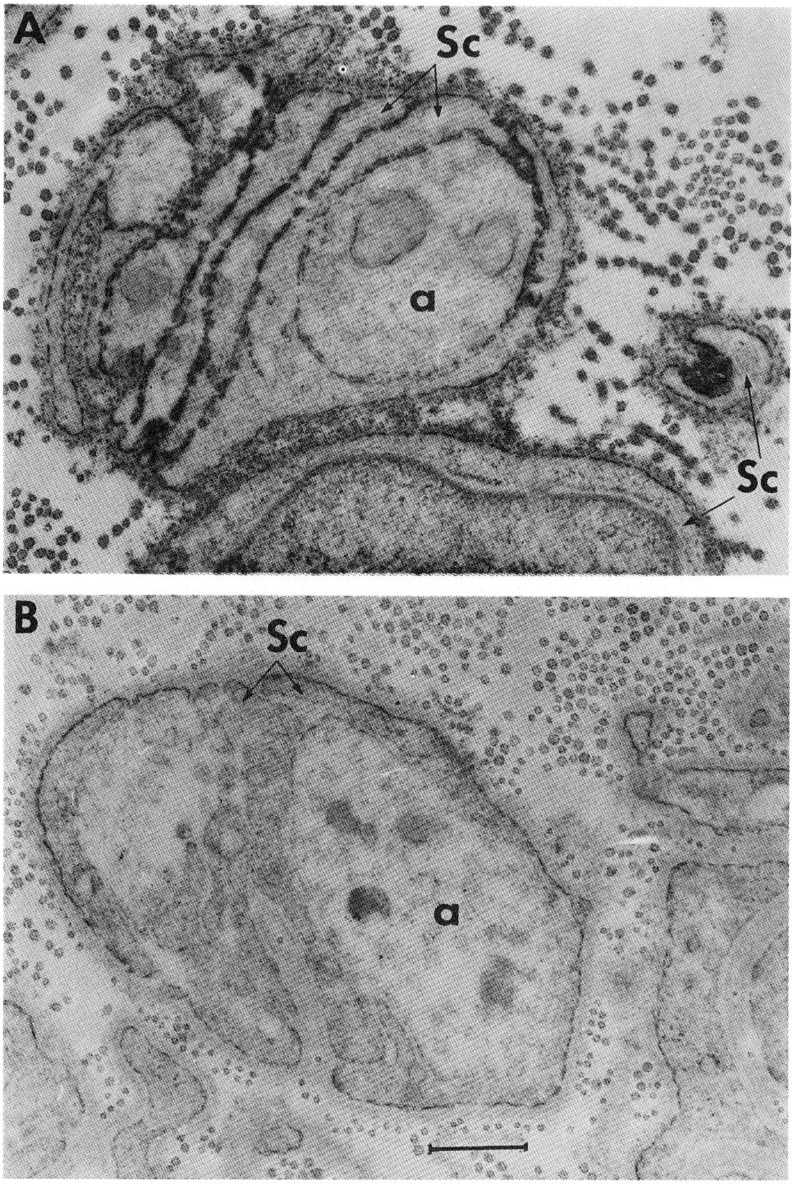

Figure 3.8 MHC class II molecules in GBS. Electron micrograph of sections from sural nerve from the same GBS patient illustrated in Figure 3.7 and immunostained for MHC class II molecules. (**A**) With primary and secondary antibodies. (**B**) Without primary antibody. a = axon, Sc = Schwann cell. Note reaction product on Schwann cell surface membrane. Bar = 1 μm

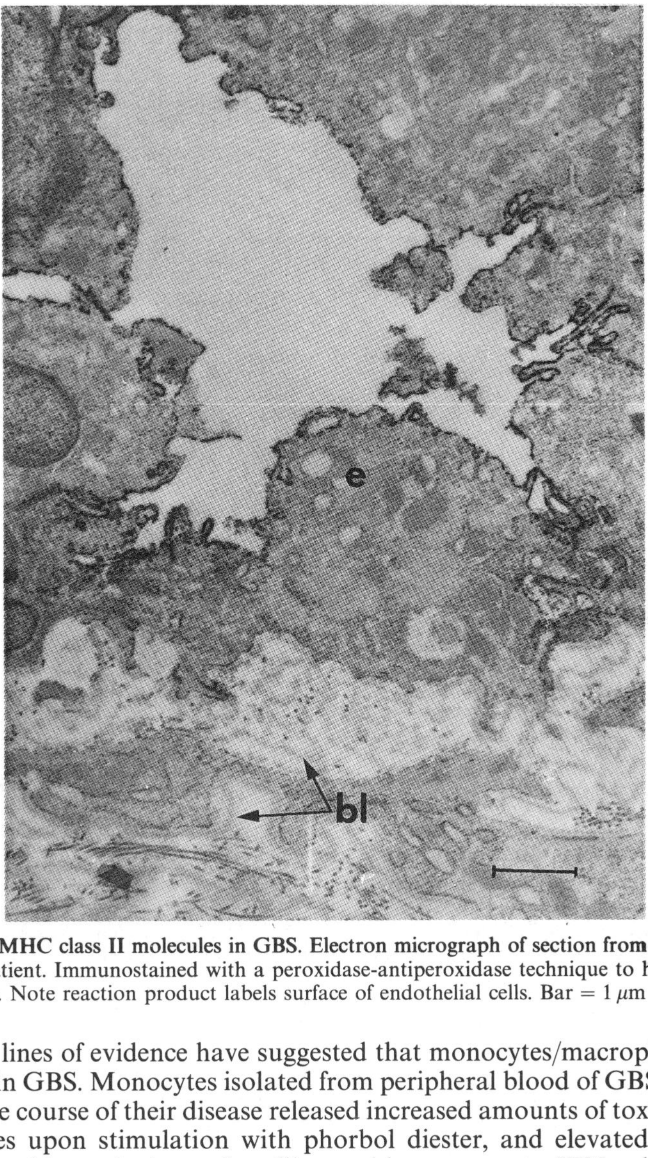

Figure 3.9 MHC class II molecules in GBS. Electron micrograph of section from sural nerve of a GBS patient. Immunostained with a peroxidase-antiperoxidase technique to human class II molecules. Note reaction product labels surface of endothelial cells. Bar = 1 μm

Several lines of evidence have suggested that monocytes/macrophages are activated in GBS. Monocytes isolated from peripheral blood of GBS patients early in the course of their disease released increased amounts of toxic oxygen metabolites upon stimulation with phorbol diester, and elevated levels of neopterin, a biosynthetic product liberated in response to IFN-γ, have been measured in GBS sera. Macrophages are activated by IFN-γ, and neopterin production mirrors the presence of this cytokine in the patients' circulation[207,220]. Studies of cytokines in the pathogenesis of GBS are summarized in Table 3.15.

The two hypotheses of a cellular or a humoral pathogenesis for GBS are, of course, not mutually exclusive. On one hand, antibodies to protein antigens are generated as a consequence of T/B cell interaction, and on the other,

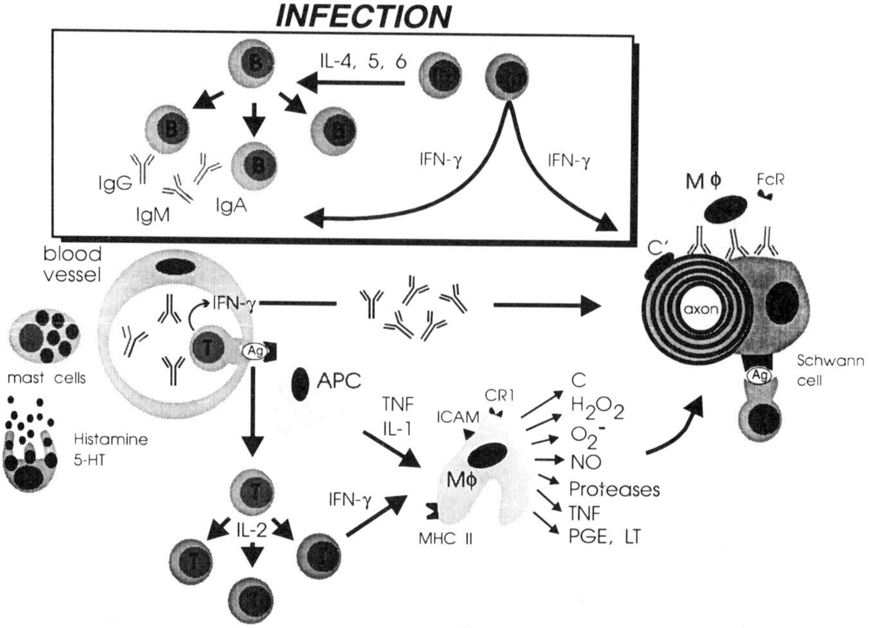

Figure 3.10 Overview of immune responses in GBS. An attempt has been made to incorporate evidence from studies in the animal model experimental autoimmune neuritis and investigations in patients with GBS to implicate immunoinflammatory reactions in the pathogenesis of GBS. The upper shaded panel represents the systemic immune compartment (peripheral blood). There, T cells circulate with specificity for myelin antigens. How they are triggered to become activated remains elusive (Table 3.16). An attractive hypothesis implies sharing of antigenic epitopes on microbes and myelin (molecular mimicry) and holds that an immune response mounted to the infectious agent is inadvertently misdirected to peripheral nerve. T cells, through release of cytokines, can either instruct B cells to proliferate and secrete myelin-directed antibodies and/or elaborate interferon (IFN)-γ which is known to enhance vascular permeability and activate macrophages. T cell independent antigens can directly stimulate B cell proliferation obviating the need for cognate T cell help. The systemic immune compartment is separated from nerve by the blood–nerve barrier. This is not complete and its function is disturbed early in inflammation when T cells are instrumental in breaching it. Subsequently, antibodies and inflammatory mediators can access peripheral nerve. Breakdown of the blood–nerve barrier also permits invasion of additional T cells, neutrophils, monocytes, and macrophages. If autoreactive T cells encounter an antigen presenting cell in nerve (endoneurial macrophage, pericyte, possibly Schwann cell) that upon stimulation by IFN-γ or tumour necrosis factor (TNF)-α expresses MHC class II gene products on its surface along with accessory recognition molecules (e.g. ICAM-1) plus the relevant autoantigen in suitably processed form, they can clonally proliferate and initiate a local immune response. Macrophages are activated by IFN-γ or TNF-α to enhanced phagocytosis and release noxious mediators that act on the myelin sheath. Myelin-directed antibodies can bind via the Fc receptor to macrophages and guide them to their target. Through activation of the complement system they effect demyelination of nerve fibres. Mast cells subserve a role in providing vasoactive amines that open the blood–nerve barrier

cooperation between T cells, macrophages and antibodies can be envisaged. Activated T cells could induce blood–nerve barrier changes, enhancing permeability and thereby allowing circulating antibodies access to the relevant antigenic structures on the myelin sheath (Figure 3.10).

Table 3.15 Involvement of cytokines in the pathogenesis of Guillain–Barré syndrome

Studies in humans
Interleukin-2 concentrations paralleling clinical disease activity in blood
Increased neopterin concentrations as a mirror of interferon-γ in blood
Increased interleukin-6 concentrations in blood
Increased tumour necrosis factor-α concentrations in blood
Evidence from studies in experimental autoimmune neuritis
Increased interferon-γ concentrations paralleling disease severity in blood
Localization *in situ* of interferon-γ and tumour necrosis factor-α immunoreactivity paralleling disease activity
Enhancement of disease by recombinant interferon-γ
Attenuation/abrogation of disease by neutralization of endogenously produced interferon-γ or tumour necrosis factor-α

Table 3.16 Possible mechanisms of immune activation in Guillain–Barré syndrome

Activation of autoreactive T cells
Molecular mimicry: cross-reactivity of myelin-specific T cells with antigenic structures on microbes
Activation of T cells by bacterial superantigens (? antigen-independent)
Polyclonal T cell activation by viral infections and antigen-nonspecific bystander inflammatory demyelination
B cell activation
Cognate T cell help
Molecular mimicry: sharing of B cell epitopes on myelin and microbes
Infection-triggered polyclonal B cell activation which raises low level 'natural' glycolipid antibodies above threshold

Initiation of the immune response

While much has been learnt about pathological events following activation of the immune system, the initiating mechanisms are yet to be elucidated. It is intriguing to implicate antecedent infections as triggers of the immune-mediated attack on peripheral nerves. A number of mechanisms may explain such a link (Table 3.16). Microbial agents may act as polyclonal activators stimulating lymphocyte proliferation, or may directly precipitate the liberation of cytokines which coordinate immune responses and exhibit inflammatory properties. In this context, induction of MHC class I and II molecules in response to IFN-γ or TNF-α, in association with self-antigens, may prime an autoreactive T cell response. So-called superantigens of microbial origin (e.g. enterotoxins) can trigger oligoclonal responses of T lymphocytes with a limited bias of their receptor usage[251]. In patients developing GBS following *C. jejuni* infection, generation of anti-GM1 antibodies may be dependent on the elaboration of the heat-labile 68 kDa enterotoxin which uses GM1 as its receptor[252]. The enterotoxin–receptor complex could then act as an antigenic carrier for the terminal Galβ(1-3)GalNac hapten. Microbes may directly infect and destroy immunocompetent cells, resulting in an altered balance between immunosuppressive and immunostimulating mechanisms. Finally, infecting organisms can contain chemical structures that mimic normal host self protein, forming the basis of molecular mimicry[253,254]. Under these circumstances, a B or T cell response initially directed towards microbial antigens may cross-react with self constituents resulting in autoimmunity. Currently available evidence suggests that polyclonal activation of B or T lymphocytes and molecular mimicry are both possible mechanisms by which a preceding microbial infection may be linked with the subsequent immune-mediated nerve damage in GBS. It has been reasoned that the presence of antiglycolipid antibodies of low and medium titre reflect polyclonal B cell stimulation[155]. Autoimmunity due to molecular mimicry can only occur when shared epitopes are different enough to break B or T cell tolerance and when the response is mounted against a self epitope of the host that carries significant biological activity[253].

With regard to molecular mimicry, computer searches have shown partial homology of amino acid sequences for cytomegalovirus, varicella zoster virus, and the P0 glycoprotein[154]. P0 is a neuritogen in rat EAN[209,255], and transient early T cell responses to this glycoprotein have been recorded in GBS patients[216]. Circulating antibodies have also occasionally been detected[152]. Recently, immunochemical evidence for a shared antigenic determinant between herpes simplex virus ribonucleotide reductase and peripheral nerve P0 with a molecular weight of 29 kDa has been produced[256]. With respect to the association between GBS and *C. jejuni* infection, a cross-reactive epitope contained in the lipopolysaccharide moiety of *C. jejuni* (PEN 19) and GM1 isolated from a GBS patient with GM1 ganglioside antibodies has been identified[257].

There is now evidence to suggest that nerve dysfunction and tissue damage in GBS result from an orchestrated action of immunocompetent cells, inflammatory cells, their soluble communication signals, and their injurious biosynthetic products (Figure 3.10). Definite proof that GBS has an autoimmune aetiology still needs to be furnished. In general, autoimmunity culminating in peripheral damage could result from a failure of mechanisms that normally operate to maintain self-tolerance, such as incomplete deletion or silencing of self-reactive clones or the aberrant stimulation or regulation of self-reactive lymphocytes that are normally anergic to self-antigens. One typical feature of autoimmune diseases, the association with particular MHC class II haplotypes, is lacking in GBS. Typical of autoimmune diseases, however, is the observation that infections often precede GBS. Nerve damage cannot be attributed to the infectious agent itself but is probably a consequence of host immune responses. The possible pathogenetic links between infection and disease include polyclonal lymphocyte activation, alterations of self-antigens to create partially cross-reactive neoantigens, and cross-reactivity to epitopes shared by nerves and microbes (molecular mimicry). Results of research over the past few years make it increasingly likely that multiple autoantigenic epitopes exist for both T and B cell responses. T and B cell responses directed against the same, or possibly different, epitopes may cooperate in launching an immune attack on peripheral nerves. The pathogenic significance of anti-glycoconjugate antibodies has yet to be established. Studies on T cell sensitization to neural antigens, examination of nerve-specific antibody repertoire, association with infections by different organisms with diverse antigenic characteristics,

Table 3.17 Treatment of Guillain–Barré syndrome

Reference	*Number of patients/ design*	*Treatment*	*Results*
273	40; open, randomized	Prednisolone ($n = 21$) vs. conventional therapy ($n = 19$)	Corticosteroid group slightly worse
39	245; open, randomized	Plasma exchange 3–5 × 40–50 ml/kg body weight vs. conventional therapy ($n = 122$)	Plasma exchange significantly superior
264	220; open, randomized	Plasmapheresis of albumin/fresh frozen plasma 4 × 100 ml/kg body weight vs. conventional therapy ($n = 109$)	Plasma exchange significantly superior in particular with early institution
263	37; open, randomized	Plasmapheresis ($n = 20$), 6 l plasma for at least 5 sessions vs. conventional therapy	Improvement in the therapy group
274	242; double-blind randomized	5 × 500 mg methylprednisolone i.v. vs. placebo	No significant difference
46	147; open, randomized	Intravenous immunoglobulin ($n = 74$) 5 × 400 mg/kg body weight vs. plasmapheresis ($n = 73$)	Immunoglobulins at least as efficient as PE, possibly superior

different clinical courses, and distinct electrophysiological changes and pathological alterations raise the possibility that Guillain–Barré syndrome may have several aetiologies.

Management

Immunotherapy

Plasma exchange

Following a number of anecdotal reports, two definite open randomized multicentre trials established the therapeutic efficacy of plasma exchange[39,45,258–264] (Table 3.17). In the North American trial published in 1985[39], 122 patients were treated with plasmapheresis while 123 received supportive therapy. Patients included were incapable of walking independently and 200–250 ml/kg body weight of plasma were exchanged over 7–14 days. Overall, patients treated with plasma exchange improved more rapidly, needed less assisted ventilation, spent less time in intensive care units, and less time in the hospital. Treatment was most efficacious when initiated within 1 week of the onset of neuropathic symptoms. If plasma exchange could not be instituted within 2 weeks of onset of symptoms, patients did not benefit. Interestingly, outcome at 6 months was the same in plasmapheresed and conventionally treated patients. These results were corroborated by the study of the French Cooperative Group[263], who treated 111 patients with plasma exchange and 109 patients with supportive measures. Plasma exchange was started within 17 days of disease onset, and comprised 4 × 2 plasma volumes. Plasmapheresed patients had a more rapid onset of recovery, shortened time to unassisted walking, and shorter duration of mechanical ventilation. This trial also demonstrated equal effects of replacing plasma with albumin or fresh frozen plasma. Since five of 52 patients who received fresh frozen plasma contracted hepatitis, these investigators advised against its use as replacement fluid. In a follow-up report[264] the French Cooperative Group recently reported the 1-year assessment of patients receiving either plasma exchange or conventional treatment. In contrast to the North American study, long-term benefit from plasmapheresis was observed as demonstrated by full recovery of muscular strength at 1 year: 71% in the plasma exchange group and 52% in the control group. However, the use of plasma did not affect the incidence of severe motor disability. These studies also served to identify predictive factors (Table 3.3). Poor outcome was associated with diminished summed compound muscle action potentials (< 20% of normal) upon distal stimulation in the North American trial[50,137,272]. Plasma exchange was still beneficial in this group. Up to 25% of patients have been reported to experience some kind of relapse approximately 1–2 weeks after plasma exchange; this usually responds to further plasmapheresis[265–271]. Relapses after plasma exchange are generally thought to result from antibody rebound, and in one study recurrence of disease after plasma exchange was indeed associated with increased levels of peripheral myelin-directed antibodies[270,271]. It is not known whether patients with less severe neuropathy (those still ambulatory) profit from plasma exchange, and whether frequent exchanges would provide more benefit. Plasma exchange is reasonably safe, but is not totally without risk, particularly in patients with conditions such a GBS, who are particularly prone to infections and autonomic disturbance. Such risks, combined with limited availability of apparatus and trained personnel, and efficacy in only 60% of patients, prompted the search for alternative treatments.

Corticosteroids

A small, open, randomized trial of oral prednisolone (60 mg/day), in the treatment of GBS showed no benefit[273]. Recently, a double-masked, multicentre trial has been completed which looked at the effects of a high-dose intravenous methylprednisolone regimen. A total of 242 patients were randomized to receive intravenous methylprednisolone 500 mg/day for 5 days or placebo within 15 days of onset of neuropathic symptoms. They were not able to run. No significant difference was noted in any outcome parameter between the 124 patients treated with high dose corticosteroids and 118 patients who received placebo, and the relapse rates were not different in the two treatment arms[274]. These results are somewhat surprising in view of the dramatic effects seen with corticosteroids in the animal model. Such treatment diminishes production of inflammatory mediators and dampens cellular reactions involved in inflammation. Several possible explanations for the lack of effect have been advanced, including interference by steroids with macrophage function in the repair phase, and suppression of Schwann cell proliferation, with consequent inhibition of remyelination. Steroids may also prevent the development of anti-idiotypic antibody or T cell suppressor mechanisms that normally control immune responses and allow recovery from GBS.

High-dose intravenous immunoglobulin (IVIG)

High-dose intravenous immunoglobulin has shown therapeutic promise in a number of disorders of a presumed autoimmune nature. Van der Meché and his colleagues recently reported the results of an open randomized trial in which patients were assigned to receive either five plasma exchanges (200–250 ml/kg body weight) or five doses of intravenous immunoglobulin (0.4 g/kg body weight/day)[46]. Treatment was initiated within less than 2 weeks and all patients were unable to walk independently. The predefined outcome measure was improvement at 4 weeks by at least one grade on a 7-point scale of motor function. The trial was stopped when an interim analysis of 150 patients revealed that 53% of the 74 patients who received immune globulin had improved by one grade or more compared with 34% of those treated with plasma exchange. Median time to improvement by one grade was 27 days with immunoglobulin therapy and 41 days with plasma exchange. Fewer patients receiving immunoglobulin required assisted ventilation, and the mean duration of intubation was 15.2 days, compared with 22.6 days in those treated by plasma exchange. This study also looked at prognostic factors that had been identified in previous trials: univariate analysis showed that old age and low distal amplitude of the compound muscle action potential was associated with a poorer prognosis (Table 3.3). However, when a multivariate logistic–regression analysis was performed only age remained statistically significant. Furthermore, serologically proven *C. jejuni* infection (36% of 129 patients examined) and the presence of antibodies to GM1 (30%) predicted a poorer outcome in this trial. While these results would suggest superiority of IVIG over plasma exchange, one has to consider that patients receiving plasma exchange in this trial fared significantly worse than in two previously published studies. A number of differences between the two treatment arms may have biased the outcome. Plasma exchange was delayed by a mean of 1 day compared with IVIG. Plasmapheresed patients were older, had been ill longer before commencement of therapy and had on average lower summed distal compound muscle action potentials. Moreover, reports are appearing that caution against the preferential use of IVIG because relapses and worsening of the disease occurred during the treatment[275,276]. There is, therefore, need for further evaluation of this treatment. A multicentre trial is underway in which patients will be randomized to receive either plasma exchange, IVIG or a combination of both therapies.

IVIG is not completely without risk: back pain, meningeal reaction, fever, tachycardia and headache during or within hours of completing the infusion

Table 3.18 Proposed mechanisms underlying therapeutic efficacy of plasma exchange and high-dose intravenous immunoglobulin therapy in Guillain–Barré syndrome

Plasma exchange
Removal of pathogenic circulating factors (antibodies, complement, cytokines, inflammatory mediators)
Immunomodulation (favouring suppressor mechanisms)
High-dose intravenous immunoglobulin
Anti-idiotypic antibodies
Blockade of Fc receptors on macrophages
Down-regulation of B cells/antibody production
Contaminating soluble HLA class II gene products and soluble CD4 molecules interfering with T cell activation
Induction of T suppressor cells

are known side-effects[277,278]. Anaphylactic reactions can occur in patients with IgA immunodeficiency and anti-IgA antibodies[279]. It may also be hazardous to administer IVIG to patients with impaired renal function[280,281]. Mechanisms by which this therapy is thought to act are summarized in Table 3.18[283–288].

General care of GBS patients

Ropper *et al.*[15] give an excellent account of the general medical management and the nursing care of patients with GBS. Immobilized patients are particularly prone to nosocomial infections (pneumonia, tracheobronchitis, urinary infections, and less commonly, sepsis), and up to 5% of bed-bound patients develop embolism as a consequence of immobilization: appropriate early antibiotic treatment and anticoagulation with heparin can prevent these complications. Pain may be particularly troublesome, and occurs in up to half of the patients. Non-steroidal analgesics or carbamazepine may be effective. Meticulous nursing care is required and, above all, psychological support. Physical therapy is of paramount importance. It includes facilitation of pulmonary toilet, range of motion exercises, appropriate limb positioning, strengthening exercises, and assisted mobilization. Later on, gait retraining and instruction in the use of orthotic devices is provided. Based on his large experience at the Massachusetts General Hospital Neurology ICU, Ropper has established criteria for admission of GBS patients to intensive care units (Table 3.19)[15].

Potentially life-threatening complications resulting from autonomic dysfunction are discussed above. Acute autonomic disturbances often resolve spontaneously, and it is not always necessary to administer blood pressure regulating drugs during hypertensive periods, since the situation often resolves within a short period of time. Fluid administration is preferred for the treatment of hypotension: sympathomimetics are best avoided because blood pressure may over-react. However, episodes of second- and third-degree atrioventricular block and severe bradycardia should prompt consideration of a (temporary) demand pacemaker to avoid progression towards asystole.

Patients should be intubated if vital capacity goes down to 12–15 ml/kg.

Table 3.19 Criteria for admitting patients with Guillain–Barré syndrome to an intensive care unit

Deteriorating vital capacity < 18–20 ml/kg: signs of diaphragmatic fatigue
Poor cough, accumulating secretions, aspiration pneumonia
Progressive weakness associated with difficulty swallowing
Major dysautonomic features (wide blood pressure and pulse fluctuations, arrhythmias, heart block, pulmonary oedema, profound ileus with risk of visceral rupture)
Hypotension precipitated by plasma exchange, or plasma exchange planned in a ventilated or unstable patient
Secondary sepsis
Chest pain

If bulbar paralysis is present, intubation is recommended at a vital capacity of 15–18 ml/kg[15,289,290].

CHRONIC INFLAMMATORY DEMYELINATING POLYRADICULONEUROPATHY (CIDP)

Diagnosis

Patients with CIDP present with evidence of polyradiculoneuropathy that evolves subacutely over more than 4 weeks or chronically over many months; the disease course may be progressive, characterized by relapses and remissions, or occasionally a subacute and monophasic course[291,292]. In a patient with the latter clinical course, the diagnosis is usually made when neurophysiological studies provide evidence of underlying demyelination, and other causes of demyelination, including malignancy, paraproteinaemia, and metabolic disorders such as diabetes or renal failure, have been excluded[291–296]. Occasional patients present acutely, as in GBS, but subsequently follow a progressive or relapsing course and the diagnosis of CIDP is made in retrospect[295]. Histological confirmation of demyelination is usually deemed appropriate since treatment of this condition may involve the use of potentially toxic immunosuppressive agents. There are no reliable incidence figures of CIDP. The prevalence has been estimated to be about 3–5/100 000 of population[292].

Clinical features

The majority of patients present with a sensorimotor peripheral neuropathy although some cases are predominantly motor; occasional patients have a predominantly sensory neuropathy and may resemble cases of sensory neuropathy associated with malignancy[291–297]. Since CIDP is a polyradiculoneuropathy, weakness is usually seen in proximal and distal muscles. Sensory symptoms and signs were evident in about 75% of the cases reported by McCombe *et al.*[295] and pain was a symptom in about one-fifth. Cranial nerve involvement has been reported in approximately 16% of patients[295], which is less than that seen in patients with GBS. Postural or intention tremor is occasionally present[298]. Two-thirds of the patients reported by McCombe and colleagues[295] followed a chronic relapsing course and one-third had a chronic progressive course or a monophasic illness with a subacute onset. These proportions have varied in other series[293,297]. The mean age of onset of the relapsing cases was 26.8 years, compared with 51 years in the non-relapsing group, a finding which provides further evidence for regarding CIDP as the peripheral nerve analogue of multiple sclerosis[299]. Other uncommon clinical features include papilloedema, nerve hypertrophy and Horner's syndrome[293].

Differential diagnosis

The most common problem in differential diagnosis is provided by the hereditary demyelinating neuropathies, particularly HMSN-I, when no family history is available. Electrophysiological changes can be very helpful. Neuropathies associated with malignancy must also be excluded. Demyelinating neuropathy may occur in association with lymphoma, carcinoma and myeloma, including POEMS (polyneuropathy, organomegaly, endocrinopathy, monoclonal gammopathy, skin changes) syndrome. Metabolic causes of demyelinating neuropathy include diabetes, uraemia, hypothyroidism and acromegaly, while drugs that may induce demyelinating neuropathy include amiodorone and perhexilene maleate. Neuropathy associated with *N*-hexane and 2,5-hexanedione (glue sniffing) may be associated with paranodal demyelination and slow motor nerve conduction[294,295a,296].

HIV infection and Lyme disease may cause neuropathy. Cerebrospinal fluid pleocytosis is commonly seen in CIDP associated with HIV infection[66].

Neuropathy may also be associated with monoclonal gammopathy of undetermined significance (MGUS). Most clinicians exclude all MGUS-associated neuropathies. However, a case can be made for including IgG- and IgA-associated neuropathies, since these are often similar in all respects to CIDP and respond to the same treatments[300]. Neuropathies associated with IgM MGUS, however, are usually slowly progressive sensorimotor polyneuropathies with mostly distal weakness and sensory abnormalities. About 50% of patients show specific binding to myelin-associated glycoprotein (MAG) and related epitopes and widened myelin lamellae on electron microscopy, and much controversy surrounds their response to treatment[301,302]. For these reasons neuropathies associated with IgM MGUS are excluded from the definition of CIDP (see Chapter 2).

Differential diagnosis also includes multifocal motor neuropathy with persistent conduction block. Lewis and co-workers[112] described five patients selected from a group of 40 with CIDP, who presented with mononeuritis multiplex with prominent motor manifestations; there were unique electrophysiological features of well localized, persistent motor conduction block and some temporal dispersion. These regions of conduction block were located at sites other than the usual sites of nerve entrapment and distal sensory action potentials were preserved. Furthermore, conduction block persisted for months or years. Parry and Clarke[303] described a further group of patients with similar findings, who presented with muscle atrophy, cramps and fasciculations, and preserved tendon reflexes, who had initially been diagnosed as having motor neurone disease. In one case, severe motor conduction block was seen in the forearm segment of the median nerve, yet the ascending mixed nerve action potential was normal. Pestronk *et al.*[167,304] and other workers have reported high titres of antibodies against GM1 and other gangliosides in some patients with lower motor neurone syndrome of the type described above. However, the specificity of these antibodies remains to be determined. Some authorities regard these cases as a CIDP variant[112,305] and others regard them as a separate entity[167,304]. This issue is unresolved at this present time.

Recurrent Guillain–Barré syndrome must also be excluded[41,48,306]. Acute recurrent episodes of this type with complete or virtually complete recovery are considered to be recurrent GBS, rather than CIDP.

Prognosis

In the series of McCombe *et al.*[295], 76 patients were reviewed at an interval of 1–41 years (mean 10.6) after disease onset. Seventy-three per cent made a good recovery with only minor degrees of disability, but 6% had died as a result of the disease. Only 2% of patients were unable to work. The prognosis was better in patients with relapsing disease than in those with progressive disease.

Autonomic symptoms in chronic inflammatory demyelinating neuropathy

Clinically relevant autonomic dysfunction is much rarer in chronic inflammatory neuropathy than it is in GBS. Correspondingly, unmyelinated fibres show only a minor degree of pathology in this disorder[29].

Clinical variants of CIDP

Chronic ataxic sensory neuropathy

Occasionally, patients present with a peripheral neuropathy without weakness; they display prominent sensory symptoms and signs, gait ataxia, depressed or absent reflexes, but no clinical evidence of muscle weakness or wasting. In some cases there is electrophysiological evidence of demyelination in motor fibres in addition to clinical, electrophysiological and pathological evidence of demyelination in sensory fibres. Other patients, however, show electrophysiological abnormalities confined to sensory fibres, and occasionally abnormalities of the sensory evoked studies only may be found, implying that the pathological changes are predominantly within the dorsal root proximal to the dorsal root ganglion. These cases should be differentiated from sensory neuropathy or neuronopathy associated with carcinoma,

Sjögren's syndrome, coeliac and amyloid disease[307]. Such cases may represent the opposite spectrum of disease to those with multifocal motor neuropathy.

Focal hypertrophic neuropathy

Cases of focal[308] and multifocal[309] hypertrophic neuropathy have been described, with pathological findings of demyelination and inflammation as in CIDP. The enlarged nerves were located within the brachial plexus and in cranial and thoracic regions. Some patients followed a relapsing course and were responsive to corticosteroid treatment.

Multifocal motor neuropathy with persistent conduction block

This neuropathy, although regarded by some authors as a separate disease entity[304], is considered by others as a CIDP variant[112,305]. Kaji and co-workers[310] have recently examined the pathological changes in a typical case, and have shown demyelination at the site of conduction block and nerve enlargement. The changes were indistinguishable from those of inflammatory demyelination.

Chronic demyelinating polyneuropathy with monoclonal gammopathy

Patients with clinical, electrophysiological and pathophysiological features of a chronic demyelinating polyneuropathy indistinguishable from CIDP may have an associated monoclonal gammopathy, particularly of the IgG or IgA class[300]. Such patients may also respond to the same treatment regimens as others with CIDP and are regarded by some authorities as a subgroup of CIDP[301].

Electrophysiology of chronic inflammatory demyelinating neuropathy (CIDP)

Electrophysiology is crucial to the diagnosis of CIDP and reveals abnormalities in almost all patients[295,297]. The electrophysiological features of CIDP are similar to those found in advanced stages of Guillain–Barré syndrome: typical signs of multifocal demyelination with or without additional axonal degeneration. Because of the longer time course of the disease, conduction slowing is more pronounced owing to the greater proportion of chronic demyelination and remyelination usually found in CIDP. As a consequence of conduction slowing there may be gross temporal dispersion of CMAP, leading to persistently small CMAP amplitudes. Unlike the situation in GBS, antecedent illness is usually lacking in CIDP, and initial symptoms may be vague so that the beginning of the disease cannot be determined precisely enough to make a proper distinction between early and late findings in CIDP. Some conclusions may, however, be drawn from evaluating the course

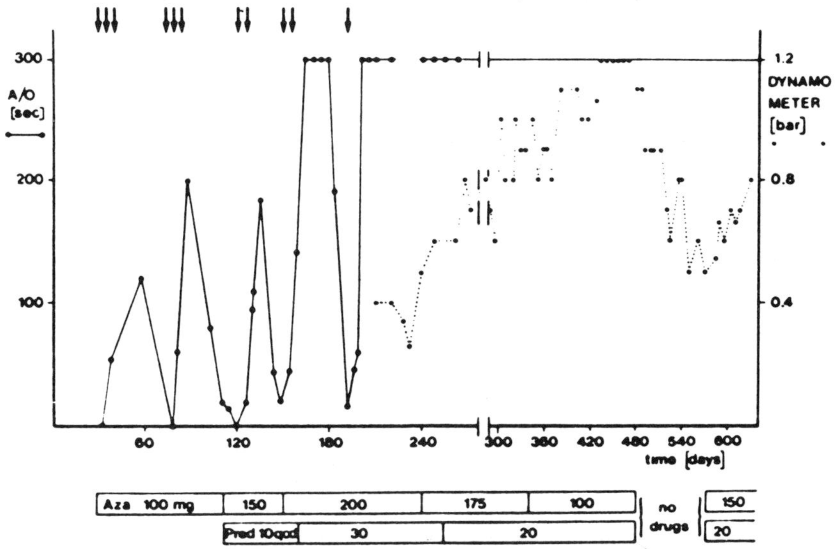

Figure 3.11 Correlation between clinical improvement with plasma exchange therapy in CIDP. Data taken from a 16-year-old girl suffering from the chronic relapsing form of CIDP. Following the deliberate discontinuation of effective long-term immunosuppressive therapy, plasma exchange therapy was administered because of a sudden severe relapse. Arm-outstretch time is depicted on the left (solid line), followed by dynamometric evaluations of hand grip strength on later check-ups (dashed line). Times of plasma exchanges are indicated by arrows above the top trace, and immunosuppressive medication is listed below the graph. Note the immediate and dramatic clinical response to plasma exchange, followed by the stabilization while under immunosuppression. Discontinuation of medication after more than 4 years was again followed by a deterioration in symptoms which was again reversed by reintroduction of immunosuppression. (From reference 358a, with permission)

of electrodiagnostic measures in the relapsing form of CIDP (Figures 3.11, 3.12).

Electrophysiological criteria for diagnosing CIDP

The electrophysiological research criteria for the diagnosis of CIDP are basically identical to those published for GBS and aim at identifying multifocal conduction block as the essential finding related to demyelination (Table 3.6). In order to prove the presence of conduction block, additional tests are required (Table 3.8). Reduction in sensory conduction velocity below 80% of the lower limit of normal and absent H reflexes lend further support to the diagnosis of CIDP[130a]. In practice, CIDP must always be considered if a patient with chronic polyneuropathy shows electrophysiological signs of demyelination, so particular effort must be made to detect slowing of nerve conduction or conduction block and temporal dispersion of CMAP or sensory nerve action potential (NAP). Conduction slowing is characteristically patchy in distribution and non-uniform along a particular nerve, a finding which is most helpful in differentiating between this acquired demyelinating neuropathy

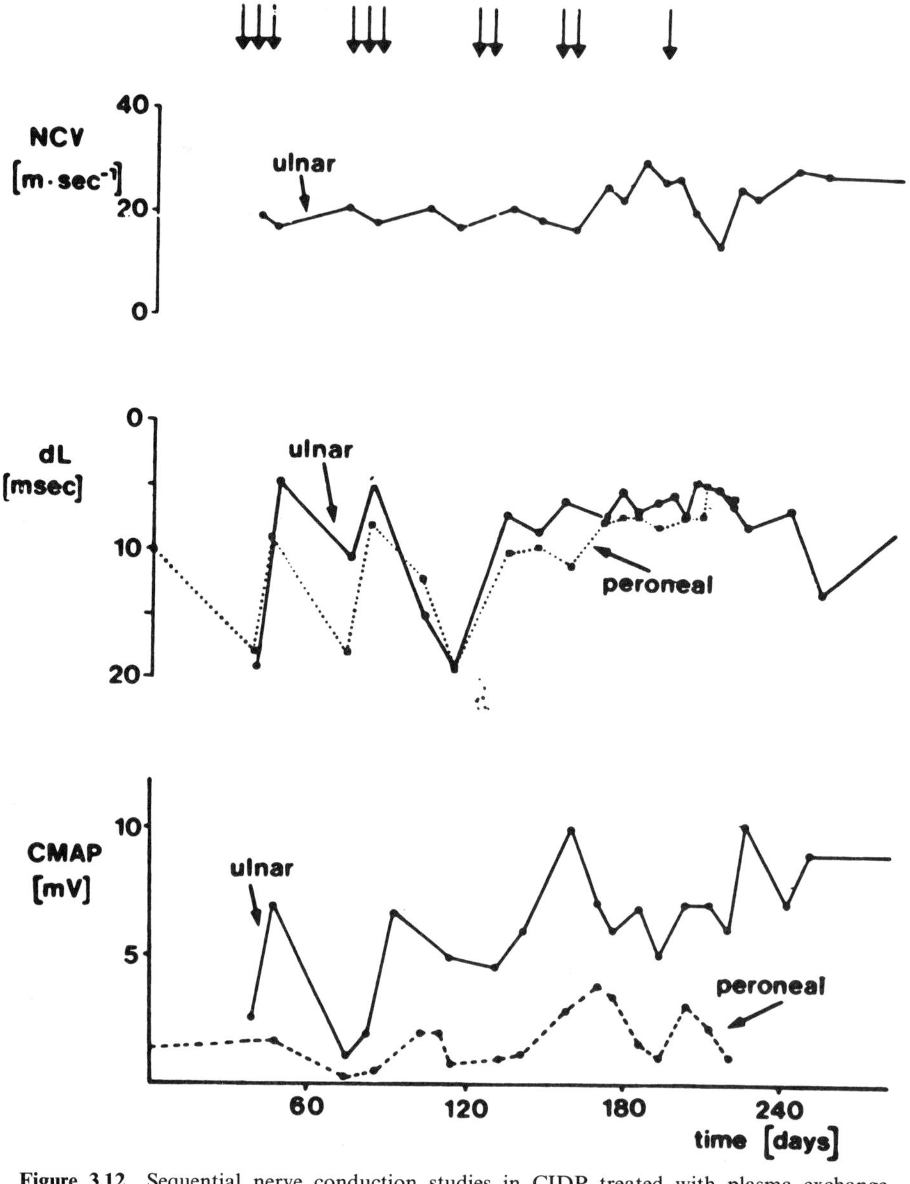

Figure 3.12 Sequential nerve conduction studies in CIDP treated with plasma exchange therapy. Ulnar (solid line) and peroneal nerve (dashed line) motor conduction velocity (NCV), distal latency (dL) and compound muscle action potential (CMAP) amplitude in the patient shown in Figure 3.11. Plasma exchanges (indicated by arrows over top trace) were clinically effective and mostly followed by an increase of CMAP amplitudes and normalization of dL while NCV remained basically unchanged. This demonstrates that distal nerve segments may be more susceptible to the immune attack in CIDP than more proximal parts of the nerve. (From reference 358a, with permission)

and hereditary neuropathies from which it may be indistinguishable clinically[311,312].

Abnormal NAP are more clearly detectable with needle recordings, but the surface technique is usually sufficient to discover abnormal dispersion or total absence of NAP. As in GBS, it is important to examine an appropriate number of nerves (at least two motor nerves in the upper limbs and two in the lower limb); sensory conduction should be examined in at least two nerves. In addition to conventional nerve conduction studies, F waves are particularly helpful and should be analysed with respect to persistence (number of F waves obtained on 10 successive stimuli), latency, and chronodispersion. Thus, F wave impersistence or absent F waves in the presence of near normal CMAP amplitudes is highly suggestive of proximal demyelination which otherwise would escape attention[124].

CMAP and NAP amplitudes are more difficult to interpret in CIDP than in many other forms of neuropathy. Owing to the wider scatter of individual nerve fibre conduction velocities in chronic demyelination, phase cancellation becomes important, and may lead to a substantial decrease in amplitude (as well as area under the curve) in the absence of any conduction block. As a result, conduction block can only be diagnosed if the area under the curve and/or CMAP amplitude are diminished by at least 50% on proximal compared to distal nerve stimulation[110,128] (Table 3.9).

Electromyography (EMG) is an indispensable complement to nerve conduction studies in CIDP. EMG is the best means to substantiate axonal lesions, which occur in more than 50% of patients with CIDP[295].

The contribution of electrophysiology in the differential diagnosis of CIDP

While acute GBS can be readily diagnosed, problems may arise if the time of onset of the disease is unclear or if relapses occur. The latter situation is rare (less than 5% in large series). The differential diagnosis requires further laboratory data because electrophysiologically, the relapsing form of acute GBS cannot be distinguished from neuropathy associated with acute intermittent porphyria[313] or in some forms of connective tissue disease, such as systemic lupus erythematosus or Sjögren's syndrome[314] where, as in other cases of vascular neuropathy[315], even focal conduction block can occur in the absence of conduction slowing.

Another difficult differential diagnosis is that of CIDP and hereditary motor and sensory neuropathy (HMSN). Here, the pattern of demyelination may help to establish the correct diagnosis. In hereditary neuropathies, demyelination (and therefore conduction slowing) is more uniformly distributed along the entire length of the nerves, while its distribution in acquired chronic polyneuritis is more likely to be patchy[311,312,317]. With proper criteria, conduction block could not be confirmed to occur in HMSN type 1 at all[312]. In both disorders, conduction slowing can be particularly pronounced at sites of physiological entrapment, such as the carpal tunnel[90,131]. However, not all patients can be properly classified by these criteria[109,317].

Multifocal conduction block in a proportion of nerve fibres within a nerve is the hallmark of chronic motor polyneuropathy associated with antibodies against ganglioside M1 (GM1 antibodies)[304]. Because of its almost exclusively motor pathology, the most important differential diagnosis of this type of neuropathy is spinal muscular atrophy, or even amyotrophic lateral sclerosis. Clinically, involvement of bulbar muscles along with clear pyramidal signs are not compatible with a diagnosis of GM1-associated polyneuropathy. GM1-associated neuropathy presents with multifocal conduction block, the focality of which should be tested for by 'inching' along individual nerves. Segments with conduction block and marked slowing have been shown to be 3–10 cm long[114]. Distal latencies are normal, but there may be more than one site of pathology along the individual nerve. Sensory conduction remains unaffected at the sites where motor fibres are blocked. Another characteristic feature of this type of chronic pure motor neuropathy is the predominant involvement of distal muscles of the upper extremities. Whether patients reported with persistent motor conduction block at the same site over years and some sensory abnormalities[112] also belong to this group or form another variant of CIDP is not clear.

Other chronic neuropathies, in particular those associated with dysproteinaemia, acquired immunodeficiency syndrome (AIDS) and neoplasia, have electrophysiological signs that are not distinctly different from CIDP. Thus, electrophysiology cannot help in separating these entities from classical CIDP[5,318].

Patients with uraemic or diabetic neuropathy may sometimes fulfil the electrodiagnostic criteria of CIDP, including conduction block[319]; this emphasizes the often neglected notion that electrodiagnostic studies help in establishing the diagnosis but are not alone sufficient to reach the diagnosis.

Central involvement in CIDP

Occasionally, patients with typical clinical and electrophysiological signs of CIDP also develop symptoms of central nervous system pathology[320]. If upper motor neurone signs are also present, studies of conduction in the CNS by magnetic cortical stimulation can reveal additional slowing in the pyramidal tract. However, it may be difficult properly to determine the latencies of CMAP elicited by magnetic stimulation because the variation in potential shape and latency tends to become much more pronounced owing to peripheral demyelination alone, not taking into account the effect of dispersed conduction in the pyramidal tract. Because of the over-riding effect of the peripheral pathology, studies of central motor conduction are not sensitive enough to detect subclinical involvement of central pathways. MRI studies have suggested central demyelination in some cases of CIDP, raising the possibility of a more than chance association between CIDP and multiple sclerosis[321,322] which has also been disputed[323].

Electrodiagnostic clues to prognosis

Prognostic indicators in CIDP electrodiagnosis have not yet been established, though it seems that the general statements made in GBS are also valid in this entity: the more pronounced axonal damage (as validated by EMG) the poorer is the general outcome. Conduction block may persist to a relevant extent and contribute to paresis, but slowed conduction itself remains functionally unimportant. Unbalanced recovery of conduction with consequential desynchronization of impulses may, however, be responsible for tendon reflexes failing to recover in spite of good recovery of muscle strength.

F-wave latencies often remain considerably prolonged, and with poor recovery F-waves remain unobtainable. Unlike the situation in GBS (see above), sensory nerve action potentials of the arm are usually not more severely affected than sural nerve NAP, probably because the longer time course has levelled out early differences.

As in GBS, needle EMG helps in determining whether low CAP amplitudes result from persistent distal conduction block or axonal degeneration. Despite appropriate treatment, denervation potentials in the affected muscles may persist for several years, but may sometimes disappear with some delay during periods of clinical recovery. Thus, spontaneous activity in the EMG still recordable years after the disease has come to a clinical standstill raises the suspicion that compensatory factors such as physical exercise may have improved the patient's condition despite further very slow progression of the disease.

Magnetic resonance imaging

Advances in MRI techniques have recently allowed accurate imaging of the cauda equina and nerve roots. MRI is currently being evaluated as an adjunct in the diagnosis of inflammatory neuropathies. Crino *et al.*[324] recently reported a patient with biopsy proven CIDP in whom abnormal enhancement of the cauda equina and spinal nerves could be demonstrated following gadolinium injection. Gadolinium enhancement is probably the consequence of blood–nerve barrier disturbance associated with inflammation. Similar findings were obtained in a patient with GBS[325].

Pathology of CIDP

Post-mortem studies have shown that inflammatory demyelinating lesions predominate within the spinal nerves, nerve roots and major plexuses, but they may be found at any level within the peripheral nervous system, including autonomic nerves and at the distal ends of motor fibres[294,326,327]. Although no abnormality may be found in sural nerve biopsies, at least one abnormality is usually detected (Table 3.20)[291,293,294]. The presence of inflammatory cells, macrophages and T cells may provide confirmatory evidence of the diagnosis (Figure 3.13). This is usually accompanied by up-regulation of MHC class I and II antigens[328]. Evidence of chronicity may

Table 3.20 Pathological features of chronic inflammatory demyelinating polyneuropathy

Endoneurial or subperineurial oedema
Demyelinated nerve fibres – large fibres devoid of myelin
Macrophage phagocytosis of myelin
T cells may be present
Thinly myelinated fibres
Axonal degeneration

be provided by 'onion bulb' formations (Figure 3.13), due to repeated segmental demyelination and remyelination of cluster formation as a result of axonal degeneration and regeneration[291,297]. The ultrastructural finding of macrophage stripping of myelin sheaths is important, since it is virtually diagnostic of inflammatory demyelinating neuropathy[141,299].

Immunopathogenesis of CIDP

Immunogenetic factors

A role for genetic factors in CIDP is suggested by its association with certain HLA antigens, unlike GBS, which has no such associations in most populations studied, with the possible exception of HLA-B35 in patients with the axonal subtype of the disease[176,179,329]. A significantly increased number of patients were HLA-B8-positive in three studies[330–332] and another class I antigen, HLA-CW7, was over-represented in the latter study. An association with HLA-DR2 was suggested by Feeney *et al.*[333], but this finding needs to be confirmed. There is also an increased frequency of the abnormal M3 allele of α1-antitrypsin, the major proteinase inhibitor, in CIDP patients.

Cell-mediated immunity

The pathological changes within nerves of patients with CIDP are highly suggestive of a delayed hypersensitivity cell-mediated immune response: myelin is removed by macrophages, the dominant inflammatory cell within the endoneurium, although $CD4^+$ and $CD8^+$ T cells may also be demonstrated within the lesions[328]. The up-regulation of MHC class I and II molecules within these lesions[230,328] provides further evidence for the presence of T cells. Additional evidence of T cell activation in CIDP has been provided by the demonstration of an increased percentage of circulating T cells positive for the DR activation marker[218] and the presence of increased serum levels of soluble IL-2 receptors[219–221]. However the antigen to which such activated T cells may be directed has not been identified: some workers have reported T cell hyper-responsiveness to crude nerve antigens or P2 basic protein, but others have not confirmed these findings[217,334,335].

Autoantibodies

Immunofluorescent studies by Dalakas and Engel[298] showed immunoglobulin bound to Schwann cell or myelin membranes in nine of 12 patients;

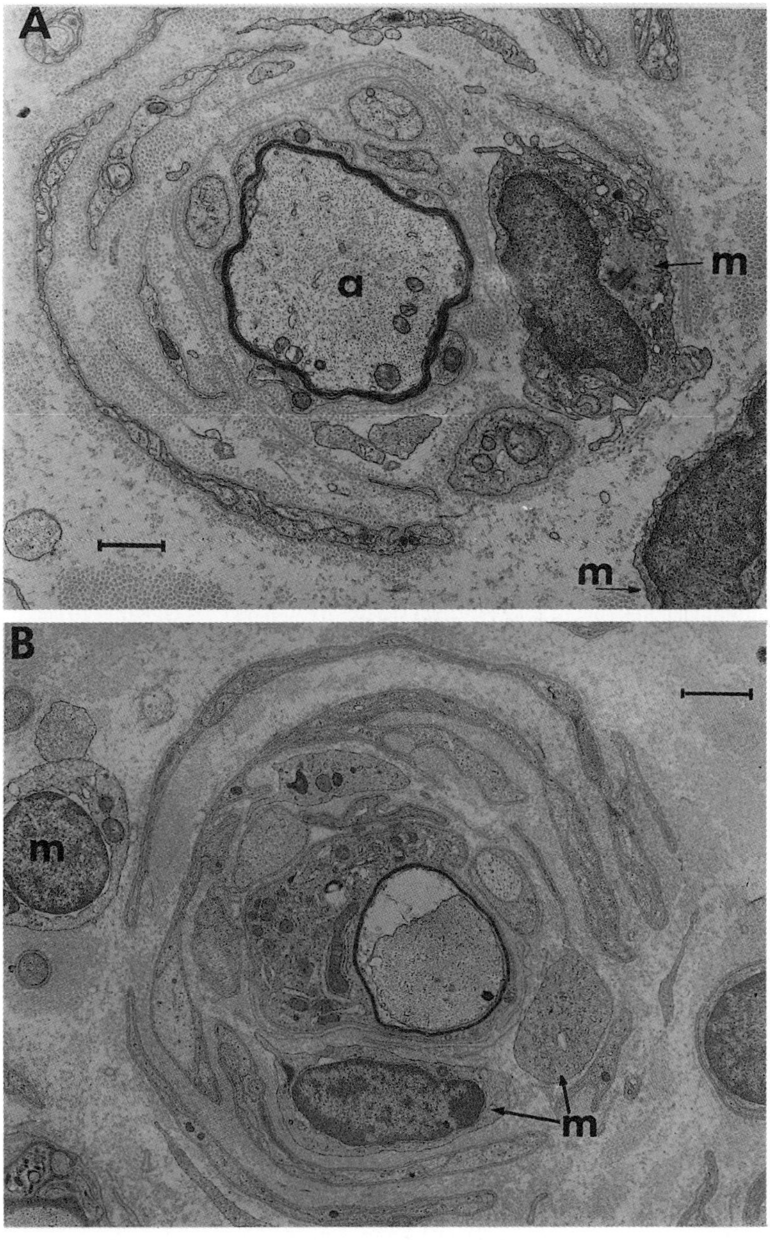

Figure 3.13 Electron micrographs of sural nerve biopsies from two patients with chronic inflammatory demyelinating polyneuropathy showing inflammatory cells within onion bulb formation. a = axon, m = mononuclear cell. Bar A = 2 μm, B = 2.5 μm

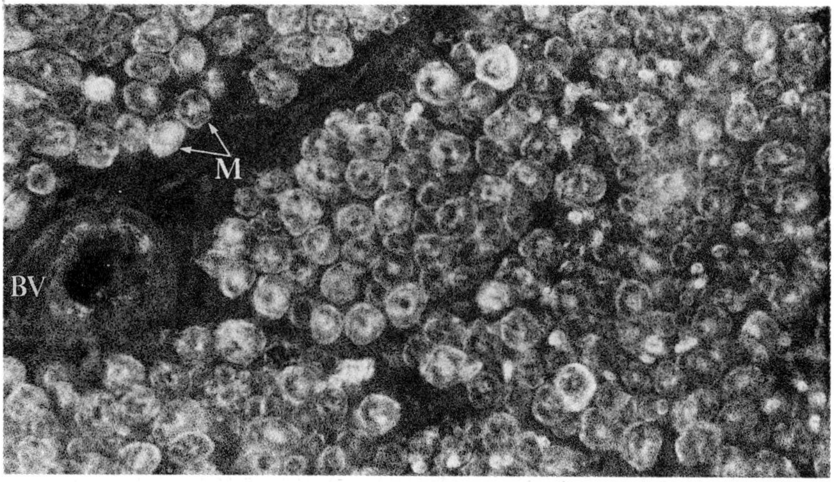

Figure 3.14 Immunofluorescent study showing binding C3 to myelin sheaths. Serum from a patient responsive to plasma exchange was incubated with normal sural nerve and then with goat anti-human antibody C3. M = myelin sheath; BV = blood vessel. Bar = 10 μm

however this high proportion of positive results has not been confirmed in recent studies of larger numbers of patients[295]. Hays and co-workers[204] reported the presence of chemotactic split products of complement on the outer portion of the myelin sheath in two of four patients with CIDP, but in only one patient was immunoglobulin also deposited at the same site (Figure 3.14). Koski and co-workers[156] found anti-myelin antibody using a complement (C1) fixation and transfer assay in the majority of GBS patients but in only three of 12 CIDP patients with progressive disease and seven patients with a relapsing disease. However, Hughes *et al.*[212], using a conventional complement fixation assay, found anti-myelin antibody in none of 11 cases, and Latov *et al.*[158] obtained positive results in only two of nine cases. Enzyme-linked immunosorbent assays used to detect antibody to defined myelin antigens P0, P2 and galactocerebroside have, with rare exceptions, failed to do so[145,212,213,217,335,336]. Studies using thin layer chromatography showed antibody to GM1 gangliosides in three of 20 CIDP patients, but these patients were said to be of the multifocal motor neuropathy subgroup, which by some workers is regarded as a different disease entity[304].

Passive transfer studies

Since many patients with CIDP respond to plasma exchange it is a reasonable assumption that the sera removed from such patients may contain a demyelinating agent, possibly antibody. Several groups have injected CIDP sera intraneurally, but most sera have not produced demyelination[336–338]. In one patient however whole serum and the IgG fraction was potently demyelinating[339]. Systemic transfer of serum or IgG into normal or tolerant mice has produced only negative results[148,338,341,342] while long-term transfer to marmoset monkeys induced a functional deficit without overt neuropathy in the recipient animals. This may speak for a species barrier pertinent to the putative demyelinating antibodies. The intact blood–nerve barrier in the recipients may have precluded the development of a clear-cut neuropathy.

It is of considerable interest that antibody plays an important role in the pathogenesis of three animal models of CIDP. In chronic EAN in the rabbit[343] the clinical course and electrophysiological findings are highly reminiscent of human CIDP, and marked hypertrophic changes are evident in nerve roots and peripheral nerve. The anti-myelin antibody level in these animals correlates to some degree with the disease course, in that stabilization of the disease by plasma exchange or plasma infusion is accompanied by a decline in antibody level[344–346]. Saida *et al.*[347] have shown that the demyelinating activity of rabbit EAN serum is largely due to anti-galactocerebroside antibody. Moreover repeated immunization of rabbits with galactocerebroside produces a chronic experimental neuritis which shares some features of human CIDP[348–350]. Finally, in chronic relapsing experimental allergic encephalomyelitis in the guinea pig, repeated episodes of demyelination occur within the nerve roots, resulting in hypertrophic change[351]. Serum from these animals produces demyelination when given into the subarachnoid space of naive animals and the demyelinating activity is due to anti-myelin oligodendrocyte glycoprotein (MOG)[352].

Synthesis

The pathological changes within nerves in CIDP suggest a major role for cell-mediated mechanisms; macrophages are clearly the major effectors in the process of demyelination, but $CD4^+$ and $CD8^+$ T cells, though more sparse, are present. There is however no clear evidence at this stage for a cytotoxic role for these T cells *in vivo*, despite evidence from *in vitro* studies regarding Schwann cell cytotoxicity by $CD4^+$ EAN-producing P2-reactive T cells[226]. In the analogous animal model, EAE, MBP-reactive T cells accumulate within perivascular regions but do not themselves penetrate the CNS parenchyma[353]. Autoreactive neural-specific $CD4^+$ T cells clearly accumulate around neural endothelium[354] and, by means of their cytokine production, recruit macrophages and increase the permeability of the blood–nerve/brain barrier. In the peripheral nervous system this process may allow circulating anti-myelin antibodies access to endoneurium, where they bind to myelin sheaths with consequent demyelination.

The effectiveness of plasma exchange in CIDP may, then, result from removal of antibody, or the soluble products of cells, such as cytokines or even proteases or free radicals produced by macrophages[200]. High dose immunoglobulin may act by blocking Fc-receptors, thus inactivating myelin

Table 3.21 Treatment of chronic inflammatory demyelinating polyneuropathy

Reference	*Number of patients/ design*	*Treatment*	*Results*
356	28; open, randomized	Prednisone (initially 120 mg; tapering over 3 months) ($n = 14$) vs. no therapy ($n = 14$)	Corticosteroids slightly better
368	27; open, randomized	Prednisone (initially 120 mg; tapering over 9 months) ($n = 13$) vs. prednisone + azathioprine ($n = 14$)	No additional benefit from azathioprine
360	17; open	Fresh frozen plasma, i.v. (100 mg/kg body weight) for 5–76 days	Patients improved for up to 4 months
359	29; double-blind, randomized	Plasma exchange (6 × in 3 weeks) ($n = 15$) vs. sham exchange ($n = 14$)	Plasma exchange superior
365	7; double-blind, randomized, placebo-controlled, cross-over	Immunoglobulin (i.v.) (400 mg/kg body weight for 5 days) vs. placebo	All improved with immunoglobulin
366	52; open	Immunoglobulin (400 mg/kg body weight i.v. for 5 days)	Improvement in 32 patients; 9 brought to remission, 21 needed regular repeats
367	18; double-blind, randomized, placebo-controlled	Immunoglobulin ($n = 15$) (400 mg/kg body weight i.v. for 5 days) vs. placebo ($n = 13$)	No difference

phagocytosis or promoting anti-idiotypic antibody interactions[282,283,285,287,292].

Management of CIDP

Several therapeutic options are available for CIDP; different centres may vary in the primary treatment used, depending upon availability and cost of the various procedures. Results of published trials are reviewed in Table 3.21.

Corticosteroids

The efficacy of these agents has been shown in many uncontrolled studies[298,355a,356]. Patients may be commenced on a daily dose of 1 mg/kg for 4 weeks and then changed to an alternate day regimen with gradual dose reduction (10 mg/month) to an acceptable maintenance level. However patients may respond to smaller starting doses, such as 0.5 mg/kg, and for some with relapsing disease, short courses of relatively low dose may be sufficient to induce a relapse. Certainly this is the cheapest and most convenient form of therapy. High doses for a prolonged period are unsatisfactory due to the serious complications associated with these agents.

Plasmapheresis

This treatment has been shown to be effective in uncontrolled studies[339,357,358,358a] and a controlled study[359]. It is preferred by some as first line therapy because of the side-effects of corticosteroids[356a]. Plasma exchange is effective in a high proportion of cases (about 75%) and is safe therapy. In our institution no serious side-effects have been encountered over a 10-year period since fresh frozen plasma was discarded as a replacement fluid. It is, however, expensive, available only in specialized centres, and cannot be used in small children. Regimens for plasmapheresis vary, depending upon plasma volumes exchanged. In severely affected patients 7–10 2-l exchanges may be given over 10–14 days, resting the patient over weekends. Out-patient therapy may then be continued once or twice weekly, gradually decreasing to a maintenance regimen of once every 3–4 weeks. Other centres exchange larger volumes; twice-weekly plasmapheresis may be given for 3 weeks then once or twice weekly for a further 3 weeks with gradual reduction to once every 3–4 weeks[294]. There is limited but convincing evidence that selective immunoadsorption of plasma to a tryptophane-polyvinyl alcohol resine (selective immunoadsorption) may also remove the putative pathogenic factors from plasma[342]; (Heininger, Borberg, Hartung, Grabensee, Toyka, unpublished observations).

High-dose intravenous immunoglobulin (IVIG)

The efficacy of this therapy was first reported by Vermeulen *et al.*[360] and subsequently in several uncontrolled studies[361–364]. A placebo-controlled crossover study in patients selected for their known response to IVIG was published by van Doorn *et al.*[365]; all patients were shown to respond to IVIG but not to placebo, thus providing evidence for the efficacy of IVIG in some patients. No controlled trial comparing IVIG to plasmapheresis or steroid has yet been published. Van Doorn and colleagues have reported their experience in 52 CIDP patients treated with IVIG[366]; 62% improved, the majority over a mean follow-up period of 4 years, but 65% of these patients needed intermittent therapy to maintain the improvement. The recommended dose is 0.4 g/kg body weight/day over 5 consecutive days. Maintenance therapy is usually 0.4 g/kg every second week, although in some patients the dose may gradually be reduced to approximately half of this. However, a randomized double-blind, placebo-controlled multicentre trial to assess the efficacy of high-dose intravenous immunoglobulin treatment on 5 consecutive days showed a similar degree of improvement of patients in the IVIG treatment group (4 of 15) and the placebo group (3 of 13) patients[367]. One has to conclude that only a subgroup of CIDP patients may benefit from intravenous immunoglobulin, and that we have to search for criteria to identify them. The advantages of IVIG include its ease of administration, few contraindications, and safety. Such advantages are clear in the treatment of small children, patients with poor venous access and cardiovascular instability, and those from remote areas. The infrequent complications of this therapy (anaphylactic reactions, particularly in individuals with IgA deficiency, thrombotic events, renal failure and aseptic meningitis) have been referred to earlier.

Immunosuppressive agents

Some patients remain unresponsive to the front-line therapies described above, and immunosuppressive therapy may be necessary. In addition, for patients responsive but dependent upon chronic plasmapheresis or human immunoglobulin, the interval between these expensive therapies may be increased by immunosuppressive treatment. No controlled trials have been reported for immunosuppressive drugs except for azathioprine; Dyck and co-workers[368] found no benefit from the addition of azathioprine to prednisone therapy.

Azathioprine nevertheless has been reported to be effective in a small number of uncontrolled studies with small numbers of patients[342,358a,369], it is given in a daily dose of 2–3 mg/kg initially with a stepwise reduction after reaching remission for a prolonged time. Full blood count and liver function should be monitored weekly for 6 weeks and then at monthly intervals.

Cyclophosphamide has been reported to be particularly effective in patients with motor neuropathy and multifocal conduction block[305]. It may be given orally in a daily dose of 2–3 mg/kg, or intravenously and used in higher dose as pulse therapy, for example 3–5 mg/kg intravenously twice weekly, or 10–15 mg/kg every 7–10 days. Adverse side-effects of cyclophosphamide treatment include haemorrhagic cystitis, alopecia, sterility, mucosal ulceration, cancer and interstitial pulmonary fibrosis. A high fluid intake and frequent voiding are recommended during its use, with regular assessment of bone marrow function[305].

Cyclosporin A (CSA) has been reported to be effective in patients who have failed to respond to other therapies[370]. It may be commenced in a dose of 8–10 mg/kg/day with reduction to 5 mg/kg by 3 months. Further gradual dose reduction may be effected as improvement occurs. Whole blood CSA level, creatinine clearance and serum creatinine levels should be monitored, and the dose regulated accordingly. Nephrotoxicity is dose-dependent and is the most serious side-effect.

Recommendations

First-line therapy will depend on the resources available, both technical and financial. Corticosteroid therapy is simple and cheap, but is acceptable only when remission is readily achieved with moderate dosage and when a reduction to a small maintenance dose is easily obtained. In practice, corticosteroid therapy may be effective in subacute cases with a monophasic course and in some relapsing cases to induce a remission. In progressive and other relapsing cases, other treatment modalities are often needed.

Since immunoglobulin therapy has not yet proven effective by an acceptable double blind, randomized trial, we recommend plasma exchange in those centres where it is available. This may be used on an out-patient basis for patients not in need of emergency hospital admission, or more intensively for patients admitted to hospital. In patients who have not responded to plasma exchange, immunoglobulin should be tried; this may be used instead of plasmapheresis in young children or patients with venous access problems or those with other contraindications.

When these therapies are not effective, immunosuppressive agents may be used. They may also play a role in the treatment of patients who need plasmapheresis frequently, or when this is not effective alone. Azathioprine is certainly associated with the least side-effects, but some find it less helpful than cyclosporin A in those patients unresponsive to the first-line therapies.

In patients suffering from multifocal motor neuropathy with conduction block, cyclophosphamide has been reported to be the most effective agent; moreover, steroids and plasmapheresis appear to be ineffective in this patient group[305]. Some of these patients may also respond to high dose immunoglobulin therapy[371,372].

References

1. Guillain G, Barré A, Strohl A. Sur un syndrome de radiculoneurite avec hyperalbuminose du liquide cephalo-rachidien sans reaction cellulaire. Remarques sur les caracteres cliniques et graphique des reflexes tendineux. Bull Soc Med Hôp Paris. 1916;40:1462–70.

1a. Asbury AK, Arnason BG, Adams RD. The inflammatory lesion in idiopathic polyneuritis. Medicine. 1969;48:173.

2. Alter M. The epidemiology of Guillain–Barré syndrome. Ann Neurol. 1990;27(suppl): S7–S12.

3. Arnason BGW, Solivan B. Acute inflammatory demyelinating polyradiculoneuropathy. In: Dyck PJ, Thomas PK, Griffin JW, Low PA, Poduslo J, editors. Peripheral Neuropathy. 3rd edn. Philadelphia: W.B. Saunders; 1993:1437–97.

4. Ropper AH. The Guillain–Barré syndrome. N Engl J Med. 1992;326:1130–6.

5. Albers JW, Kelly JJ. Acquired inflammatory demyelinating polyneuropathies. Clinical and electrodiagnostic features. Muscle Nerve. 1989;12:435–51.

6. Haymaker W, Kernohan JW. The Landry–Guillain–Barré syndrome. A clinicopathological report of fifty fatal cases and a critique of the literature. Medicine. 1949;28:59–141.

7. Kennedy RH, Danielson MA, Mulder DW, Kurland LT. Guillian–Barré syndrome: a 42-year epidemiologic and clinical study. Mayo Clin Proc. 1978;53:93–9.

8. Löffel NB, Rossi LN, Mumenthaler M, Lutschg J, Ludin HP. The Landry–Guillain–Barré syndrome: complications, prognosis, and natural history in 123 cases. J Neurol Sci. 1977;33:71–9.

9. Masucci EF, Kurtzke JE. Diagnostic criteria of the Guillain–Barré syndrome: an analysis of 50 cases. J Neurol Sci. 1971;13:483–501.

10. McFarland HR, Heller GL. Guillain–Barré disease complex: a statement of diagnostic criteria and analysis of 100 cases. Arch Neurol. 1966;14:196–201.

11. Parry GJ. Guillain–Barré Syndrome. New York: Thième Medical Publishers, 1993.

12. Ravn H. The Landry–Guillain–Barré syndrome: a survey and a clinical report of 127 cases. Acta Neurol Scand. 1967;43(suppl 30):1–64.

13. Ropper AH, Shahani BT. Pain in Guillain–Barré syndrome. Arch Neurol. 1984;45:511–14.

14. Ropper AH. Unusual clinical variants and signs in Guillain–Barré syndrome. Arch Neurol. 1986;43:1150–2.

15. Ropper AH, Wijdicks EFM, Truax BT, eds. Guillain–Barré Syndrome. Philadelphia: F.A. Davis, 1991.
16. Wiederholt WC, Mulder DW, Lambert EH. The Landry–Guillain–Barré–Strohl syndrome or polyradiculoneuropathy: historical review, report on 97 patients and present concepts. Mayo Clin Proc. 1964;39:427–51.
17. Winer JB, Hughes RAC, Osmond C. A prospective study of acute idiopathic neuropathy. I. Clinical features and their prognostic value. J Neurol Neurosurg Psychiatry. 1988;51: 605–12.
18. Asbury AK, Cornblath DR. Assessment of current diagnostic criteria for Guillain–Barré syndrome. Ann Neurol. 1990;27(suppl):S21–4.
19. Truax BT. Autonomic disturbances in the Guillain–Barré syndrome. Semin Neurol. 1984;4:462–8.
20. Truax BT. Autonomic disturbances in the Guillain–Barré syndrome. Acta Neurol Scand. 1988;77:270–1.
21. Lichtenfeld P. Autonomic dysfunction in the Guillain–Barré syndrome. Am J Med. 1971;50:772–80.
22. Bolgert F, Carayon A, Josse MO, Brunet P, Laplane D. Inappropriate secretion of atrial natriuretic factor (ANF) complicating the Guillain–Barré syndrome. Neurology. 1991;41(suppl.1):391.
23. Wijdicks EFM, Ropper AH, Nathanson JA. Atrial natriuretic factor and blood pressure fluctuation in Guillain–Barré syndrome. Ann Neurol. 1990;27:337–8.
24. Tuck RR, Pollard JD, McLeod JG. Autonomic neuropathy in experimental allergic neuritis. Brain. 1981;104:187–208.
25. Eiben RM, Gersony WM. Recognition, prognosis and treatment of the Guillain–Barré syndrome (acute idiopathic polyneuritis). Med Clin North Am. 1963;47:1371–80.
26. Krone A, Reuther P, Fuhrmeister U. Autonomic dysfunction in polyneuropathies: a report on 106 cases. J Neurol. 1983;230:111–12.
27. Singh NK, Jaiswal AK, Misra S, Srivastava PK. Assessment of autonomic dysfunction in Guillain–Barré syndrome and its prognostic implications. Acta Neurol Scand. 1987;75: 101–5.
28. Gunreben G, Englert D, Hassel W, Seybold D. Computer-gestützte Analyse der Herzfrequenzvariation bei Patienten mit Guillain–Barré-Syndrom. Intensivmed. 1985;22:446–9.
29. Ingall TJ, McLeod JG, Tamura N. Autonomic function and unmyelinated fibres in chronic inflammatory demyelinating polyradiculoneuropathy. Muscle Nerve. 1990;13:70–6.
30. McLeod JG. Autonomic dysfunction in peripheral nerve disease. Muscle Nerve. 1992;15: 3–13.
31. Dalos NP, Borel C, Hanley DF. Cardiovascular autonomic dysfunction in Guillain–Barré syndrome. Arch Neurol. 1988;45:115–17.
32. Winer JB, Hughes RAC. Identification of patients at risk of arrhythmia in the Guillain–Barré syndrome. Q J Med. 1988;68:735–9.
33. Sohn YH, Sunwoo IN, Chi JG. Acute postganglionic dysautonomia with polyneuropathy. Muscle Nerve. 1991;14:474–6.
34. Ferrer X, Vital C, Lagueny A, Brechenmacher C, Ellie E, Julien J. Neuropathie sensitive et dysautonomique subaigue. Etude clinique et pathologique. Rev Neurol (Paris). 1991;14: 663–7.
35. Feldman EL, Bromberg MB, Blaivas M, Junck L. Acute pandysautonomic neuropathy. Neurology. 1991;41:746–8.
36. Stoll G, Thomas C, Reiners K, Schober R, Hartung H-P. Encephalo-myelo-radiculoganglionitis presenting as pandysautonomia. Neurology. 1991;41:723–6.
37. Hughes RAC, Sanders E, Hall S, Atkinson P, Colchester A, Payan P. Subacute idiopathic demyelinating polyradiculoneuropathy. Arch Neurol. 1992;49:612–16.
38. Gibbels E, Giebisch U. Natural course of acute and chronic monophasic inflammatory demyelinating polyneuropathy (IDP). Acta Neurol Scand. 1992;85:282–91.
39. Guillain–Barré Syndrome Study Group: Plasmapheresis and acute Guillain–Barré syndrome. Neurology. 1985;35:1096–104.
40. Hall J, Bredkjaer C, Friis ML. Guillain–Barré syndrome: diagnostic criteria, epidemiology, clinical course and prognosis. Acta Neurol Scand. 1988;78:118–22.
41. Hughes RAC. Guillain–Barré syndrome. London: Springer Verlag, 1990.

42. Kleyweg R, van der Meché FGA, Loonen MCB, de Jonge J, Knip B. The natural history of the Guillain–Barré syndrome in 18 children and 50 adults. J Neurol Neurosurg Psychiatry. 1989;52:853–6.
43. Marshall J. The Landry–Guillain–Barré syndrome. Brain. 1963;86:55–66.
44. Raphael JC, Masson C, Morice Y, *et al.* Le syndrome de Landry–Guillain–Barré: étude des facteurs prognostique dans 223 cas. Rev Neurol (Paris). 1986;142:613–24.
45. Smith GDP, Hughes RAC. Plasma exchange treatment and prognosis of Guillain–Barré syndrome. Q J Med. 1992;85:751–60.
46. van der Meché FGA, Schmitz PIM, The Dutch Guillain–Barré Study Group. A randomized trial comparing intravenous immune globulin and plasma exchange in Guillain–Barré syndrome. N Engl J Med. 1992;326:1123–9.
47. Wijdicks EFM, Ropper AH. Acute relapsing Guillain–Barré syndrome after long asymptomatic intervals. Arch Neurol. 1990;47:82–4.
48. Grand'Maison F, Feasby TE, Hahn AF, Koopman WJ. Recurrent Guillain–Barré syndrome. Brain. 1992;115:1093–106.
49. Al-Hakim M, Cohen M, Daroff RB. Postmortem examination of relapsing acute Guillain–Barré syndrome. Muscle Nerve. 1993;16:173–6.
50. McKhann GM, Griffin JW, Cornblath DR, *et al.* Plasmapheresis and Guillain–Barré-syndrome: Analysis of prognostic factors and the effect of plasmapheresis. Ann Neurol. 1988;23:347–53.
51. Fisher M. An unusual variant of acute idiopathic polyneuritis (syndrome of ophthalmoplegia, ataxia and areflexia). N Engl J Med. 1956;255:57–65.
52. Al-Din AN. The nosological position of the ophthalmoplegia, ataxia, and areflexia syndrome: 'The spectrum hypothesis'. Acta Neurol Scand. 1987;75:287–94.
53. Dehaene I, Martin JJ, Greens K, Cras P. Guillain–Barré syndrome with ophthalmoplegia: clinicopathological study of the central and peripheral nervous system, including the oculomotor nerves. Neurology. 1986;36:851–4
54. Jamal GA, Ballantyne JP. The localization of the lesion in patients with acute ophthalmoplegia, ataxia and areflexia (Miller–Fisher syndrome): a serial multimodal neurophysiological study. Brain. 1988;111:95–114.
55. Petty RKH, Duncan R, Jamal GA, Hadley D, Kennedy PGE. Brainstem encephalitis and the Miller Fisher syndrome. J Neurol Neurosurg Psychiatry. 1993;56:201–3.
56. Ropper AH. Three patients with Fisher's syndrome and normal MRI. Neurology. 1988;38: 30–1.
57. Sauron B, Bouche P, Cathala H-P, Chain F, Castaigne P. Miller–Fisher syndrome: clinical and electrophysiological evidence of peripheral origin in 10 cases. Neurology. 1984;34: 953–6.
58. Brown WF, Feasby TE, Hahn AF. Electrophysiological changes in the acute 'axonal' form of Guillain–Barré syndrome. Muscle Nerve. 1993;16:200–5.
59. Feasby TE, Gilbert JJ, Brown WF, *et al.* An acute axonal form of Guillain–Barré polyneuropathy. Brain. 1986;109:1115–26.
60. Kanda T, Hayashi H, Tanabe H, Tsubaki T, Oda M. A fulminant case of Guillain–Barré syndrome: topographic and fibre size related analysis of demyelinating changes. J Neurol Neurosurg Psychiatry. 1989;52:857–64.
61. van der Meché FGA, Meulstee J, Kleyweg RP. Axonal damage in Guillain–Barré syndrome. Muscle Nerve. 1991;14:997–1002.
62. Ramos-Alvarez M, Bessudo L, Sabin AB. A paralytic syndrome associated with non-inflammatory cytoplasmic or nuclear neuronopathy. Acute paralytic disease in Mexican children neuropathologically distinguishable from Landry–Guillain–Barré syndrome. J Am Med Assoc. 1969;207:1481–92.
63. McKhann GM, Cornblath DR, Ho T, *et al.* Clinical and electrophysiological aspects of acute paralytic disease of children and young adults in northern China. Lancet. 1991;338: 593–7.
64. McKhann GM, Cornblath DR, Griffin JW, *et al.* Acute motor axonal neuropathy: a frequent cause of acute flaccid paralysis in China. Ann Neurol. 1993;33:333–42.
65. Cornblath DR, McArthur JC, Kennedy PGE, Witte AS, Griffin JW. Inflammatory demyelinating peripheral neuropathies associated with human T cell lymphotrophic virus Type III infection. Ann Neurol. 1987;21:32–40.

66. Cornblath DR, McArthur JC, Parry GJ. Peripheral neuropathies in human immunodeficiency virus infection. In: Dyck PJ, Thomas PK, Griffin JW, Low PA, Poduslo J, editors. Peripheral Neuropathy. 3rd edn. Philadelphia: W.B. Saunders, 1993:1343–53.
67. Lipkin I, Parry G, Kiprov D, Abrams D. Inflammatory neuropathy in homosexual men with lymphadenopathy. Neurology. 1985;35:1479–83.
68. Winer JB, Hughes RAC, Anderson MJ, Jones DM, Kangro H, Watkins RPF. A prospective study of acute idiopathic neuropathy. II. Antecedent events. J Neurol Neurosurg Psychiatry. 1988;51:613–18.
69. Dowling PC, Cook SD. Role of infection in Guillain–Barré syndrome: laboratory confirmation on herpes virus in 41 cases. Ann Neurol. 1981;9(suppl):44–55.
70. Enders U, Karch H, Toyka KV, *et al.* The spectrum of immune responses to *Campylobacter jejuni* and glycoconjugates in Guillain–Barré syndrome and in other neuroimmunological disorders. Ann Neurol. 1993;34:136–44.
71. Gruenewald R, Ropper AH, Lior H, Chan J, Lee R, Molinary VS. Serologic evidence of *Campylobater jejuni/coli* enteritis in patients with Guillain–Barré syndrome. Arch Neurol. 1991;48:1080–2.
72. Kaldor J, Speed BR. Guillain–Barré syndrome and *Campylobacter jejuni.* Br Med J. 1984;288:1867–70.
73. Kuroki S, Saida T, Nukina M, *et al. Campylobacter jejuni* strains from patients with Guillain–Barré syndrome belong mostly to Penner serogroup 19 and contain β-N-acetylglucosamine residues. Ann Neurol. 1993;33:243–7.
74. Mishu B, Ilyas AA, Koski CL, *et al.* Serologic evidence of preceding *Campylobacter jejuni* infection in patients with Guillain–Barré syndrome. Ann Intern Med. 1993;118:947–53.
75. Vriesendorp FJ, Mishu B, Blaser M, Koski CL. Serum antibodies to GM1, GD1b, peripheral nerve myelin, and *Campylobacter jejuni* in patients with Guillain–Barré syndrome and controls: correlation and prognosis. Ann Neurol. 1993;34:130–135.
76. Walsh FS, Cronin M, Koblar S, *et al.* Association between glycoconjugate antibiotics and *Campylobacter* infection in patients with Guillain–Barré syndrome. J Neuroimmunol. 1991;34:43–51.
77. Fujimoto S, Yuki N, Itoh T, Amako K. Specific serotype of *Campylobacter jejuni* associated with Guillain–Barré syndrome. J Infect Dis. 1992;165:183.
78. Breman JG, Hayner NS. Guillain–Barré syndrome and its relationship to swine influenza vaccination in Michigan 1976–1977. Am J Epidemiol. 1984;119:880–9.
79. Kaplan JE, Schonberger LB, Hurwitz ES, Katona P. Guillain–Barré syndrome in the United States, 1978–1981: additional observations from the national surveillance system. Neurology. 1983;33:633–7.
80. Langmuir AF, Bregman DJ, Kurland LT, Nathanson N, Victor M. An epidemiological and clinical evaluation of Guillain–Barré syndrome reported in association with the administration of swine influenza vaccines. Am J Epidemiol. 1984;119:841–79.
81. Safranek TJ, Lawrence DN, Kurland LT, *et al.* Reassessment of the association between Guillain–Barré syndrome and receipt of swine influenza vaccine in 1976–1977: result of a two-state study. Am J Epidemiol. 1991;133:940–51.
82. Cabrera J, Griffin DE, Johnson RT. Unusual features of the Guillain–Barré syndrome after rabies vaccine prepared in suckling mouse brain. J Neurol Sci. 1987;81:239–45.
83. Hemachudha T, Phanuphak P, Johnson RT, *et al.* Neurologic complications of Semple type rabies vaccine: clinical and immunological studies. Neurology. 1987;37:550–6.
84. Hemachudha T, Griffin DE, Chen WW, Johnson RT. Immunologic studies of rabies vaccination-induced Guillain–Barré syndrome. Neurology. 1988;38:375–8.
85. Kinnunen E, Färkkilä M, Hovi T, Juntunen J, Weckström P. Incidence of Guillain–Barré syndrome during a nationwide oral poliovirus vaccine campaign. Neurology. 1989;39: 1034–6.
86. Ropper AH, Wijdicks EMW, Shahani BT. Electrodiagnostic abnormalities in 113 consecutive patients with Guillain–Barré syndrome. Arch Neurol. 1990;47:881–7.
86a. Cornblath DR. Electrophysiology in Guillain–Barré syndrome. Ann Neurol. 1990;27(suppl 1): S17–20.
87. Bostock H, Sears TA. Continuous conduction in demyelinated mammalian nerve fibres. Nature. 1976;263:786–7.
88. Bostock H, Sears TA. The internodal axon membrane: Electrical excitability and continuous

conduction in segmental demyelination. J Physiol (Lond.). 1978;280:273–301.
89. Bostock H, Feasby TE, Sears TA. Continuous conduction in regenerating myelinated nerve fibres. J Physiol. 1977;269:88P.
90. Brown WF, Feasby TE. Conduction block and denervation in Guillain–Barré polyneuropathy. Brain. 1984;107:219–39.
91. Rudge P, Ochoa J, Gilliatt RW. Acute peripheral nerve compression in the baboon. J Neurol Sci. 1974;23:403–20.
92. Feasby TE, Brown WF, Gilbert JJ, Hahn AF. The pathological basis of conduction block in human neuropathies. J Neurol Neurosurg Psychiatry. 1985;48:239–44.
93. McDonald WI. The effects of experimental demyelination on conduction in peripheral nerves: A histological and electrophysiological study: I. Clinical and histological observations. Brain. 1963;86:481–500.
94. Cragg BG, Thomas PK. Changes in nerve conduction in experimental allergic neuritis. J Neurol Neurosurg Psychiatry. 1964;27:106–15.
95. Brown WF, Ferguson GG, Jones MW, Yates SK. The location of conduction abnormalities in human entrapment neuropathies. Can J Neurol Sci. 1976;3:111–22.
96. Ochoa J, Fowler TJ, Gilliatt RW. Changes produced by a pneumatic tourniquet. In: Desmedt JE, editor. New developments in electromyography and clinical neurophysiology. Vol. 2. Basel: Karger, 1973:174–180.
97. Lehmann HJ, Tackmann W. Die Übermittlung frequenter Impulsserien in demyelinisierten und in degenerierenden Nervenfasern. Arch Psychiatr Nervenkr. 1970;213:215–27.
98. McDonald WI, Sears TA. The effects of experimental demyelination on conduction in the central nervous system. Brain. 1970;93:583–98.
99. Smith KJ, Hall SM. Nerve conduction during demyelination and remyelination. J Neurol Sci. 1980;48:201–19.
100. Rasminsky M. The effects of temperature on conduction in demyelinated single nerve fibres. Arch Neurol. 1973;28:287–92.
101. Rasminsky M. Ectopic generation of impulses and cross-talk in spinal nerve roots of dystrophic mice. Ann Neurol. 1978;3:351–7.
102. Brick JF, Gutmann L, McComas CF. Calcium effect on generation and amplification of myokymic discharges. Neurology. 1982;32:618–22.
103. Daube JR, Kelly JJ, Martin RA. Facial myokymia with polyradiculoneuropathy. Neurology. 1979;29:662–9.
104. Korczyn AD, Kuritzky A, Sandbank U. Muscle hypertrophy with neuropathy. J Neurol Sci. 1978;38:399–408.
105. Valenstein E, Watson RT, Parker JL. Myokymia, muscle hypertrophy and percussion 'myotonia' in chronic recurrent polyneuropathy. Neurology. 1978;28:1130–4.
106. Albers JW. Inflammatory demyelinating polyneuropathy. In: Brown WF, Bolton CF, editors. Clinical electromyography. Boston: Butterworth, 1987:209–44.
107. Gilliatt RW, Hopf HC, Rudge P, Baraitser M. Axonal velocities of motor units in the hand and foot muscles of the baboon. J Neurol Sci. 1976;29:249–58.
108. Feasby TE, Hahn AF, Brown WF, Bolton CF, Gilbert JJ, Koopman WJ. Severe axonal degeneration in acute Guillain–Barré syndrome: evidence of two different mechanisms. J Neurol Sci. 1993;116:185.
109. Hoogendijk JE, de Visser M, Jennekens FGI, Ongerboer BW. Conduction block in hereditary motor and sensory neuropathy type I. Muscle Nerve. 1992;15:520–1.
110. Rhee RK, England JD, Sumner AJ. Computer simulation of conduction block: Effects produced by actual block versus interphase cancellation. Ann Neurol. 1990;28:146–56.
111. Albers JW, Donofrio PD, McGonagle TK. Sequential electrodiagnostic abnormalities in acute inflammatory demyelinating polyneuropathy. Muscle Nerve. 1985;8:528–39.
112. Lewis RA, Sumner AJ, Brown MJ, Asbury AK. Multifocal demyelinating neuropathy with persisting conduction block. Neurology. 1982;32:958–64.
113. Cornblath DR, Sumner AJ, Daube J, *et al.* Conduction block in clinical practice. Muscle Nerve. 1991;14:869–71.
114. Krarup C, Stewart MB, Sumner AJ, Pestronk A, Lipton SA. A syndrome of asymmetric limb weakness with motor conduction block. Neurology. 1990;40:118–27.
115. Sumner AJ. The physiological basis for symptoms of the Guillain–Barré syndrome. Ann Neurol. 1981;9(suppl.):28–30.

116. Heininger K, Stoll G, Linington C, Toyka KV, Wekerle H. Conduction failure and nerve conduction slowing in experimental allergic neuritis induced by P2-specific T cell lines. Ann Neurol. 1986;19:44–9.
117. Ropper AH, Chiappa KH. Evoked potentials in Guillain–Barré syndrome. Neurology. 1986;36:587–90.
118. McLeod JG, Wray SH. An experimental study of the F wave in the baboon. J Neurol Neurosurg Psychiatry. 1966;29:196–200.
119. Kimura J, Yanagisawa H, Yamada T, Mitsudome A, Sasaki H, Kimura A. Is the F-wave elicited in a selected group of motoneurons? Muscle Nerve. 1984;7:392–9.
120. Kimura J, Butzer JF. F-wave conduction velocity in Guillain–Barré syndrome. Arch Neurol. 1975;32:524–9.
121. Walsh JC, Yiannikas C, McLeod JG. Abnormalities of proximal conduction in acute idiopathic polyneuritis: Comparison of short latency somatosensory evoked potentials and F-waves. J Neurol Neurosurg Psychiatry. 1984;47:197–200.
122. Olney RK, Aminoff MJ. Electrodiagnostic features of the Guillain–Barré syndrome: The relative sensitivity of different techniques. Neurology. 1990;40:471–5.
123. Reiners K, Jackowski M, Toyka KV. F response latency determinations. Muscle Nerve. 1984;7:338.
124. Fraser JL, Olney RK. The relative diagnostic sensitivity of different F-wave parameters in various polyneuropathies. Muscle Nerve. 1992;15:912–18.
125. McLeod JG, Walsh JC, Prineas JW, Pollard JD. Acute idiopathic polyneuritis: a clinical and electrophysiological follow-up study. J Neurol Sci. 1976;27:145–62.
126. Mills KR, Murray NMF. Proximal conduction block in early Guillain–Barré syndrome. Lancet. 1985;II:659.
127. Reiners K, Herdmann J, Freund H-J. Altered mechanisms of muscular force generation in lower motor neuron disease. Muscle Nerve. 1989;12:647–59.
128. Lange DJ, Trojaborg W, Latov N, *et al.* Multifocal motor neuropathy with conduction block: Is it a distinct clinical entity? Neurology. 1992;42:497–505.
129. McQuillen MP. Idiopathic polyneuritis: Serial studies of nerve and immune functions. J Neurol Neurosurg Psychiatry. 1971;34:607–15.
130. Baneji NK, Millar JHD. Guillain–Barré syndrome in children, with special reference to serial nerve conduction studies. Dev Med Child Neurol. 1972;14:56–63.
130a. Cornblath DR, Asbury AK, Albers JW, *et al.* Research criteria for diagnosis of chronic inflammatory demyelinating polyneuropathy (CIDP). Neurology. 1991;41:617–18.
131. Lambert EH, Mulder DW. Nerve conduction in the Guillain–Barré syndrome. Electroencephalogr Clin Neurophysiol. 1964;17:86.
132. Murray NWF, Wade DT. The sural sensory action potential in Guillain–Barré syndrome. Muscle Nerve. 1980;3:444.
133. Fross RD, Daube JR. Neuropathy in the Miller Fisher syndrome: clinical and electrophysiological findings. Neurology. 1987;37:1493–8.
134. Jamal GA, McLeod WN. Electrophysiologic studies in Miller–Fisher syndrome. Neurology. 1984;34:685–8.
135. Kimura J. An evaluation of the facial and trigeminal nerves in polyneuropathy: electrodiagnostic study in Charcot–Marie–Tooth disease, Guillain–Barré syndrome, and diabetic neuropathy. Neurology. 1971;21:745–52.
135a. Bredshaw DY, Jones HR Jr. Guillain–Barré syndrome in children: clinical course, electrodiagnosis, and prognosis. Muscle Nerve. 1992;15:500–6.
136. Berger AR, Logigian EL, Shahani BT. Reversible proximal conduction block underlies rapid recovery in Guillain–Barré syndrome. Muscle Nerve. 1988;11:1039–42.
137. Cornblath DR, Mellits ED, Griffin JW, *et al.* Motor conduction studies in Guillain–Barré syndrome: description and prognostic value. Ann Neurol. 1988;23:354–9.
138. McDonald WI, Kocen RS. Diphtheric neuropathy. In Dyck PJ, Thomas PK, Griffin JW, Low PA, Poduslo JF, editors. Peripheral neuropathy. 3rd edn. Philadelphia: W.B. Saunders; 1993:1412–7.
138a. Hall SM, Hughes RAC, Atkinson PF, McColl I, Gale A. Motor nerve biopsy in severe Guillain–Barré syndrome. Ann Neurol. 1992;31:441–4.
139. Hughes RAC, Atkinson P, Coates P, Halls S, Leibowitz S. Sural nerve biopsy in Guillain–Barré syndrome: axonal degeneration and macrophage-associated demyelination and

absence of cytomegalovirus genome. Muscle Nerve. 1992;15:568–75.

140. Brechenmacher C, Vital C, Deminiere C, *et al.* Ultrastructural study of peripheral nerve in Guillain–Barré syndrome: 65 patients. Clin Neuropathol. 1987;6:19–24.
141. Prineas JW. Acute idiopathic polyneuritis. An electron microscope study. Lab Invest. 1972;26:133–46.
142. Prineas JW. Pathology of the Guillain–Barré syndrome. Ann Neurol. 1981;9(suppl):6–19.
143. Ropper AH. Severe acute Guillain–Barré syndrome. Neurology. 1986;36:429–32.
144. Ropper AH, Adelman L. Early Guillain–Barré syndrome without inflammation. Arch Neurol. 1992;49:979–81.
145. Hartung HP, Stoll G, Toyka KV. Immune reactions in the peripheral nervous system. In: Dyck PJ, Thomas PK, Griffin J, Low PA, Poduslo JF, editors. Peripheral Neuropathy, 3rd edn. Philadelphia: W.B. Saunders, 1993:418–44.
146. Honavar M, Tharakan JKJ, Hughes RAC, Leibowitz S, Winer JB. A clinicopathological study of the Guillain–Barré syndrome: Nine cases and literature review. Brain. 1991;114:1245–69.
147. Hartung HP, Heininger K, Schäfer B, Fierz W, Toyka KV. Immune mechanisms in inflammatory polyneuropathy. Ann NY Acad Sci. 1988;540:122–61.
148. Toyka KV, Hartung HP. Circulating immune factors. In: Asbury AK, McKhann GM, McDonald WI, editors. Diseases of the Nervous System, 2nd edn. Philadelphia: W.B. Saunders, 1992:1396–409.
149. Harrison BM, Hansen LA, Pollard JD, McLeod JG. Demyelination induced by serum from patients with Guillain–Barré syndrome. Ann Neurol. 1984;15:163–70.
150. Oomes PG, van der Meché FGA, Markus-Silvis L, Meulstee J, Kleyweg RP. *In vivo* effects of sera from Guillain–Barré subgroups: An electrophysiological and histological study on rat nerves. Muscle Nerve. 1991;14:1013–20.
151. Cook SD, Dowling PC. The role of autoantibody and immune complexes in the pathogenesis of Guillain–Barré syndrome. Ann Neurol. 1980;9(suppl):70–9.
152. Quarles RH, Ilyas AA, Willison JH. Antibodies to gangliosides and myelin proteins in Guillain–Barré syndrome. Ann Neurol. 1990;27(suppl):S48–52.
153. Connolly AM, Pestronk A, Trotter JL, Feldman EL, Cornblath DR, Olney RK. High-titer selective serum anti-β-tubulin antibodies in chronic inflammatory demyelinating polyneuropathy. Neurology. 1993;43:557–62.
154. Linington C, Brostoff SW. Peripheral nerve antigens. In: Dyck PJ, Thomas PK, Griffin JW, Low PA, Poduslo J, editors. Peripheral Neuropathy, 3rd edn. Philadelphia: W.B. Saunders, 1993:404–17.
155. Svennerholm L, Fredman P. Antibody detection in Guillain–Barré syndrome. Ann Neurol. 1990;27(suppl.):S36–40.
156. Koski CL, Humphrey R, Shin ML. Anti-peripheral myelin antibody in patients with demyelinating neuropathy: quantitative and kinetic determination of serum antibody in complement component 1 fixation. Proc Natl Acad Sci USA. 1985;82:905–9.
157. Koski CL. Characterization of complement-fixing antibodies to peripheral nerve myelin in Guillain–Barré syndrome. Ann Neurol. 1990;27(suppl):S44–7.
158. Latov N, Gross RB, Kastelman J, *et al.* Complement-fixing antiperipheral nerve myelin antibodies in patients with inflammatory polyneuritis and polyneuropathy and paraproteinemia. Neurology. 1981;31:1530–4.
158a. Ilyas AA, Mithen FA, Chen ZW, Cook SD. Search for antibodies to neutral glycolipids in sera of patients with Guillain–Barré syndrome. J Neurol Sci. 1991;102:67–75.
159. Adams D, Kuntzer T, Burger D, *et al.* Predictive value of anti-GM1 ganglioside antibodies in neuromuscular diseases: a study of 180 sera. J Neuroimmunol. 1991;32:223–30.
160. Fredman P, Vedeler C, Nyland H, *et al.* Antibodies in sera from patients with inflammatory demyelinating polyradiculoneuropathy react with ganglioside LM1 and sulphatide of peripheral nerve myelin. J Neurol. 1991;238:75–9.
161. Garcia-Guijo C, Garcia-Merino A, Rubio G, Guerrero A, Cruz Martinz A, Arpa J. IgG anti-ganglioside antibodies and their subclass distribution in two patients with acute and chronic motor neuropathy. J Neuroimmunol. 1992;37:141–8.
162. Gregson NA, Koblar S, Hughes RAC. Antibodies to gangliosides in Guillain–Barré syndrome: specificity and relationship to clinical features. Q J Med. 1993;86:111–17.
163. Ilyas AA, Willison HJ, Quarles RH. Serum antibodies to gangliosides in Guillain–Barré

syndrome. Ann Neurol. 1988;23:440–7.

164. Ilyas AA, Mithen FA, Dalakas MC, *et al.* Antibodies to sulfated glycolipids in Guillain–Barré syndrome. J Neurol Sci. 1991;105:108–17.
165. Ilyas AA, Mithen FA, Chen ZW, Cook SD. Anti-GM1 IgA antibodies in Guillain–Barré syndrome. J Neuroimmunol. 1992;36:69–76.
166. Ilyas AA, Mithen FA, Dalakas MC, Chen ZW, Cook SD. Antibodies to acidic glycolipids in Guillain–Barré syndrome and chronic inflammatory demyelinating polyneuropathy. J Neurol Sci. 1992;107:111–21.
167. Pestronk A. Motor neuropathies, motor neuron disorders, and antiglycolipid antibodies. Muscle Nerve. 1991;14:927–36.
168. Quarles RH, Ilyas AA, Willison JH. Antibodies to glycolipids in demyelinating diseases of the human peripheral nervous system. Chem Phys Lipids. 1986;42:235–49.
169. Simone IL, Annunziata P, Maimone D, Liguori M, Leante R, Livrea P. Serum and CSF anti-GM1 antibodies in patients with Guillain–Barré syndrome and chronic inflammatory demyelinating polyneuropathy. J Neurol Sci. 1993;114:49–55.
170. van den Berg LH, Marrink J, de Jaeger AEJ, *et al.* Anti-GM1 antibodies in patients with Guillain–Barré syndrome. J Neurol Neurosurg Psychiatry. 1992;55:8–11.
171. Yuki N, Yoshino H, Sato S, Miyatake T. Acute axonal polyneuropathy associated with anti-GM1 antibodies following *Campylobacter enteritis*. Neurology. 1990;40:1900–2.
172. Yuki N, Yoshino H, Sato S, Shinozawa K, Miyatake T. Severe acute axonal form of Guillain–Barré syndrome associated with IgG anti-GD1a antibodies. Muscle Nerve. 1992;15:899–903.
173. Yuki N, Yamada M, Sato S, *et al.* Association of IgG anti-GD1a antibody with severe Guillain–Barré syndrome. Muscle Nerve. 1993;16:642–7.
174. Nobile-Orazio E, Carpo M, Meucci N, *et al.* Guillain–Barré syndrome associated with high titers of anti-GM1 antibodies. J Neurol Sci. 1992;109:200–6.
175. Marcus DM. Measurement and clinical importance of antibodies to glycolipids. Ann Neurol. 1990;27(suppl):S53–S55.
176. Yuki N, Sato S, Itoh T, Miyatake T. HLA-B35 and acute axonal polyneuropathy following campylobacter infection. Neurology. 1991;41:1561–3.
177. Yuki N, Sato S, Fujimoto S, *et al.* Serotype of *Campylobacter jejuni*, HLA, and the Guillain–Barré syndrome. Muscle Nerve. 1992;15:968–9.
178. Yuki N, Sato S, Tsuji S, Ohsawa T, Miyatake T. Frequent presence of anti-GQ1b antibody in Fisher's syndrome. Neurology. 1993;43:414–17.
179. Winer JB, Briggs D, Welsh K, Hughes RAC. HLA antigens in the Guillain–Barré syndrome. J Neuroimmunol. 1988;18:13–16.
180. Chiba AM, Kusinoki S, Shimizu T, Kanazawa I. Serum IgG antibody to ganglioside GQ1b is a possible marker of Miller Fisher syndrome. Ann Neurol. 1992;31:677–9.
181. Willison HJ, Veitch J, Paterson G, Kennedy PGE. Miller Fisher syndrome is associated with serum antibodies to GQ1b ganglioside. J Neurol Neurosurg Psychiatry. 1993;56: 204–6.
182. Mithen FA, Ilyas AA, Birchem R, Cook SD. Effects of Guillain–Barré sera containing antibodies against glycolipids in cultures of rat Schwann cells and sensory neurons. J Neurol Sci. 1992;112:223–32.
183. Willison HJ, Kennedy PGE. Gangliosides and bacterial toxins in Guillain–Barré syndrome. J Neuroimmunol. 1993;46:105–12.
184. Gallo P, Piccinno MG, Tavolato B, *et al.* Effect of parenteral administration of GM1 on cytokines and antiganglioside antibody patterns. Preliminary report in normal individuals. J Neuroimmunol. 1992;36:81–6.
185. Figueras A, Morales-Olivas FJ, Capella D, Palop V, Laporte J-R. Bovine gangliosides and acute motor polyneuropathy. Br Med J. 1992;305:1330–1.
186. Latov N, Koski CL, Walicke PA. Guillain–Barré syndrome and parenteral gangliosides. Lancet. 1991;338:757.
187. Granieri E, Casetta I, Govoni V, Tola MR, Paolino E, Rocca WA. Ganglioside therapy and Guillain–Barré syndrome. Neuroepidemiology. 1991;10:161–9.
188. Ponzin D, Menegus AM, Kirschner G, *et al.* Effects of gangliosides upon the expression of autoimmune demyelination in the peripheral nervous system. Ann Neurol. 1991;30: 678–85.

188a. Yuki N, Sato S, Tsuji S, Ogawa K, Miyataka T. Human leukocyte antigens in Fisher's syndrome. Ann Neurol. 1993;33:655–67.
189. Wiethölter H, Schabet M, Stevens A, Melms A, Sommer N, Weller M. Influence of gangliosides on experimental allergic neuritis. J Neuroimmunol. 1992;38:221–8.
190. Zielasek J, Jung S, Schmidt B, Ritter G, Hartung H-P, Toyka KV. Effects of ganglioside administration on experimental autoimmune neuritis induced by peripheral nerve myelin or P2-specific T cell lines. J Neuroimmunol. 1993;43:103–12.
191. Chaudhry V, Pestronk A. Different patterns of glycolipid antibody reactivity: lower motor neuron syndromes vs. immunization. J Neuroimmunol. 1992;36:127–34.
192. Santoro M, Uncini A, Corbo M, *et al.* Experimental conduction block induced by serum from a patient with anti-GM1 antibodies. Ann Neurol. 1992;31:385–90.
193. Vitetta ES, Berton MT, Burger C, Kepron M, Lee WT, Yin XM. Memory B and T cells. Annu Rev Immunol. 1991;9:193–217.
194. Sander VM, Vitetta ES. Collaboration between T and B cells. In: Callard RE, editor. Cytokines and B Lymphocytes. London: Academic Press, 1990:143–72.
195. Snapper CM, Mond JJ. Towards a comprehensive view of immunoglobulin class switching. Immunol Today. 1993;14:15–17.
196. Banchereau J, Rousset F. Human B lymphocytes: phenotype, proliferation, and differentiation. Adv Immunol. 1992;52:125–62.
197. Ishioka GY, Lamont AG, Thomson D, *et al.* MHC interaction and T cell recognition of carbohydrates and glycopeptides. J Immunol. 1992;148:2446–51.
198. Ladisch S, Becker H, Ulsh L. Immunosuppression by human gangliosides: I. Relationship of carbohydrate structure to the inhibition of T cell responses. Biochim Biophys Acta. 1992;1125:180–8.
199. Hartung HP, Schwenke C, Bitter-Suermann D, Toyka KV. Guillain–Barré syndrome: activated complement components C3a and C5a in CSF. Neurology. 1987;37:1006–9.
200. Hartung HP, Jung S, Stoll G, Zielasek J, Schmidt B, Archelos JJ, Toyka KV. Inflammatory mediators in demyelinating disorders of the CNS and PNS. J Neuroimmunol. 1992;40: 197–210.
201. Koski CL, Sanders ME, Swoveland PT, *et al.* Activation of terminal components of complement in patients with Guillain–Barré syndrome and other demyelinating neuropathies. J Clin Invest. 1987;80:1492–7.
202. Koski CL, Chou EHK, Jungalwala FB. Anti-peripheral nerve myelin antibodies in Guillain–Barré syndrome bind to a neutral glycolipid of peripheral myelin and cross-react with Forssman antigen. J Clin Invest. 1989;84:280–7.
203. Sanders ME, Koski CL, Robbins D, *et al.* Activated terminal complement in cerebrospinal fluid in Guillain–Barré syndrome and multiple sclerosis. J Immunol. 1986;136:4456–9.
204. Hays AP, Lee SSL, Latov N. Immune reactive C3d on the surface of myelin sheaths in neuropathy. J Neuroimmunol. 1988;18:231–44.
205. Stoll G, Schmidt B, Jander S, Toyka KV, Hartung HP. Presence of the terminal complement complex (C5b-9) precedes myelin degradation in immune-mediated demyelination of the rat peripheral nervous system. Ann Neurol. 1991;30:147–55.
206. Burton DR, Woof JM. Human antibody effector function. Adv Immunol. 1992;51:1–84.
207. Hartung HP, Toyka KV. T cell and macrophage activation in experimental autoimmune neuritis and Guillain–Barré syndrome. Ann Neurol. 1990;27(suppl.):S57–63.
208. Linington C, Izumo S, Suzuki M, *et al.* A permanent rat T cell line that mediates experimental allergic neuritis in the Lewis rat in vivo. J Immunol. 1984;133:1946–50.
209. Linington C, Lassmann H, Ozawa K. Kosin S, Mongan L. Cell adhesion molecules of the immunoglobulin supergene family as tissue-specific autoantigens: induction of experimental allergic neuritis (EAN) by P0 protein-specific T cell lines. Eur J Immunol. 1992;22: 1813–17.
210. Rostami A, Burns B, Brown MJ, *et al.* Transfer of allergic neuritis with P2-reactive T cell lines. Cell Immunol. 1985;91:354–61.
211. Hartung SP, Schäfer B, Diamantstein T, Fierz W, Heininger K, Toyka KV. Suppression of P2 T cell line-mediated experimental autoimmune neuritis by interleukin-2 receptor targeted monoclonal antibody ART18. Brain Res. 1989;489:120–8.
212. Hughes RAC, Gray IA, Gregson NA, *et al.* Immune responses to myelin antigens in Guillain–Barré syndrome. J Neuroimmunol. 1984;6:303–12.

213. Iqbal A, Oger JJF, Arnason BGW. Cell-mediated immunity in idiopathic polyneuritis. Ann Neurol. 1981;9(suppl):65–9.
214. Winer JB, Gray IA, Gregson NA, *et al.* A prospective study of acute idiopathic neuropathy. III. Immunologic studies. J Neurol Neurosurg Psychiatry. 1988;51:619–25.
215. Taylor WA, Brostoff SW, Hughes RAC. P2-specific lymphocyte transformation in Guillain–Barré syndrome and chronic idiopathic demyelinating polyradiculoneuropathy. J Neurol Sci. 1991;104:52–5.
216. Khalili-Shirazi A, Hughes RAC, Brostoff SW, Linington C, Gregson N. T cell responses to myelin proteins in Guillain–Barré syndrome. J Neurol Sci. 1992;111:200–3.
217. Zweiman B, Rostami A, Lisak RP, Moskowitz AR, Pleasure DE. Immune reactions to P2 protein in human inflammatory demyelinative neuropathies. Neurology. 1983;33:234–7.
218. Taylor WA, Hughes RAC. T lymphocyte activation antigens in Guillain–Barré syndrome and chronic idiopathic demyelinating polyradiculoneuropathy. J Neuroimmunol. 1989;24:33–9.
219. Bansil S, Mithen FA, Cook SD, Sheffet A, Rohowsky-Kochan C. Clinical correlation with serum soluble interleukin-2 receptor levels in Guillain–Barré syndrome. Neurology. 1991;41:1302–5.
220. Bansil S, Mithen FA, Singhal BS, Cook SD, Rohowsky-Kochan C. Elevated neopterin levels in Guillain–Barré syndrome. Arch Neurol. 1992;49:1277–80.
221. Hartung HP, Hughes RAC, Taylor WA, *et al.* T cell activation in the Guillain–Barré syndrome and in MS. Elevated serum levels of soluble IL-2 receptors. Neurology. 1990;40:215–18.
222. Hartung HP, Reiners K, Schmidt B, Stoll G, Toyka KV. Serum interleukin-2 concentrations in Guillain–Barré syndrome and chronic idiopathic demyelinating polyradiculoneuropathy: Comparison with other neurological diseases of presumed immunopathogenesis. Ann Neurol. 1991;30:48–53.
223. Archelos JJ, Mäurer M, Jung S, Toyka KV, Hartung H-P. Suppression of experimental autoimmune neuritis by antibodies to the intercellular adhesion molecule-1. Brain. 1993;116:1043–58.
224. Hartung HP. Immune-mediated demyelination. Ann Neurol. 1993;33:563–7.
225. Stoll G, Jander S, Jung S, *et al.* Macrophages and endothelial cells express intercellular adhesion molecule-1 immune-mediated demyelination but not in Wallerian degeneration of the rat peripheral nervous system. Lab Invest. 1993;68:637–44.
226. Argall K, Armati PJ, Pollard JD, Bonner J. Interaction between $CD4^+$ T cells and rat Schwann cells *in vitro*. 2. Cytotoxic effects of P_2 specific $CD4^+$ T cell lines in Lewis rat Schwann cells. J Neuroimmunol. 1992;40:19–29.
227. Hughes RAC, Aslan S, Giray IA. Lymphocyte subpopulations and suppressor cell activity in acute polyradiculoneuritis (Guillain–Barré syndrome). Clin Exp Immunol. 1983;51: 448–54.
228. Griffin JW, Stoll G, Li CY, Tyor W, Cornblath DR. Macrophage responses in inflammatory demyelinating neuropathies. Ann Neurol. 1990;27(suppl):S64–8.
229. Monaco S, Gehrmann J, Raivich G, Kreutzberg G. MHC-positive, ramified macrophages in the normal and injured rat peripheral nervous system. J Neurocytol. 1992;21:623–34.
230. Mancardi GL, Cadoni A, Zicca A, *et al.* HLA-DR Schwann cell reactivity in peripheral neuropathies of different origins. Neurology. 1988;38:848–51.
231. Mitchell GW, Williams GS, Bosch EP, Hart MN. Class II antigen expression in peripheral neuropathies. J Neurol Sci. 1991;102:170–6.
233. Scarpini E, Lisak RP, Beretta S. Quantitative assessment of class II molecules in normal and pathological nerves. Immunocytochemical studies *in vivo* and in tissue culture. Brain. 1990;113:659–75.
234. Schmidt B, Stoll G, Hartung HP, Heininger K, Schäfer B, Toyka KV. Macrophages but not Schwann cells express Ia antigen in experimental autoimmune neuritis. Ann Neurol. 1990;28:70–7.
235. Atkinson PF, Perry ME, Hall SM, Hughes RAC. Immunoelectronmicroscopical demonstration of major histocompatibility class II antigen: expression on endothelial and perivascular cells but not Schwann cells in human neuropathy. Neuropathol Appl Neurobiol. 1993;19:22–30.
236. Stoll G, Hartung HP. The role of macrophages in degeneration and immune-mediated

demyelination of the peripheral nervous system. Adv Neuroimmunol. 1992;2:163–79.
237. Cammer W, Brosnan CF, Bloom BR, Norton WT. Degradation of the P_0, P_1, and P_r proteins in peripheral nervous system myelin by plasmin: Implications regarding the role of macrophages in demyelinating diseases. J Neurochem. 1981;36:1506–14.
238. Halliwell B, Gutteridge JMC, Cross CE. Free radicals, antioxidants, and human disease: Where are we now? J Lab Clin Med. 1992;119:598–620.
239. Hartung HP, Schäfer B, Heininger K, Stoll G, Toyka KV. The role of macrophages and eicosanoids in the pathogenesis of experimental allergic neuritis. Serial clinical, electrophysiological, biochemical, and morphological observations. Brain. 1988;111: 1039–59.
240. Pollard JD, Baverstock J, McLeod JG. Class II antigen expression and inflammatory cells in the Guillain–Barré syndrome. Ann Neurol. 1987;21:337–41.
241. Hartung HP, Schäfer B, Heininger K, Toyka KV. Suppression of experimental autoimmune neuritis by the oxygen radical scavengers superoxide dismutase and catalase. Ann Neurol. 1988;23:453–60.
242. Heininger K, Schäfer B, Hartung HP, Fierz W, Linington C, Toyka KV. The role of macrophages in experimental autoimmune neuritis induced by a P2-specific T cell line. Ann Neurol. 1988;23:326–31.
243. Schmidt B, Stoll G, van der Meide PH, Jung S, Hartung HP. Transient cellular expression of interferon-gamma in experimental autoimmune neuritis. Brain. 1992;115:1633–46.
244. Sobue G, Yamamoto S, Hirayama M, Matsuoka Y, Uematsue H, Sobue I. The role of macrophages in demyelination in experimental allergic neuritis. J Neurol Sci. 1982;56: 75–87.
245. Hartung HP, Schäfer B, van der Meide PH, Fierz W, Heininger K, Toyka KV. The role of interferon-gamma in the pathogenesis of experimental autoimmune disease of the peripheral nervous system. Ann Neurol. 1990;27:247–57.
246. Strigard K, Holmdahl R, van der Meide P, Klareskog L, Olsson T. *In vivo* treatment of rats with monoclonal antibodies against gamma interferon: effects on experimental allergic neuritis. Acta Neurol Scand. 1989;80:201–5.
247. Stoll G, Jung S, Jander S, van der Meide P, Hartung H-P. Tumor necrosis factor-alpha in immune-mediated demyelination and Wallerian degeneration of the rat peripheral nervous system. J Neuroimmunol. 1993;45:175–82.
248. Cammer W, Brosnan C, Basile C, Bloom B, Norton W. Complement potentiates the degradation of myelin proteins by plasmin: implications for a mechanism of inflammatory demyelination. Brain Res. 1986;364:91–101.
249. Chia LS, Thompson JE, Moscarello MA. Disorder in human myelin induced by superoxide radical: an in vitro investigation. Biochem Biophys Res Commun. 1983;117:141–6.
249a. Sharief MK, Zeman A, McLean B, Thompson EJ. Elevated serum levels of tumor necrosis factor-alpha in Guillain–Barré syndrome. Ann Neurol. 1993;33:591–6.
250. Selmaj K, Raine CS. Tumor necrosis factor mediates myelin and oligodendrocyte damage *in vitro*. Ann Neurol. 1988;23:339–46.
251. Herman A, Kappler JW, Marrack P, Pullen AM. Superantigens: mechanism of T-cell stimulation and role in immune responses. Annu Rev Immunol. 1991;9:745–72.
252. Daikotu T, Kawaguchi M, Takami K, Suzuki S. Partial purification and characterization of the enterotoxin produced by *Campylobacter jejuni*. Infect Immunol. 1990;58:2414–19.
253. Barnett LA, Fujinami RS. Molecular mimicry: a mechanism for autoimmune injury. FASEB J. 1992;6:840–4.
254. Jahnke U, Fischer EH, Alvord EC. Sequence homology between certain viral proteins and proteins related to encephalomyelitis and neuritis. Science. 1985;229:282–4.
255. Milner P, Lovelidge CA, Taylor WA, Hughes RAC. P0 myelin protein produces experimental allergic neuritis in Lewis rats. J Neurol Sci. 1987;79:275–85.
256. Höjeberg B, Ingermarsson R, Kristensson K, *et al.* A monoclonal antibody against HSV type 1 ribonucleotide reductase reacts with the P0 protein of peripheral nerve myelin. J Neurol Sci. 1991;106:91.
257. Yuki N, Hand S, Taki T, *et al.* Cross-reactive antigen between nervous tissue and a bacterium elicits Guillain–Barré syndrome: Molecular mimicry between ganglioside GM1 and lipopolysaccharide from Penner's serotype 19 of *Campylobacter jejuni*. Biomed Res. 1991;13:451–3.

258. Consensus Conference. The utility of therapeutic plasmapheresis for neurological disorders. J Am Med Assoc. 1986;256:1333–7.
259. Greenwood RJ, Newsom-Davis J, Hughes RA, *et al.* Controlled trial of plasma exchange in acute inflammatory polyradiculoneuropathy. Lancet. 1984;1:877–9.
260. Gross MLP, Sweny P, Legg NJ. Successful plasmapheresis in the Miller-Fisher syndrome. Br Med J. 1981;282:1394.
261. Jones HR, Bradshaw DY. Guillain–Barré syndrome and plasmapheresis in childhood. Ann Neurol. 1991;29:688–9.
262. Osterman PO, Fagius J, Säfwenberg J, Danersund A, Wallin BG, Nordesjo L-O. Treatment of the Guillain–Barré syndrome by plasmapheresis. Arch Neurol. 1982;39:148–54.
263. French Cooperative Group on Plasma Exchange in Guillain–Barré syndrome. Efficiency of plasma exchange in Guillain–Barré syndrome: role of replacement fluids. Ann Neurol. 1987;22:
264. French Cooperative Group on Plasma Exchange in Guillain–Barré Syndrome. Plasma exchange in Guillain–Barré syndrome: one-year follow-up. Ann Neurol. 1992;32:94–7.
265. Kleyweg R, van der Meché FGA. Treatment related fluctuations in Guillain–Barré syndrome after high-dose immunoglobulins or plasma-exchange. J Neurol Neurosurg Psychiatry. 1991;54:957–60.
266. Osterman PO, Fagius J, Säfwenberg J, Danielson BG, Wikström B. Early relapses after plasma exchange in acute inflammatory polyradiculoneuropathy. Lancet. 1986;2:1161.
267. Osterman PO, Fagius J, Säfwenberg J, Wikström BG. Early relapses of acute inflammatory polyradiculoneuropathy after successful treatment with plasma exchange. Acta Neurol Scand. 1988;77:273–7.
268. Färkkila M, Kinnumen E, Haapanen E, Iivanainen M. Guillain–Barré syndrome: quantitative measurement of plasma exchange therapy. Neurology. 1987;37:837–40.
269. Osterman PO, Vedeler CA, Ryberg B, Fagius J, Nyland H. Serum antibodies to peripheral nerve tissue in acute Guillain Barré syndrome in relation to outcome of plasma exchange. J Neurol. 1988;235:285–9.
270. Ropper AH, Albers JW, Addison R. Limited relapse in Guillain–Barré syndrome after plasma exchange. Arch Neurol. 1988;45:314–15.
271. Vriesendorp FJ, Mayer RF, Koski CL. Kinetics of anti-peripheral nerve myelin antibody in patients with Guillain–Barré syndrome treated and not treated with plasmapheresis. Arch Neurol. 1991;48:858–61.
272. Guener G, Bosch EP, Strauss RG, Klugman M, Kimura J. Prediction of early beneficial response to plasma exchange in Guillain–Barré syndrome. Arch Neurol. 1987;44:295–8.
273. Hughes RAC, Newsom-Davis J, Perkin GD, Pierce JM. Controlled trial of prednisolone in acute polyneuropathy. Lancet. 1978;2:750–3.
274. Guillain–Barré Syndrome Steroid Trial Group: Double-blind trial of intravenous methylprednisolone in Guillain–Barré syndrome. Lancet. 1993;341:586–90.
275. Castro LHM, Ropper AH. Gammaglobulin infusion in acute Guillain–Barré syndrome: Worsening during and after treatment. Neurology. 1993;43:1034–6.
276. Irani DN, Cornblath DR, Chaudhury V, Borel C, Hanley DF. Relapse in Guillain–Barré syndrome after treatment with human immune globulin. Neurology. 1993;43:872–5.
277. Casteels-Van Daele M, Wijndaele L, Huminck K. Intravenous immune globulin and acute aseptic meningitis. N Engl J Med. 1990;323:614–15.
278. Vera-Ramirez M, Charlet M, Parry GJ. Recurrent aseptic meningitis complicating intravenous immunoglobulin therapy for chronic inflammatory polyradiculoneuropathy. Neurology. 1992;42:1636–7.
279. Burks AQ, Sampson HA, Buckley RH. Anaphylactic reactions after gamma globulin administration in patients with hypogammaglobulinaemia. N Engl J Med. 1986;314: 560–4.
280. Tan E, Hajinazarian MO, Bay W, Neff J, Mendell JR. Acute renal failure resulting from intravenous immunoglobulin G therapy. Arch Neurol. 1993;50:137–9.
281. Thornton CA, Ballow M. Safety of intravenous immunoglobulin. Arch Neurol. 1993;50: 135–6.
282. Dietrich G, Kaveri SV, Kazatchkine MD. Modulation of autoimmunity by intravenous immune globulin through interaction with the function of the immune/idiotypic network. Clin Immunol Immunopathol. 1992;62:S73–81.

283. Dwyer JM. Manipulating the immune system with immune globulin. N Engl J Med. 1992;326:107–16.
284. Grosse-Wilde H, Blascyk R, Westhoff U. Soluble HLA class I and class II concentrations in commercial immunoglobulin preparations. Tissue Antigens. 1992;39:74–7.
285. Lundquist I, van Doorn PA, Vermeulen M, van Lint M, van Rood JJ, Brand A. Regulation of autoantibodies in inflammatory demyelinating polyneuropathy: spontaneous and therapeutic. Immunol Rev. 1989;110:105–17.
286. van Doorn PA, Brand A, Vermeulen M. Anti-neuroblastoma cell line antibodies in inflammatory demyelinating polyneuropathy: inhibition *in vitro* and *in vivo* by i.v. immunoglobulin. Neurology. 1988;38:1592–5.
287. van Doorn PA, Rossi F, Brand A, van Lint M, Vermeulen M, Kazatchkine MD. On the mechanism of high-dose intravenous immunoglobulin treatment of patients with chronic inflammatory demyelinating polyneuropathy. J Neuroimmunol. 1990;29:57–64.
288. Blasczyk R, Westhoff U, Grosse-Wilde H. Soluble CD4, CD8, and HLA molecules in commercial immunoglobulin concentrations. Lancet. 1993;341:789–90.
289. Ropper AH, Kehne SM. Guillain–Barré syndrome: management of respiratory failure. Neurology. 1985;35:1662–5.
290. Sunderrajan EV, Davenport J. The Guillain–Barré syndrome: pulmonary–neurologic correlations. Medicine. 1985;64:333–41.
291. Prineas JW, McLeod JG. Chronic relapsing polyneuritis. J Neurol Sci. 1976;27:427–58.
292. Pollard JD, McLeod JG. Inflammatory demyelinating neuropathies. Rec Adv Neurol. 1992;7:155–74.
293. Dyck PM, Lais AC, Ohta M, Bastron JA, Okazaki H, Groover RV. Chronic inflammatory polyradiculoneuropathy. Mayo Clin Proc. 1975;50:621–37.
294. Dyck PJ, Prineas JW, Pollard JD. Chronic inflammatory demyelinating polyradiculoneuropathy. In: Dyck PJ, Thomas PK, Griffin J, Low PA, Poduslo J, editors. Peripheral Neuropathy, 3rd edn. Philadelphia: W.B. Saunders, 1993:1498–517.
295. McCombe PA, Pollard JD, McLeod JG. Chronic inflammatory demyelinating polyradiculoneuropathy. A clinical and electrophysiological study of 92 cases. Brain. 1987;110: 1617–30.
295a. McLeod JG. Peripheral neuropathy associated with lymphomas, leukemias and polycythemia nerve. In: Dyck PJ, Thomas PK, Griffin J, Low PA, Poduslo JF, editors. Peripheral Neuropathy, 3rd edn. Philadelphia: W.B. Saunders, 1993:1591–8.
296. McLeod JG. Paraneoplastic neuropathies. In: Dyck PJ, Thomas PK, Griffin J, Low PA, Poduslo JF, editors. Peripheral Neuropathy, 3rd edn. Philadelphia: W.B. Saunders, 1993;1583–91.
297. Bahron RJ, Kissel JT, Warmolts, Mendell JR. Chronic inflammatory demyelinating polyradiculoneuropathy, clinical characteristics, course and recommendations for diagnostic criteria. Arch Neurol. 1989;14:878–84.
298. Dalakas MC, Engel WK. Chronic relapsing (dysimmune) polyneuropathy: pathogenesis and treatment. Ann Neurol. 1981;9:134–45.
299. Prineas JW. Demyelination and remyelination in recurrent idiopathic polyneuropathy. An electron microscope study. Acta Neuropathol (Berlin). 1971;18:34–57.
300. Bleasel AF, Hawke SHB, Pollard JD, McLeod JG. IgG monoclonal paraproteinemia and peripheral neuropathy. J Neurol Neurosurg Psychiatry. 1993;56:52–7.
301. Thomas PK. Separating motor neuron diseases from pure motor neuropathies: clinical clues and definitions. Adv Neurol. 1991;56:381–4.
302. Pollard JD. Neurological complications of the plasma cell dyscrasias. In: Vinken PJ, Bruyn GW, Klawans HL, editors. Handbook of Clinical Neurology. Amsterdam: Elsevier Press, 1993, Vol. 63: 391–411.
303. Parry GJ, Clarke S. Multifocal acquired demyelinating neuropathy masquerading as motor neuron disease. Muscle Nerve. 1988;11:103–7.
304. Pestronk A, Cornblath DR, Ilyas AA, *et al.* A treatable multifocal motor neuropathy with antibodies to GM1 ganglioside. Ann Neurol. 1988;24:73–8.
305. Parry GJ. Motor neuropathy with multifocal conduction block. In: Dyck PJ, Thomas PK, Griffin J, Low PA, Poduslo JF, editors. Peripheral Neuropathy, 3rd edn. Philadelphia: W.B. Saunders, 1993:1518–24.
306. Thomas PK, Lascelles RG, Hallpike JF, Hewer RL. Recurrent and chronic relapsing

Guillain–Barré polyneuritis. Brain. 1969;92:589–606.
307. Smith BE, Windebank AJ, Dyck PJ. Nonmalignant sensory polyganglionopathy. In: Dyck PJ, Thomas PK, Griffin J, Low PA, Poduslo JF, editors. Peripheral Neuropathy, 3rd edn. Philadelphia: W.B. Saunders, 1993:1525–31.
308. Cusimano MD, Bilbao JM, Cohen SM. Hypertrophic brachial plexus neuritis: a pathological study of two cases. Ann Neurol. 1988;9:134–45.
309. Adams RK, Asbury AK, Michelsen JJ. Multifocal pseudohypertrophic neuropathy. Trans Am Neurol Assoc. 1965;90:30–4.
310. Kaji R, Oka N, Tsuji T, *et al.* Pathological findings at the site of conduction block in multifocal motor neuropathy. Ann Neurol. 1993;33:152–8.
311. Lewis RA, Sumner AJ. The electrodiagnostic distinction between chronic familial and acquired demyelinative neuropathies. Neurology. 1982;32:592–6.
312. Parry GJ, Malamut R, Lupski JR, Patel PI, Garcia CA. Nerve conduction studies in hereditary motor and sensory neuropathy, type 1. Muscle Nerve. 1991;14:891.
313. Albers JW, Robertson WC, Daube JR. Electrodiagnostic findings in acute porphyric neuropathy. Muscle Nerve. 1978;1:292–6.
314. Peyronnard JM, Charron L, Beaudet F, Couture F. Vasculitic neuropathy in rheumatoid disease and Sjögren syndrome. Neurology. 1982;32:839–45.
315. Hömberg V, Reiners V, Toyka KV. Reversible conduction block in human ischemic neuropathy after ergotamine abuse. Muscle Nerve. 1992;15:467–70.
316. Brown WF, Snow R. Patterns and severity of conduction abnormalities in Guillain–Barré syndrome. J Neurol Neurosurg Psychiatry. 1991;54:768–74.
317. Oh SJ. Conduction block in hereditary motor sensory neuropathy, type I: Case report. Muscle Nerve. 1992;15:521–2.
318. Bromberg MB, Feldman EL, Albers JW. Chronic inflammatory demyelinating polyradiculoneuropathy: Comparison of patients with and without an associated monoclonal gammopathy. Neurology. 1992;42:1157–63.
319. Abu-Shakra SR, Cornblath DR, Avila OL, *et al.* Conduction block in diabetic neuropathy. Muscle Nerve. 1991;14:858–62.
320. Brashear HR, Bonnin JM, Login IS. Encephalomyeloneuritis simulating Guillain–Barré syndrome. Neurology. 1985;35:1146–51.
321. Mendell JR, Kolkin S, Kissel JT, Weiss KL, Chakeres DW, Rammohan KW. Evidence for central nervous system demyelination in chronic inflammatory demyelinating polyradiculoneuropathy. Neurology. 1987;37:1291–4.
322. Thomas P, Walker R, Rudge P, *et al.* Chronic demyelinating peripheral neuropathy associated with multifocal central nervous system demyelination. Brain. 1987;110:53–76.
323. Feasby TE, Hahn AF, Koopman WJ, Lee DH. Central lesions in the chronic inflammatory demyelinating polyneuropathy: An MRI study. Neurology. 1990;40:476–8.
324. Crino PB, Grossman RI, Rostami A. Magnetic resonance imaging of the cauda equina in chronic inflammatory demyelinating polyneuropathy. Ann Neurol. 1993;33:311–13.
325. Morgan GW, Barohn RJ, Bazan C, *et al.* Nerve root enhancement with MRI in inflammatory demyelinating polyradiculoneuropathy. Neurology. 1993;43:618–20.
326. Hyland HH, Russell WR. Chronic progessive polyneuritis with report of a fatal case. Brain. 1930;53:278–9.
327. Krücke W. Erkrankungen des peripheren Nervensystems. In: Lubarsch O, Henke F, Rössle R, editors. Handbuch der speziellen pathologischen Anatomie und Histologie. Vol. 13, part 5, Berlin: Springer-Verlag, 1955:164–83.
328. Pollard JD, McCombe PA, Baverstock J, Gatenby PA, McLeod JG. Class II antigen expression and T lymphocyte subsets in chronic inflammatory demyelinating polyneuropathy. J Neuroimmunol. 1986;13:123–4.
329. Gorodetzky C, Varela B, Castro-Escobar LE, Chavez-Negrete A, Escobar-Gutierrez A, Martinez-Mata J. HLA-DR antigens in Mexican patients with Guillain–Barré syndrome. J Neuroimmunol. 1983;4:1–7.
330. Adams D, Festenstein H, Gibson JD, *et al.* HLA antigens in chronic relapsing idiopathic inflammatory polyneuropathy. J Neurol Neurosurg Psychiatry. 1979;42:184–6.
331. Stewart GJ, Pollard JD, McLeod JG, Wolnizer CM. HLA antigens in the Landry–Guillain–Barré syndrome and chronic relapsing polyneuritis. Ann Neurol. 1978;4:285–9.
332. Vaughan R, Adam AM, Gray IA, *et al.* Major histocompatibility complex class I and

class II polymorphism in chronic idiopathic demyelinating polyradiculoneuropathy. J Neuroimmunol. 1990;27:149–53.
333. Feeney DJ, Pollard JD, McLeod JG, Stewart GJ, Doran TJ. HLA antigens in chronic inflammatory demyelinating polyneuropathy. J Neurol Neurosurg Psychiatry. 1990;53: 170–2.
334. Sheremata W, Colby S, Karkhanis Y, Eylar EH. Cellular hypersensitivity to basal myelin (P2) protein in the Guillain–Barré syndrome. Can J Neurol Sci. 1975;2:78–90.
335. Korn-Lubetzki I, Abramsky O. Acute and chronic demyelinating inflammatory polyradiculoneuropathy. Association with autoimmune diseases and lymphocyte response to human neuritogenic protein. Arch Neurol. 1986;3:604–8.
336. McCombe PA, Pollard JD, McLeod JG. Chronic inflammatory demyelinating polyradiculoneuropathy. In: Assal J-PL, Lininger C, editors. Peripheral neuropathies. What is significantly new? Fidia Research Series. Padova: Liviana Press, 1988:546–57.
337. Saida T, Saida K, Lisak RP, Brown MJ, Silberberg DH, Asbury AK. *In vivo* demyelinating activity of sera from patients with Guillain–Barré syndrome. Ann Neurol. 1982;11:69–75.
338. Tandon DS, Griffin JW, Drachman DB, Price DL, Coyle PL. Studies on the humoral mechanisms of inflammatory demyelinating neuropathies. Neurology. 1980;30:362.
339. Pollard JD. A critical review of therapies in acute and chronic demyelinating polyneuropathies. Muscle Nerve. 1987;10:214–21.
340. Heininger K, Liebert UG, Toyka KV, *et al.* Chronic inflammatory polyneuropathy. Reduction of nerve conduction velocities in monkeys by systemic passive transfer of immunoglobulin G. J Neurol Sci. 1984;66:1–14.
341. Server AC, Lefkowith J, Braine H, McKhann GM. Treatment of chronic relapsing inflammatory polyradiculoneuropathy by plasma exchange. Ann Neurol. 1979;6:258–61.
342. Toyka KV, Heininger K. Humoral factors in peripheral nerve disease. Muscle Nerve. 1987;10:222–32.
343. Harvey GK, Pollard JD, Schindhelm K, Antony J. Chronic experimental allergic neuritis. An electrophysiological and histological study in the rabbit. J Neurol Sci. 1987;81: 215–25.
344. Harvey GK, Schindhelm K, Antony J, Pollard JD. Membrane plasma exchange in experimental allergic neuritis: effect on antibody levels and clinical course. J Neurol Sci. 1988;88:207–18.
345. Harvey GK, Pollard JD, Schindhelm K, McLeod JG. Experimental allergic neuritis: effect of plasma infusion. Clin Exp Immunol. 1989;76:452–7.
346. Harvey GK, Schindhelm K, Pollard JD. IgG immunoadsorption in experimental allergic neuritis: effect on antibody levels and clinical course. J Neurol Neurosurg Psychiatry. 1989;52:865–70.
347. Saida T, Saida K, Silberberg DH, Brown MJ. Transfer of demyelination with experimental allergic neuritis serum by intraneural injection. Nature. 1978;272:629–41.
348. Saida T, Saida K, Dorfman SH *et al.* Experimental allergic neuritis induced by sensitization with galactocerebroside. Science. 1979;204:1103–6.
349. Saida T, Saida K, Silberberg DH, Brown MJ. Experimental allergic neuritis induced by galactocerebroside. Ann Neurol. 1981;9(suppl):87–101.
350. Stoll G, Schwendemann G, Heininger K, *et al.* Relation of clinical, serological, morphological and electrophysiological findings in galactocerebroside-induced experimental allergic neuritis. J Neurol Neurosurg Psychiatry. 1986;49:258–64.
351. Lassmann H, Sternberger H, Kitz K, Wisniewski HM. *In vivo* demyelinating activity of sera from animals with chronic relapsing experimental allergic encephalomyelitis. Antibody nature of the demyelinating factor and the role of complement. J Neurol Sci. 1983;59: 123–37.
352. Linington C, Lassmann H. Antibody responses in chronic relapsing experimental allergic encephalomyelitis: correlation of serum demyelinating activity with antibody titre to myelin/oligodendrocyte glycoprotein (MOG). J Neuroimmunol. 1987;17:61–9.
353. Cross AH, Cannella B, Brosnan CF, Raine CS. Homing to central nervous system vasculature by antigen-specific lymphocytes. Lab Invest. 1990;63:162–70.
354. Ludowyk PA, Willenborg DA, Parish CR. Selective localisation of neurospecific T lymphocytes in the central nervous system. J Neuroimmunol. 1992;37:237–50.
355. Austin JH. Recurrent polyneuropathies and their cortisone treatment. With five-year

observation of a placebo-controlled case treated with corticotrophin, cortisone, and prednisolone. Brain. 1958;81:157–92.

355a. Oh SJ. Subacute demyelinating polyneuropathy responding to corticosteroid treatment. Arch Neurol. 1978;35:509–16.

356. Dyck PJ, O'Brien PC, Oviatt KF, *et al.* Prednisone improves chronic inflammatory demyelinating polyradiculoneuropathy more than no treatment. Ann Neurol. 1982;11: 136–41.

356a. Pollard JD, McLeod JG, Gatenby P, Kronenberg H. Prediction of response to plasma exchange in chronic relapsing polyneuropathy. J Neurol Sci. 1983;58:269–87.

357. Gross MLP, Thomas PK. The treatment of chronic relapsing and chronic progressive idiopathic inflammatory polyneuropathy by plasma exchange. J Neurol Sci. 1981;52: 69–78.

358. Levy RL, Newkirk R, Ochoa J. Treating chronic relapsing Guillain–Barré syndrome by plasma exchange. Lancet. 1979;i:259–60.

358a. Toyka KV, Augspach R, Wiethölter H, *et al.* Plasma exchange in chronic inflammatory polyneuropathy: evidence suggestive of a pathogenic humoral factor. Muscle Nerve. 1982;5:479–84.

359. Dyck PJ, Daube J, O'Brien P, *et al.* Plasma exchange in chronic inflammatory demyelinating polyradiculoneuropathy. N Engl J Med. 1986;314:461–5.

360. Vermeulen M, van der Meché FGA, Speelman JD, Weber A, Busch HFM. Plasma and gamma-globulin infusion in chronic inflammatory polyneuropathy. J Neurol Sci. 1985;70:317–26.

361. Albama M, McNamara ME, Sokol M, Wijshock E. Improvement of neurological function in chronic inflammatory demyelinating polyradiculoneuropathy following intravenous gammaglobulin infusion. Arch Neurol. 1987;44:148–9.

362. Cook JD, Delgado MR, Soutter-Glass D. Treatment of childhood autoimmune polyneuropathy: IV. Gamma globulin. Neurology. 1987;37(suppl 1):253.

363. Curro-Dossi B, Tezzon F. High-dose intravenous gammaglobulin for chronic inflammatory demyelinating polyneuropathy. Ital J Neurol Sci. 1987;8:321–6.

364. Faed JM, Day B, Pollock M, Taylor PK, Nukada H, Hammond-Tooke GD. High-dose intravenous human immunoglobulin in chronic inflammatory demyelinating polyneuropathy. Neurology. 1989;39:422–5.

365. van Doorn PA, Brand A, Strengers PFW, Meulstee J, Vermeulen M. High-dose intravenous immunoglobulin treatment in chronic inflammatory demyelinating polyneuropathy: a double blind placebo-controlled cross over study. Neurology. 1990;40:209–12.

366. van Doorn PA, Vermeulen M, Brand A, Mulder PGH, Busch HFM. Intravenous immunoglobulin treatment in patients with chronic inflammatory demyelinating polyneuropathy. Clinical and laboratory characteristics associated with improvement. Arch Neurol. 1991;48:217–20.

367. Vermeulen M, van Doorn PA, Brand A, Strengers PFW, Jennekens FGI, Busch HFM. Intravenous immunoglobulin treatment in patients with chronic inflammatory demyelinating polyneuropathy: a double blind, placebo controlled study. J Neurol Surg Psychiatry. 1993;56:36–9.

368. Dyck PJ, O'Brien P, Swanson C, Low P, Daube J. Combined azathioprine and prednisone in chronic inflammatory demyelinating polyneuropathy. Neurology. 1985;35:1173–6.

369. Walker GL. Progressive polyradiculoneuropathy: treatment with azathioprine. Aust NZ J Med. 1979;9:184.

370. Hodgkinson SJ, Pollard JD, McLeod JG. Cyclosporin A in the treatment of chronic inflammatory demyelinating polyradiculoneuropathy. J Neurol Neurosurg Psychiatry. 1990;53:327–30.

371. Chaudhry V, Corse AM, Cornblath DR, Kuncl RW, Drachman DB, Freimer ML, Miller RG, Griffin JW. Multifocal motor neuropathy: response to human immune globulin. Ann Neurol. 1993;33:237–42.

372. Nobile-Orazio E, Meucci N, Barbieri S, Carpo M, Scarlato G. High-dose intravenous immunoglobulin therapy in multifocal motor neuropathy. Neurology. 1993;43:537–44.

4
Peripheral neuropathy due to vasculitis: immunopathogenesis, clinical features and treatment

J. T. KISSEL and J. R. MENDELL

INTRODUCTION

In the 15 years that have elapsed since the publication of Fauci *et al.*'s seminal view on vasculitis[1], there has been significant growth in our understanding of this enigmatic group of disorders. Advances in basic and clinical research have resulted in new concepts concerning the aetiology, immunology, and pathophysiology of the vasculitides, and new proposals for the diagnosis and classification of these diseases. More importantly, new and innovative therapies have been proposed based on current formulations of the immunopathogenesis of the blood vessel damage. Most of this information is immediately relevant for the practising clinician, who is faced with the formidable task of diagnosing and treating these difficult patients. This review will summarize our current understanding of vasculitis affecting the peripheral nervous system and outline the diagnosis and clinical management of these patients.

DEFINITION AND EPIDEMIOLOGY

The vasculitides are a heterogeneous group of disorders, all of which are characterized by inflammation and necrosis of blood vessel walls, with secondary ischaemia in affected tissues[1,2]. Vasculitis may be a primary disease or may occur secondary to some other disease process, such as an infection, toxin, connective tissue disease or neoplasm. Precise figures concerning the incidence of vasculitic neuropathy are unavailable. However, some idea of the frequency of these disorders can be gleaned from a recent report of the American College of Rheumatology Subcommittee on Classification of Vasculitis[3,4]. In this project, rheumatologists from 48 medical centres throughout North America submitted their cases of vasculitis to a central co-ordinating centre (Mayo Clinic) for precise classification. Over a $5\frac{1}{2}$ year period, 1000 new cases of vasculitis were submitted for analysis. Since peripheral neuropathy occurs in up to 75% of patients with primary vasculitis in most series[5–8], this would indicate approximately 750 new cases of vasculitis neuropathy in the 48 centres over the study period. This translates to roughly three cases per year per centre, a figure very close to that of several published series of vasculitic neuropathy, including that from our own centre[9–11]. Vasculitic neuropathy is, therefore, relatively uncommon; nevertheless, it is important to the clinician as a challenging diagnostic problem and a potentially treatable cause of neurological disability.

PATHOGENESIS

Although all of the vasculitides are assumed to have an autoimmune pathogenesis, the precise sequence of immunological events causing vessel injury is not well understood. The events that trigger the immune reaction and the antigens that serve as targets for the autoimmune processes have not been identified for most of these disorders. The factors involved in determining the size of the blood vessels affected and their organ distribution, both factors crucial in determining the clinical expression of the disease, also remain unknown. In fact, most of the evidence for the autoimmune origin of vasculitis is indirect, derived from analyses of the inflammatory infiltrates in affected tissue and the clinical response to immunosuppressive drugs.

A growing consensus has emerged that three predominantly humoral mechanisms (vascular deposition of circulating immune complexes, direct antibody attack on blood vessels, and antibody-induced degranulation of neutrophils causing passive endothelial cell damage) and one predominantly cell-mediated mechanism (direct endothelial cell destruction by cytotoxic T cells) are responsible for most primary vasculitides in humans.

Humoral mechanisms

The most extensively studied and perhaps best understood pathogenic mechanism for vasculitis is the passive deposition of circulating immune complexes. According to this model (Figure 4.1), antibodies interact with circulating antigens that have been processed by antigen-presenting cells to form complexes of varying size, usually under conditions of antigen excess[1,2,12]. These immune complexes activate complement and become coated with C3b and C4b, triggering host regulatory and defence mechanisms. The erythrocyte C3b receptor (CR1) is particularly important, binding the antigen–antibody–C3b complexes for transport to the liver, where they are cleared from the circulation[12–17]. Insufficient host regulatory mechanisms allow complexes to be deposited in vessel walls, a reaction facilitated by the

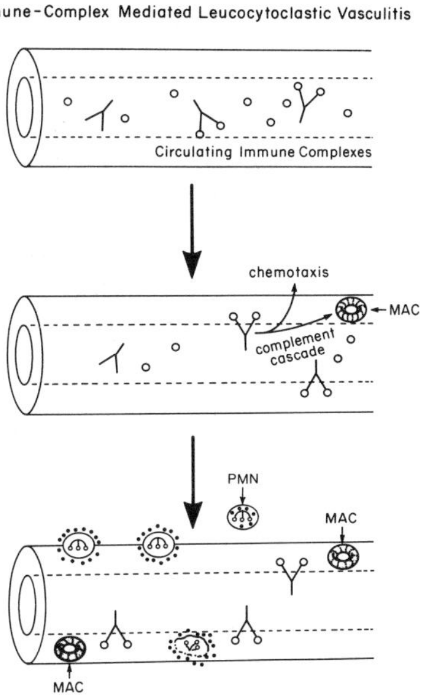

Figure 4.1 Schematic representation of immune complex/leucocytoclastic model of vasculitis. Antigen–antibody complexes, formed in the circulation, deposit in vessel walls and activate complement. Chemotactic factors are generated that recruit polymorphonuclear leucocytes (PMN) which release intracytoplasmic enzymes. Complement C5b-9 membrane attack complex (MAC), a ring-shaped membranolytic structure, is also generated contributing to vessel wall damage (see text for details).

action of histamine and bradykinin[16]. Local deposits of immune complexes activate the complement system, generating factors chemotactic for neutrophils such as C3a and C5a. The immune complexes are phagocytosed through the interaction of neutrophil Fc receptors with the Fc portion of the complexed antibody[12,18]. The neutrophils release proteolytic enzymes, free radicals, and various inflammatory and chemotactic peptides which damage the vessel walls directly in the so-called leucocytoclastic reaction[1,12,19]. These processes secondarily recruit macrophages and lymphocytes that also infiltrate the vessel wall. The complement membrane attack complex (C5b-9) which is formed as the result of complement activation probably also contributes to the vessel wall injury (Figure 4.2)[12,20]. As part of the process the coagulation system is activated by the procoagulant effects of damaged endothelium, the action of C5b-9 (which increases platelet prothrombinase activity) and the binding of coagulation factors Va and Xa to the endothelial cell membrane[12,16,17,21,22].

The final result of this cascade of events is compromise of the blood vessel lumen, resulting in reduction of blood flow and ischaemic damage in the distribution of the involved vessels. The exact vessels targeted by the process are determined by additional factors, including properties of the inciting antigen (such as type, size, and quantity), characteristics of the immune complexes (i.e. whether formed in antigen or antibody excess), physiochemical properties of the blood vessels, and the genetic susceptibility of the host[12,16,17,19].

These classic forms of immune complex reaction have been studied most extensively in animal models of vasculitis, especially in experimental acute and chronic serum sickness and the Arthus reaction[1,2,16]. In man, the clearest

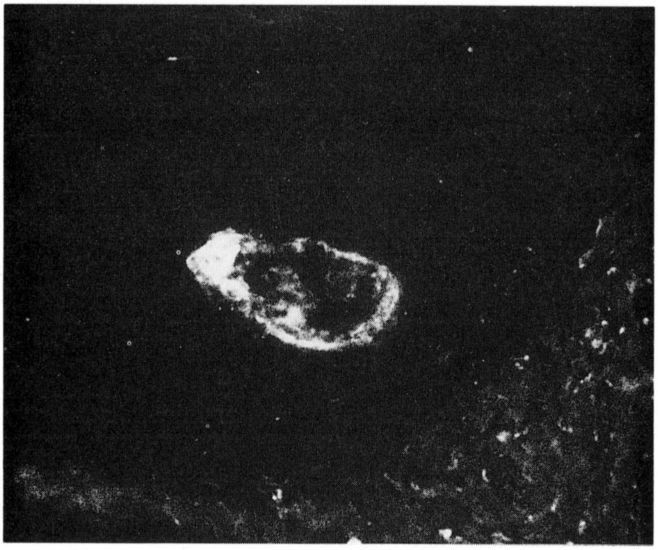

Figure 4.2 Sural nerve specimen from a patient with peripheral nerve vasculitis immunostained for complement membrane attack complex showing intense transmural deposits in a single epineurial vessel[20] (indirect immunofluorescent technique × 250)

evidence favouring immune complex-mediated vasculitis occurs in patients with hepatitis B antigenaemia, in whom circulating and vascular deposits can be demonstrated; such patients account for one-third of cases of polyarteritis nodosa[1,16]. Immune complexes may also be important in many of the secondary vasculitides, where the inciting agent may be an infectious organism, an exogenous toxin (usually a systemic drug), or a neoplasm.

Support for immune complex-mediated peripheral nerve vasculitis is based on the consistent demonstration of deposits of immunoglobulin, complement, or both in the epineurial vessels of nerve biopsies from patients with vasculitic neuropathy (Figure 4.2)[11,20,23]. In one study, the pattern of immunofluorescence was assessed to be 'granular' or inhomogeneous in seven of 23 patients (33%); this pattern is characteristic of that seen in other immune complex diseases, particularly those affecting the kidney[23].

An immune complex vasculitis need not necessarily involve circulating antigen–antibody complexes. An alternative possibility involves antibody directed against antigens within the microvasculature. Endothelial cells can serve as antigen-presenting cells for either exogenous or autologous antigens[17,24]. This might explain organ specificity, since particular endothelial cells expressing tissue-specific antigens could be altered by an inciting event[17,25]. This mechanism is supported by the demonstration of anti-endothelial cell antibodies (or AECA) in several autoimmune disorders, including systemic lupus erythematosus, rheumatoid arthritis, Kawasaki disease, scleroderma, and the systemic necrotizing vasculitides of Wegener's granulomatosis and polyarteritis nodosa[26–30]. In one series, 18 of 21 patients (86%) with a proven systemic vasculitis had detectable AECA[26], although the incidence has not been that high in other series[27–30]. There is some suggestion that the level of AECA may correlate with disease activity. Presumably these antibodies lead to endothelial cell damage through complement-mediated or antibody-dependent cell-mediated cytotoxic mechanisms; direct evidence for either of these mechanisms, however, has not been established. The putative antigens against which the AECA are directed have not been precisely identified for any of the vasculitic syndromes.

Recently, the discovery of the anti-neutrophil cytoplasmic autoantibody (ANCA), has provided another potentially important humoral mechanism for mediating vessel damage in the vasculitides[31]. ANCA was initially described in 1982 in patients with systemic vasculitis and necrotizing glomerulonephritis. Subsequently ANCA has been demonstrated in patients with Wegener's granulomatosis, classic and microscopic polyarteritis, Churg–Strauss syndrome and 'small vessel' vasculitis[27,29,31–36]. Using indirect immunofluorescent staining, ANCA produces either a 'cytoplasmic' (C-ANCA) or a 'perinuclear' (P-ANCA) staining pattern related to two different antigens[29,31]. C-ANCA is produced by antibody reactivity to proteinase-3, a neutral serine proteinase; the P-ANCA pattern results from antibody to myeloperoxidase. Both are enzymes of the neutrophil primary granule. Many studies have reported sensitivities and specificities of 90–95% for C-ANCA in patients with Wegener's granulomatosis[30–32]. More importantly, there is provocative evidence that the ANCA titre may correlate with disease activity, falling below detectable levels with treatment and rising significantly prior to a clinical relapse[31,33,37].

ANCA has a wide range of actions, including the ability to activate neutrophils and release reactive oxygen species that can damage endothelial cells[36]. These antibodies induce neutrophil degranulation and also bind to neutrophil proteases, inhibiting their inactivation by protease inhibitors and allowing them to remain active in the circulation[27].

The role of both AECA and ANCA in the pathogenesis of vasculitis neuropathy is unknown. A single recent study found AECA in only two of 12 patients with vasculitic neuropathy, including one of five patients with isolated peripheral nerve vasculitis[38]. In a separate clinicopathological study, a single vasculitis patient with an IgG-κ paraprotein was found to have a homogeneous pattern of immune deposition in epineurial vessels on nerve biopsy. This pattern was judged to be similar to the glomerular basement membrane pattern deposition seen in Goodpasture's syndrome, and suggested that the antibody was an AECA[23]. Further studies are required to determine the importance of both AECA and ANCA in the vasculitic neuropathies.

Cellular mechanisms

Despite the experimental and pathological studies which support a humorally-mediated, immune complex mechanism for some types of vasculitis, it is clear that other immunopathogenic processes are more significant in many other types, particularly those affecting peripheral nerves. The presence of granulomatous changes in Wegener's granulomatosis, Churg–Strauss syndrome and giant cell arteritis supports a role of cell-mediated mechanisms in these disorders. Recent immunohistological studies of peripheral nerve vasculitis also provide evidence for this concept. Studies from our laboratory using quantitative cell typing on the infiltrates in 22 nerve biopsies from 14 patients with systemic vasculitis and eight patient with isolated peripheral nerve vasculitis demonstrated cellular infiltrates composed primarily of T cells (71% of cells) and macrophages (28%)[20]. Two-thirds of the T cells were of the CD8 cytotoxic/suppressor subset. Although immunoglobulin and complement deposits were seen in 80% of the biopsy specimens, B cells were extremely rare (only 2% of cells) and neutrophils were never observed. These observations, which have been confirmed by other investigators[11,23], suggest that the classic leucocytoclastic reaction is not the primary process in patients with vasculitic neuropathy. Similar immunohistological studies in other vasculitic syndromes, including temporal arteritis[39] and Wegener's granulomatosis[40], have demonstrated a predominance of macrophages and $CD8^+$ lymphocytes. Other investigations have demonstrated circulating levels of lymphocyte-secreted cytokines, such as interferon-α and interleukin (IL)-1B and 2, in patients with vasculitis[24,41–43]. Cytotoxic T lymphocytes specific for class 2 major histocompatibility complex (MHC) antigens have also been shown to lyse endothelial cells in culture after exposure to interferon-γ[24]. These observations support a role for a cell-mediated, cytotoxic process in vasculitis.

The endothelial cell appears to play a vital role in cell-mediated vasculitis. Endothelial cells express class 1 MHC antigens and can be induced to express class 2 antigens[24], a finding well demonstrated in patients with peripheral nerve vasculitis[44]. Endothelial cells can serve as antigen-presenting cells and can be induced to secrete prostaglandin, chemotactic factors and a number of cytokines (including IL-1, IL-6 and intercellular adhesion molecule)[24,38,41–43] all of which act to recruit and activate lymphocytes, perpetuating the cycle of immune damage in vasculitis.

It is highly unlikely that a single immunological mechanism can explain the wide variety of clinical and pathological manifestations of the different vasculitic diseases. While many, if not most, of the vasculitic syndromes may arise from a combination of humoral and cellular mechanisms, acting either sequentially or simultaneously, some immunological specificity must develop to explain the widely differing clinical, serological and histological findings that are often found in patients with distinct vasculitic diseases.

PATHOLOGY

Irrespective of the immune mechanisms involved, the final outcome for all vasculitic syndromes is compromise of the vessel lumen with resulting ischaemia in the distribution of the involved vessels. Peripheral nerve vasculitis affects the 50–300 μm vessels of the vasa nervorum. Peripheral nerve ischaemia causes axonal degeneration as the major pathological process; selective demyelination is unusual[45–47]. Because of the rich anastomotic vascular supply of nerve fascicles and the random, focal nature of the

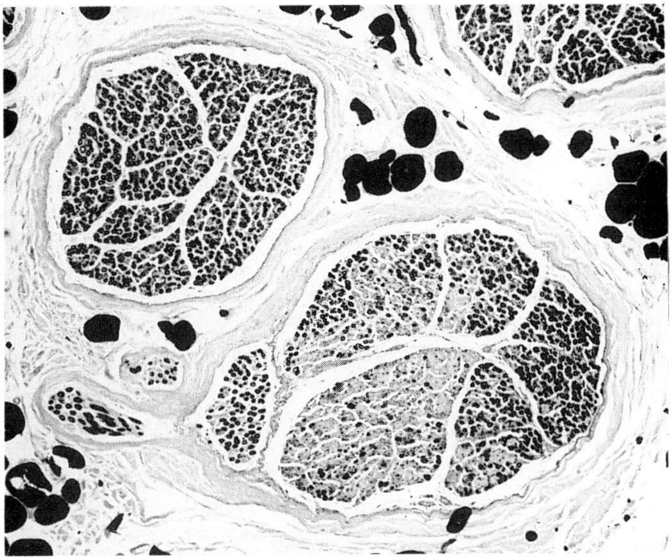

Figure 4.3 Two fascicles from a sural nerve biopsy performed in a patient with isolated peripheral nerve vasculitis. The smaller fascicle on the left is essentially unaffected while that on the right shows severe myelinated fibre loss, particularly on the left side of the fascicle (paraffin-embedded and osmicated; × 200)

vasculitis process, axonal degeneration is characteristically asymmetrical between and within individual fascicles (Figure 4.3)[9,46,48]. This asymmetrical involvement is most prominent in proximal nerves, while distally the branching and intermixing of nerve fibres can result in a homogeneous pattern[9,47]. Recent morphometric studies by Fujimura *et al.* have demonstrated that myelinated fibres are more susceptible to ischaemia than are unmyelinated fibres, and larger myelinated fibres ($> 7\,\mu m$) are particularly vulnerable to damage[47]. Nevertheless, unmyelinated fibres and even Schwann cells are susceptible to ischaemia. We have observed biopsy specimens of nerve in which facsicles have demonstrated nearly complete loss of intrafascicular cellular components within the intact perineurium. This loss of cellular components would impede axonal regeneration, as observed by Fujamuri *et al.*[47].

CLINICAL PRESENTATION

The extent and temporal progression of the ischaemia in peripheral nerves determines the type and pattern of neuropathic disease in patients with vasculitic neuropathy. The classic pattern is a multiple mononeuropathy (or mononeuritis multiplex), where involvement of individual nerves can be clinically identified. Recent series, however, have revealed this to be the presenting pattern in only 10–15% of patients with vasculitic neuropathy[9,10,46]. More commonly, the tempo and extent of the disease process obscures the involvement of individual nerves, producing an overlapping multiple mononeuropathy. The process may superficially appear symmetrical but careful examination reveals asymmetry between sides. This pattern occurs in 50–60% of patients and results from the summated effects of multiple individual nerves being involved in an affected limb. Finally, a distal symmetric 'stocking–glove' polyneuropathy can arise when vasculitic disease at multiple levels of individual nerve trunks leads to overlapping distal involvement, resulting in a symmetrical pattern of deficits[49,50]. This pattern, which occurs in 30–40% of patients, may be difficult to distinguish from other types of distal axonopathies[9,10].

Burning, dysaesthetic pain in the distribution of involved nerves is found in 70–80% of patients[9]. Most often, ischaemia affects motor and sensory fibres, causing both sensory loss and muscle weakness. Rarely, vasculitis can selectively damage cutaneous sensory nerves[10].

Peripheral neuropathy in a patient with multi-organ systemic disease (including kidney, lungs, bowel, skin, or central nervous system) suggests a systemic necrotizing vasculitis (Group 1, see discussion below). Approximately 50% of patients presenting to a neurologist have an isolated peripheral nerve vasculitis (Group 4). Patients with hypersensitivity vasculitis (Group 2) and giant cell arteritides (Group 3) rarely have involvement of the peripheral nerves. In any patient with vasculitis, including those in whom involvement is restricted to peripheral nerves, non-specific constitutional symptoms such as fever, malaise, and weight loss are common. The presence of any of these symptoms in a patient without neuropathy should raise a strong suspicion of an underlying vasculitis.

DIAGNOSIS

The diagnostic evaluation of a patient with a suspected peripheral nerve vasculitis should include studies specifically directed toward identifying an underlying disorder or serological abnormality pointing toward a vasculitic syndrome or connective tissue disease. These studies include renal function studies, liver enzymes, urinalysis, erythrocyte sedimentation rate (ESR), antinuclear antibody titre, extractable nuclear antigens, rheumatoid factor, ANCA and AECA assays, serum complement, cryoglobulins, hepatitis B antigen and antibody, and total peripheral eosinophil count. We have not found assays for immune complexes helpful in individual patients; if they are performed, an entire battery of screening tests must be obtained since each test (e.g. Raji cell assay, C1q binding assay, latex fixation test) detects immune complexes of differing sizes and morphology[13].

In patients with isolated peripheral nerve vasculitis, all serum and urine tests are usually normal, although the ESR is frequently mildly elevated (< 50 mm/h)[9]. Normal results of laboratory studies should not direct attention away from a vasculitis if the clinical picture warrants this consideration.

Electromyographic (EMG) and nerve conduction studies are important in

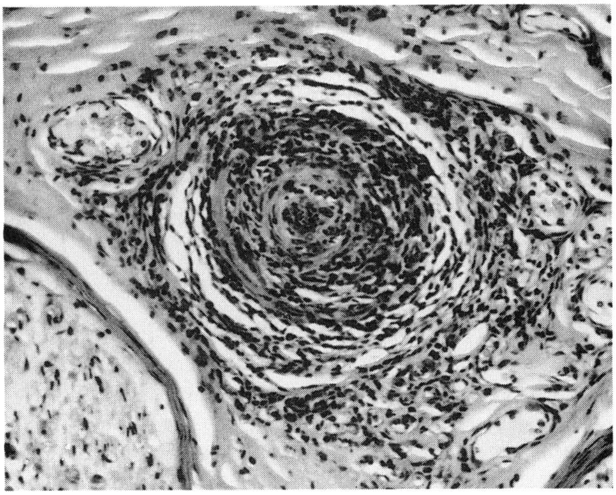

Fig. 4.4 High power view of sural nerve biopsy from a patient with isolated peripheral nerve vasculitis showing intense mononuclear cell infiltration through this epineurial vessel wall with resultant necrosis (haematoxylin and eosin, × 650)

demonstrating the distribution and severity of peripheral nerve disease[51,52]. Not only can the physiological changes demonstrate subclinical sensory or motor involvement but, more importantly, these studies can indicate a multiple mononeuropathy which has escaped clinical detection. The electromyographic findings of fibrillations, sharp potentials, and motor unit dropout reflect the degree of axonal destruction and the tempo of the process. EMG evidence of reinnervation can also be helpful in following the patients for signs of recovery. Nerve conduction studies often demonstrate unevokable sensory or motor action potentials, and conduction block is occasionally seen[53,54].

Serological and electrodiagnostic studies can suggest an underlying vasculitis, but definitive diagnosis rests on the demonstration of vascular inflammation and necrosis in a tissue specimen (Figure 4.4). Nerve biopsies are usually restricted to the cutaneous sensory nerves, specifically the sural, superficial peroneal and superficial radial. Motor nerves, even the deep motor branch to the peroneus brevis, are not easily accessible and biopsies carry the risk of causing muscle weakness. Of the cutaneous nerves, biopsy of the superficial peroneal nerve is preferred since a simultaneous muscle biopsy of peroneus brevis can be obtained through the same incision. A simultaneous sampling of both nerve and muscle will provide a higher diagnostic yield. In a study by Said *et al.*[46] the vasculitis was confirmed more frequently in the peroneus brevis muscle (80% of patients) than in the superficial peroneal nerve (only 55% of patients). Details concerning the technical aspects of the superficial peroneal nerve biopsy procedure and appropriate preparation of nerve specimens have recently been summarized[55].

A pathological diagnosis of vasculitis requires the presence of transmural mononuclear cells, and evidence of vessel wall necrosis (Figure 4.4). Inflammatory infiltration restricted to the perivascular regions, and not invading the vessel wall, is not sufficient for diagnosis but can be suggestive in the appropriate clinical and laboratory setting. Immunofluorescent staining reveals immunoglobulin and complement deposits in the vessel wall in over 80% of patients[11,20,23]. In older, partially healed lesions, fibrin deposition and recanalization of vessels may be seen. As discussed above, an asymmetrical pattern of nerve fibre loss, even in severely affected nerves, is often observed[9,46,48].

CLASSIFICATION AND TREATMENT

Precise classification of the vasculitic process has implications beyond an academic exercise. Accurate classification provides a conceptual framework for understanding underlying immunopathogenic mechanisms and helps guide therapeutic decisions. The traditional approach to classification has been based on clinical features and size of affected blood vessels. More recently, investigators have proposed newer schemes based on recent serological findings, such as the 'ANCA-associated vasculitides'[31]. Our present knowledge of immunopathogenic mechanisms for most of the vasculitides is not adequate to permit a complete classification in this manner.

We have found a useful clinical scheme to be a modification of that initially proposed by Scott[56]. This divides the vasculitides into four principal groups:

(1) Systemic necrotizing vasculitis
- Classical polyarteritis nodosa (PAN)
- Allergic angiitis and granulomatosis (Churg–Strauss disease)
- Wegener's granulomatosis
- Vasculitis with connective tissue disease
- Overlap syndromes

(2) Hypersensitivity vasculitis
- Henoch–Schönlein purpura
- Serum sickness
- Vasculitis associated with infections
- Drug-induced vasculitis (amphetamines, heroin, cocaine)
- Vasculitis associated with malignancy
- Vasculitis with connective tissue disease

(3) Giant cell arteritis
- Temporal arteritis
- Takayasu's arteritis

(4) Localized vasculitis
- Isolated peripheral nervous system vasculitis (non-systemic vasculitic neuropathy)
- Isolated angiitis of the central nervous system

This scheme serves principally to emphasize the distinction between the hypersensitivity vasculitides (Group 2), which usually affect the skin and tend to arise secondary to some other underlying illness or process, and the systemic vasculitides which are primary disorders (Groups 1, 3 and 4) that cause major organ failure. A detailed discussion of the clinical, radiological, and laboratory features of each of the diseases in this classification is beyond the scope of this review. The American College of Rheumatology has recently published diagnostic criteria for seven of the common types of vasculitis listed in the classification, including polyarteritis nodosa, Churg–Strauss syndrome, Wegener's granulomatosis, hypersensitivity vasculitis, Henoch–Schönlein purpura, temporal arteritis and Takaysu's arteritis[3,4]. These criteria are based on an analysis of over 800 patients with vasculitis and should be consulted when trying to diagnose and classify a patient. It is important to remember, however, that a significant number of patients (16% in the American College of Rheumatology Study) will not fit neatly into any specific disease category, and must be classified as having an 'overlap syndrome' or 'non-specific vasculitis'. These patients must simply be classified in the most appropriate category and managed accordingly.

IMMUNOSUPPRESSIVE THERAPY

Once vasculitis has been confirmed by biopsy and the patient's syndrome has been classified as accurately as possible, an appropriate therapeutic regimen can be planned based on a consideration of the underlying pathophysiological mechanism. For example, in patients with peripheral nerve involvement due to a hypersensitivity vasculitis (Group 2), the initial step in treatment is to remove any inciting antigen that might be triggering immune complex formation and secondary damage to the blood vessel[57]. This approach is most effective for vasculitides related to drug use, but also applies to many of the infectious vasculitides. Unfortunately, this group represents only a small minority of patients with peripheral nerve vasculitis, and in patients in groups 1, 3 and 4, no inciting antigen can be identified. Patients with peripheral nerve involvement as part of a systemic necrotizing vasculitis (Group 1) are treated with a combination regimen involving corticosteroids and a cytotoxic agent. The rare patient with peripheral nerve vasculitis due to a giant cell arteritis (Group 3) can often be managed with corticosteroid monotherapy. Patients with isolated peripheral nerve vasculitis (Group 4) represent a special group, since they do not have a life-threatening disease but the immunopathogenic lesion appears identical to the peripheral nerve vasculitis of Group 1. Recommendations regarding this group are discussed separately below.

A typical combination regimen for systemic necrotizing vasculitis consists of oral prednisone, 1.5 mg/kg/day and oral cyclophosphamide (2 mg/kg/day). Prednisone is give as a single, morning dose for 2–4 weeks and then as an alternate day regimen at the same dose. In fulminant, severe cases we recommend initiating corticosteroids with a 'pulse' of intravenous methylprednisolone (1 g every other day for six doses) followed by institution of the every other day oral regimen. Combined drug therapy is continued until significant improvement occurs and the clinical condition has stabilized. At this time, prednisone can be tapered at a rate no faster than 5 mg every 2 weeks. If a relapse of symptoms occurs during the tapering of the prednisone, a bolus of oral prednisone, and occasionally with intravenous methylprednisolone, is the treatment of choice. Cyclophosphamide is continued for approximately 1 year and then stopped if there is no evidence of active disease.

Careful monitoring is crucial in these patients to avoid side-effects[58,59]. Weight and blood pressure should be monitored closely. Steroid-induced hyperglycaemia usually occurs early in the course of administration. Patients should also be monitored for potassium loss, especially if they require a diuretic for blood pressure control. Ocular evaluations for development of cataracts and glaucoma should be performed. Patients must be warned of and agree to the risk of osteonecrosis of the head of the femur[60]. A low sodium, low simple sugar, low calorie diet supplemented with vitamin D and calcium may limit weight gain and the development of osteoporosis. We strongly recommend single daily or alternate day, morning doses of prednisone since this is usually as effective as split-dose therapy. Oral hydration (at least eight glasses of water per day) is encouraged to prevent the haemorrhagic cystitis which occurs in approximately 15% of patients receiving cyclophosphamide[61,62]. A complete blood count is obtained monthly, and the drug dose is adjusted to keep the total white count above $3000/mm^3$ and the neutrophil count above $1000/mm^3$.

The purine analogue azathioprine is our drug of choice in patients who cannot tolerate cyclophosphamide; it is used in an analogous fashion to cyclophosphamide[63,64]. The principal side-effects of azathioprine include leukopenia and an allergic-type reaction (fever, arthralgias, nausea or vomiting); this occurs in about 10% of patients[63]. Rechallenge with azathioprine at lower doses causes identical symptoms and always precludes further use of the drug. Chemical hepatitis can also occur with azathioprine. Other immune-modifying therapies, including plasma exchange and pharmacological agents such as cyclosporin, colchicine, dapsone, and methotrexate have found only anecdotal use in the vasculitides and their present role in treating these diseases is uncertain[65].

In addition to immunosuppression, other therapeutic modalities must often be employed in these patients to minimize the morbidity of the disease. Aggressive physical and occupational therapy programmes are often helpful in improving range of motion and maintaining strength. This latter benefit is particularly important since many of these patients require prolonged prednisone therapy and are at risk for developing steroid myopathy. Judicious use of agents such as carbamazepine, clonazepam and amitriptyline may be effective in treating neuropathic pain.

PROGNOSIS

There have been no prospective studies assessing the long-term prognosis of patients with peripheral nerve vasculitis, either as an isolated entity or combined with an underlying systemic disease. Support for the use of prednisone and cyclophosphamide has been demonstrated in prior retrospective studies of systemic necrotizing vasculitis, not necessarily involving peripheral nerves. For example, several studies demonstrated that the untreated 5-year survival rate for patients with polyarteritis nodosa was less than 15%, improving to 40% with corticosteroid treatment alone. When cyclophosphamide was added to the regimen, however, long-term remissions were induced in 90% of patients, and therapy could eventually be discontinued in most of these patients[66,67]. Similar results were demonstrated for Wegener's granulomatosis, where complete remission rates above 90% were reported with combination prednisone/cyclophosphamide therapy[68].

Dyck *et al.* recently reviewed the Mayo Clinic experience with 65 patients (45 with an underlying systemic necrotizing vasculitis and 20 with nonsystemic vasculitic neuropathy) over a 20-year period[10]. Approximately one-third of patients with systemic vasculitis died (within a median time of 1.5 years of presentation) while none of their patients with isolated peripheral nerve vasculitis had died after a mean follow-up time of 11.5 years. This markedly different prognosis may justify the separation of patients with isolated peripheral nerve vasculitis from those with an underlying systemic disease. A similar poor prognosis for peripheral neuropathy complicating systemic necrotizing vasculitis was reported by Hawke *et al.*[11]; 50% of patients in this series died within a mean of 36 months of presentation and the 5-year survival was only 37%, despite aggressive treatment. All patients received prednisone, either alone or in combination with plasma exchange or other immunosuppressive agents (azathioprine, chlorambucil, or cyclophosphamide). Neurological disability improved with treatment in the majority of the patients despite a poor outcome due to involvement of other organ systems. An interesting finding in their study was that no patient treated adequately with cyclophosphamide died within a mean follow-up time of 25 months[11].

FUTURE THERAPIES

Future work must focus on prospective studies of the natural history and effects of combination immunosuppressive regimens in patients with all types of vasculitic neuropathy, particularly those with isolated peripheral nerve vasculitis. In addition, controlled trials must be performed comparing the standard combination cyclophosphamide/prednisone regimen to other immunosuppressive agents, such as cyclosporin, colchicine, methotrexate and dapsone.

A second area for future investigation concerns the value of intravenous immunoglobulin (IVIg) in treating patients with peripheral nerve vasculitis. IVIg has found widespread use in the treatment of many immunodeficiency and autoimmune disorders, particularly idiopathic thrombocytopenic purpura and Kawasaki disease[69–71]. It is currently undergoing active investigation in diseases such as inflammatory muscle disease, inflammatory demyelinating neuropathy, and myasthenia gravis. The mechanism of action of IVIg may involve the presence of anti-idiotype antibodies in the IVIg which react with the pathogenic antibodies in the patient. Alternatively, the IVIg might compete for Fc receptors on effector cells, disrupt B cell maturation and T-helper cell/B cell interaction, or inhibit activated complement intermediates[69–71].

In one provocative study, IVIg was given to seven patients with systemic vasculitis, all of whom had ANCA. All seven had a significant clinical improvement, and five went into a full clinical remission. This improvement was mirrored by a fall in the ANCA titres, which were reduced to a mean of 51% of the pretreatment values within 6 weeks of therapy. These authors also found anti-idiotype antibodies in IVIg that reacted with idiotypes on the ANCA, providing a theoretical reason for the clinical improvement in these patients[72]. Further studies will be needed to establish whether IVIg is applicable to a wider group of patients with systemic vasculitis, including ANCA-negative patients and those with isolated peripheral nerve vasculitis.

Another fundamental goal is an improved understanding of the immunopathogenic mechanisms underlying peripheral nerve vasculitis, including the identification of inciting antigens and precise definition of the immunopathogenic mechanisms. This information will lead to the development of target-specific therapies. In this regard, preliminary work has begun on several novel concepts of therapy for these diseases.

The first concept involves a more specific consideration of vessel thrombosis as a contributing factor to organ damage in vasculitic lesions. This aspect of vasculitic injury has received relatively little attention. Conn has presented a hypothesis that glucocorticoids may contribute to the ischaemic damage, despite their anti-inflammatory properties[73]. This hypothesis is based on glucocorticoid inhibition of prostacyclin production by endothelial cells with preservation of the platelet thromboxane–prostaglandin system. Both systems are known to be activated by the immune processes of vasculitis, but glucocorticoids may inhibit the beneficial effects of the prostacyclin system while letting the platelet thromboxane system act unopposed to promote vasoconstriction and thrombus formation. Further experimental and clinical studies such as the use of anti-platelet agents, will be necessary to assess the potential role of glucocorticoid-inhibition of prostacyclins in the pathogenesis and treatment of vasculitic neuropathy. Currently it is probably appropriate to add an anti-platelet agent to the regimen of a patient who is neurologically deteriorating or showing signs of peripheral ischaemia despite aggressive immunosuppressive therapy[73].

A second area of future investigation will be directed towards the clinical use of monoclonal antibodies. Genetically engineered monoclonal antibodies[74] could be generated to block specific pathways of the immune system, or may even be directed against endothelial cell antigens that might trigger the vasculitic process. Such antibodies could be designed to more easily cross through the blood–nerve barrier. A recent report by Mathieson *et al.*[75] described the successful use of two monoclonal antibodies in a patient with intractable systemic vasculitis. Both were rat monoclonal antibodies; one was directed against the human CD4 molecule of T helper cells. The second monoclonal was directed against human lymphocytes and was genetically engineered by transfecting the hypervariable regions of the rat antibody onto normal human immunoglobulin genes. This eliminated immune complex-mediated serum sickness due to the development of anti-rat antibodies in the human host. The therapy proved effective, inducing remission lasting 12 months in a patient previously refractory to treatment. No anti-idiotypic antibodies to the engineered monoclonal antibodies were detected, a potent side-effect of this strategy of therapy observed in the treatment of allograft rejection. In the future, improved methods to generate human monoclonal antibodies may eliminate this problem.

References

1. Fauci AS, Haynes BF, Katz P. The spectrum of vasculitis. Clinical, pathologic, immunologic, and therapeutic considerations. Ann Intern Med. 1978;89:660–76.
2. Cupps TR, Fauci AS. The vasculitides. In: Smith LM, ed. Major problems in internal medicine. Vol. 21. Philadelphia: WB Saunders, 1981:6–19.
3. Hunder GG, Arend WP, Block DA, *et al.* The American College of Rheumatology 1990 criteria for the classification of vasculitis. Arthritis Rheum. 1990;33:1065–7.
4. Bloch DA, Michel BA, Hunder GG, *et al.* The American College of Rheumatology 1990 criteria for the classification of vasculitis. Patients and methods. Arthritis Rheum. 1990;33:1068–73.
5. Moore PM, Cupps TR. Neurologic complications of vasculitis. Ann Neurol. 1983;14: 155–67.
6. Cohen SB, Hurd ER. Neurological complications of connective tissue and other 'collagen-vascular' diseases. Semin Arthritis Rheum. 1981;11:190–212.
7. Moore PM, Fauci AS. Neurologic manifestations of systemic vasculitis. A retrospective and prospective study of the clinicopathologic features and responses to therapy in 25 patients. Am J Med. 1981;71:517–24.
8. Sigal LH. The neurologic presentation of vasculitis and rheumatologic syndromes. Medicine. 1987;66:157–80.
9. Kissel JT, Slivka AP, Warmolts JR, *et al.* The clinical spectrum of necrotizing angiopathy of the peripheral nervous system. Ann Neurol. 1985;18:251–7.
10. Dyck PJ, Benstead TJ, Conn DL, *et al.* Nonsystemic vasculitic neuropathy. Brain. 1987;110:843–54.
11. Hawke SHB, Davies L, Pamphlett R, Guo Y-P, Pollard JD, McLeod JG. Vasculitic neuropathy. A clinical and pathological study. Brain. 1991;114:2175–90.
12. Smiley JD, Moore SE. Immune complex vasculitis: role of complement and IgG-Fc receptor functions. Am J Med Sci. 1989;298:267–77.
13. McDougal JS, McDuffie FC. Immune complexes in man: detection and clinical significance. Adv Clin Chem. 1985;24:1–60.
14. Cornacoff JB, Hebert LA, Smead WL, *et al.* Primate erythrocyte-immune complex-clearing mechanism. J Clin Invest. 1983;71:236–47.
15. Becherer JD, Alsenz J, Servic C, *et al.* Cell surface proteins reacting with activated complement components. Complement Inflamm. 1989;6:142–65.
16. Fauci AS. The vasculitic syndromes. In: Wilson JD, Braunwald E, Issellbacher KJ, *et al.* (eds). Harrison's Principles of Internal Medicine. New York: McGraw Hill, 1991;1456–63.
17. Savage COS, Ng YC. The aetiology and pathogenesis of major systemic vasculitides. Postgrad Med J. 1986;62:627–36.
18. Hogg N. The structure and function of Fc receptors. Immunol Today. 1988;9:185–7.
19. Moore PM. Immune mechanisms in the primary and secondary vasculitides. J Neurol Sci. 1989;93:129–45.
20. Kissel JT, Riethman JL, Omerza J, *et al.* Peripheral nerve vasculitis: immune characterization of the vascular lesions. Ann Neurol. 1989;25:291–7.
21. Wiedmer T, Esmon CT, Sims PJ. Complement proteins C5b-9 stimulate procoagulant activity through platelet prothrombinase. Blood. 1986;4:875–80.
22. Ryan US. The endothelial surface and responses to injury. Fed Proc. 1986;45:101–8.
23. Pangyres PK, Blumbergs PC, Leong AS-Y, Bourne AJ. Vasculitis of peripheral nerve and skeletal muscle: clinicopathological correlation and immunopathic mechanisms. J Neurol Sci. 1990;100:193–202.
24. Pober JS, Cotran RS. Cytokines and endothelial cell biology. Physiol Rev. 1990;70:427–51.

25. Cavender DE. Organ-specific and non-organ-specific lymphocyte receptors for vascular endothelium. J Invest Dermatol. 1990;94(suppl.):41–85.
26. Brasile L, Kremer JM, Clarke JL. Identification of an autoantibody to vascular endothelial cell-specific antigens in patients with systemic vasculitis. Am J Med. 1989;87:74–80.
27. Frampton G, Jayne DRW, Perry GJ *et al.* Autoantibodies to endothelial cells and neutrophil cytoplasmic antigens in systemic vasculitis. Clin Exp Immunol. 1990;82:227–32.
28. Editorial. Antibodies to endothelial cells. Lancet. 1991;337:649–50.
29. Gaskin G, Savage COS. Immune markers in vasculitis. Br J Hosp Med. 1991;46:104–6.
30. Ferraro G, Meroni PL, Tincani A *et al.* Anti-endothelial cell antibodies in patients with Wegener's granulomatosis and micropolyarteritis. Clin Exp Immunol. 1990;79:47–53.
31. Goeken JA. Antineutrophil cytoplasmic antibody – a useful serological marker for vasculitis. J Clin Immunol. 1991;11:161–74.
32. Parlevliet KJ, Henzen-Logmans SC, Oe PL, *et al.* Antibodies to components of neutrophil cytoplasm: a new diagnostic tool in patients with Wegener's granulomatosis and systemic vasculitis. Q J Med. 1988;66:55–63.
33. Egner W, Chapel HM. Titration of antibodies against neutrophil cytoplasmic antigens is useful in monitoring disease activity in systemic vasculitides. Clin Exp Immunol. 1990;82: 244–9.
34. Lai KN, Jayne DRW, Brownlee A, Lockwood CM. The specificity of anti-neutrophil cytoplasm antibodies in systemic vasculitides. Clin Exp Immunol. 1990;82:233–7.
35. Bleil L, Manger B, Winkler TH, *et al.* The role of antineutrophil cytoplasm antibodies, anticardiolipin antibodies, von Willebrand factor antigen, and fibronectin for the diagnosis of systemic vasculitis. J Rheumatol. 1991;18:1199–206.
36. Ewert BH, Jennette JC, Falk RJ. The pathogenic role of antineutrophil cytoplasmic autoantibodies. Am J Kidney Dis. 1991;18:188–95.
37. Nolle B, Specks U, Lüdemann J *et al.* Anticytoplasmic antibodies: their immunodiagnostic value in Wegener's granulomatosis. Ann Intern Med. 1989;111:28–40.
38. Panegyres PK, Faull RJ, Russ GR, Appleton SL, Wangel AG, Blumbergs PC. Endothelial cell activation in vasculitis of peripheral nerve and skeletal muscle. J Neurol Neurosurg Psychiatry. 1992;55:4–7.
39. Shuki H, Shimokama T, Watanabe T. Temporal arteritis. Cell composition and the possible pathogenetic role of cell-mediated immunity. Hum Pathol. 1989;20:1057–64.
40. Gephardt GN, Ahmad M, Tubbs RR. Pulmonary vasculitis (Wegener's granulomatosis). Immunohistochemical study of T and B cell markers. Am J Med. 1983;74:700–4.
41. Grau GE, Roux-Lombard P, Gysler C *et al.* Serum cytokine changes in systemic vasculitis. Immunology. 1989;68:196–8.
42. Grau GE, Piguet PF, Vassalli P, Lambert PH. Involvement of tumour necrosis factor and other cytokines in immune-mediated vascular pathology. Int Arch Allergy Appl Immunol. 1989;88:34–9.
43. Braquet P, Hosford D, Braquet M, *et al.* Role of cytokines and platelet-activating factor in microvascular immune injury. Int Arch Allergy Appl Immunol. 1989;88:88–100.
44. Mancardi GL, Cadoni A, Zicca A *et al.* HLA-DR Schwann cell reactivity in peripheral neuropathies of different origins. Neurology. 1988;38:848–51.
45. Nukada H, Dyck PJ. Acute ischemia causes axonal stasis, swelling, attenuation and secondary demyelination. Ann Neurol. 1987;22:311–18.
46. Said G, Laxroix-Ciaudo C, Fujimura H *et al.* The peripheral neuropathy of necrotizing arteritis: a clinicopathological study. Ann Neurol. 1988;23:461–5.
47. Fujimura H, Lacroix C, Said G. Vulnerability of nerve fibers to ischaemia. A quantitative light and electron microscope study. Brain. 1991;114:1929–42.
48. Dyck P, Conn DL, Okazaki H. Necrotizing angiopathic neuropathy: three-dimensional morphology of fiber degeneration related to sites of occluded vessels. Mayo Clin Proc. 1972;47:461–75.
49. Wees SJ, Sunwoo IN, Oh SJ. Sural nerve biopsy in systemic necrotizing vasculitis. Am J Med. 1981;71:525–32.
50. Harati Y, Niakan E. The clinical spectrum of inflammatory-angiopathic neuropathy. J Neurol Neurosurg Psychiatry. 1986;49:1313–16.
51. Bouche P, Leger JM, Travers MA *et al.* Peripheral neuropathy in systemic vasculitis: clinical and electrophysiologic study of 22 patients. Neurology. 1986;36:1598–602.

52. Olney RK. Neuropathies in connective tissue disease. Muscle Nerve. 1992;15:531–42.
53. Ropert A, Metral S. Conduction block in neuropathies with necrotizing vasculitis. Muscle Nerve. 1990;13:102–5.
54. Jamieson PW, Guiliani MJ, Martinez AJ. Necrotizing angiopathy presenting with multifocal conduction blocks. Neurology. 1991;41:442–4.
55. Kissel JT, Mendell JR. Vasculitic neuropathy. Neurol Clin. 1992;10:761–81.
56. Scott DGI. Classification and treatment of systemic vasculitis. Br J Rheumatol. 1988;27: 251–7.
57. Haynes BF, Allen NB, Fauci AS. Diagnostic and therapeutic approach to the patient with vasculitis. Med Clin North Am. 1986;70:355–68.
58. Axelrod L. Glucocorticoids. In: Kelley WN, Harris ED, Ruddy S *et al.*, editors. Textbook of Rheumatology. New York: WB Saunders, 1989;845–61.
59. Dalakas M. Pharmacologic concerns of corticosteroids in the treatment of patients with immune-related neuromuscular diseases. Neurol Clin. 1990;8:93–118.
60. Mankin HJ. Nontraumatic necrosis of bone (osteonecrosis). N Engl J Med. 1992;326: 1473–9.
61. Stillwell TJ, Benson RC, DeRemee RA *et al.* Cyclophosphamide-induced bladder toxicity in Wegener's granulomatosis. Arthritis Rheum. 1988;31:465–70.
62. Katz P, Fauci AS. Immunosuppressives and immunoadjuvants. In: Samter M, Talmage DW, Frank MM *et al.*, editors, Immunological Disease. Boston: Little Brown, 1988: 675–98.
63. Kisel JT, Levy RJ, Mendell JR, Griggs RC. Azathioprine toxicity in neuromuscular disease. Neurology. 1986;36:35–9.
64. Yazici H, Pazarli H, Barnes CG *et al.* A controlled trial of azathioprine in Behçet's syndrome. N Engl J Med. 1990;322:281–5.
65. Kissel JT, Rammohan KW. Pathogenesis and therapy of nervous system vasculitis. Clin Neuropharmacol. 1991;14:28–48.
66. Fauci AS, Katz P, Haynes BF, *et al.* Cyclophosphamide therapy of severe systemic necrotizing vasculitis. N Engl J Med. 1979;301:235–8.
67. Leib ES, Restivo C, Paulus HE. Immunosuppressive and corticosteroid therapy of polyarteritis nodosa. Am J Med. 1979;67:941–7.
68. Fauci AS, Haynes BF, Katz P *et al.* Wegener's granulomatosis: prospective and therapeutic experience with 85 patients for 21 years. Ann Intern Med. 1983;98:76–85.
69. Ballow M. Mechanisms of action of intravenous immunoglobulin therapy and potential use in autoimmune connective tissue diseases. Cancer. 1991;68:1430–6.
70. Schwartz SA. Intravenous immunoglobulin (IVIG) in the therapy of autoimmune disorders. J Clin Immunol. 1990;10:81–9.
71. Dwyer JM. Manipulating the immune system with immune globulin. N Engl J Med. 1992;326:107–16.
72. Jaynes DRW, Davies MJ, Fox CJV, Black CM, Lockwood CM. Treatment of systemic vasculitis with pooled intravenous immunoglobulin. Lancet. 1991;337:1137–9.
73. Conn DL. Update on systemic necrotizing vasculitis. Mayo Clin Proc. 1989;64:535–43.
74. Huse WD, Lakshmi S, Iverson SA *et al.* Generation of a large combinatorial library of the immunoglobulin repertoire in phage lambda. Science. 1989;246:1275–81.
75. Mathieson PW, Cobbold SP, Hale G *et al.* Monoclonal antibody therapy in systemic vasculitis. N Engl J Med. 1990;323:250–4.

5
Autoimmune-mediated models of peripheral nerve disease

C. LININGTON

Autoimmune responses to peripheral nerve autoantigens are believed to play a major role in the pathogenesis of several inflammatory demyelinating diseases of the peripheral nervous system (PNS). This concept is based on the observation that autoimmune responses to peripheral nerve tissue induce an experimental autoimmune neuritis (EAN) in laboratory animals that has clinical, electrophysiological and histopathological similarities to the Guillain–Barré syndrome (GBS)[1,2]. EAN is used extensively as an animal model for GBS, but modifications to the original immunization protocols also provide animal models for chronic idiopathic demyelinating polyneuropathy (CIDP)[3–6] and paraproteinaemia-associated neuropathies (PAN)[7].

The immunopathogenesis of each variant of EAN is mediated by a unique mixture of autoimmune responses and immune effector mechanisms. In each case disease is initiated by an autoimmune response directed against peripheral nerve myelin. The identity of the autoantigen concerned determines the clinical course, immunopathology and severity of the subsequent disease. The detailed analysis of the autoimmune response to PNS myelin has therefore provided a large body of data relevant to the immunopathogenesis and treatment of a range of human diseases. This chapter will review the present status of models of peripheral nerve disease mediated by myelin-specific immune responses and their clinical relevance. However, it should be pointed out that the myelin sheath is not the only potential target for autoimmune attack in the PNS. Immune responses directed against neuronal/axonal components are receiving increasing attention with respect to their potential involvement in motor neuron disease[8].

IMMUNE REACTIVITY WITHIN THE PERIPHERAL NERVOUS SYSTEM

The pathogenesis of any tissue-specific autoimmune disease is dependent upon the ability of the tissue to interact with components of the immune system. In autoantibody-mediated diseases, the induction of a pathological response is determined primarily by the accessibility of the autoantigen within the target tissue to the autoantibody in the peripheral blood. Tissue damage is then a consequence of either the activation of complement or cell-dependent immune effector mechanisms; alternatively the autoantibody may interfere directly with physiological function of the target cell. All three of these mechanisms operate, to varying extents, in myasthenia gravis, the classical example of a human autoantibody-mediated disease[9].

The situation in T cell-mediated autoimmune disease is, however, more complicated. The induction of a tissue-specific inflammatory response is dependent on the local, antigen-specific activation of a T cell by an antigen-presenting cell (APC). T cells do not respond directly to intact antigens, but to small peptides derived from the parent antigen by proteolysis[10]. Moreover full activation of the T cell via its specific T cell receptor (TcR) requires the peptide to be associated with an appropriate major histocompatibility complex (MHC) molecule on the surface of the APC[11]. In this respect, $CD4^+$ T cells have an absolute requirement for class II MHC gene products, whilst $CD8^+$ T cells require the peptide to be associated with a class I MHC gene product[11]. Activation of T cells, therefore, involves a trimolecular interaction involving MHC, peptide and TcR complex[10]. This interaction is central to the immunopathogenesis of all T cell-mediated diseases and is of great interest as a potential target for antigen specific immunotherapies[12,13].

In the peripheral nervous system the endothelial blood–nerve barrier limits the free exchange of both cells and proteins between the blood and nerve. Circulating antibody is therefore generally excluded from the body of the nerve, although some passive leakage of antibody may occur at the level of the nerve roots and root entry zones. In contrast to the passive and limited diffusion of antibody into the PNS, immunosurveillance of the nervous system by T cells is believed to be an active process. This hypothesis is based on studies of T cell traffic into the CNS[14–16], which indicate that only activated T cells can penetrate the endothelial blood–nerve barrier. The initial interaction of the activated T cell with the vascular surface of the endothelium is mediated by cell adhesion molecules and their appropriate ligands expressed on the interacting cell surfaces[17,18]. Thereafter, penetration into the parenchyma requires in addition the expression of appropriate enzymes enabling the T cell to degrade extracellular matrix and basement membrane[19,20]. These steps are independent of the antigen specificity of the T cell. However, once within the nerve the antigen-specific activation of the T cell by a resident APC is an absolute prerequisite for the generation of a local inflammatory response. Immunohistochemical studies have identified a small number of pericytes in the PNS that express high levels of class II MHC on their surface[21]. These cells probably represent the crucial population of APCs that present PNS autoantigens to T cells within the nerve *in vivo*.

In addition, Schwann cells can also be induced to express MHC antigens *in vitro* following exposure to interferon-γ[22,23]. These class II MHC$^+$ Schwann cells can then also act as fully competent APCs, processing and presenting both foreign and endogenous antigens to T cells *in vitro*[22–25]. In addition, MHC$^+$ Schwann cells can also act as targets for cytotoxic CD4$^+$ and CD8$^+$ T cells *in vitro*, although it is uncertain whether these interactions are of significance *in vivo*. Whatever the identity of the APC with which the T cell interacts *in vivo*, the immediate consequence will be the local production of cytokines, which will then orchestrate the subsequent inflammatory response in the nerve[26].

THE COMPOSITION AND MOLECULAR ORGANIZATION OF PERIPHERAL NERVE MYELIN

The pathophysiology of autoimmune-mediated diseases of peripheral nerve is dependent upon the function and structural organization of the antigenic target, which in EAN is the PNS myelin sheath. Myelin is synthesized in the PNS by Schwann cells, which enwrap a defined length of an axon with a spiral extension of their plasma membrane; this subsequently compacts to form multilammellar myelin. The compacted membrane remains in direct continuity with the Schwann cell plasma membrane which forms the outermost surface of the myelin sheath. The function of the sheath is to increase nerve conduction velocity, by inducing saltatory conduction between the nodes of Ranvier. Any disruption of the sheath and its interaction with the axon leads to a decrease in the conduction velocity and ultimately to conduction block (see references 27 and 28 for reviews of the ultrastructural organization and physiology of the PNS).

X-ray diffraction studies have revealed that the compacted myelin membrane consists of a regular repeating unit with a periodicity of 18 nm. During the formation of compact internodal myelin virtually all fluid is removed from the extracellular and cytoplasmic compartments leaving an extracellular water space about 5 nm wide, while the intracellular space between the apposing cytoplasmic surfaces is reduced to only 4 nm. This compacted membrane structure accounts for 90–95% of the entire length of the myelin sheath. However, at its proximal and distal ends the intracellular space expands to form tongues of cytoplasm, the paranodal loops, which contain mitochondria and other organelles. The paranodal cytoplasm is connected with the cytoplasm surrounding the Schwann cell nucleus by a network of cytoplasmic channels that extend both laterally and radially throughout the compact sheath. In view of the dimensions of the myelin sheath, which in large motor axons may reach a length of more than 1 mm and consist of 100 layers of compacted membrane, these channels probably play an important role in the metabolic maintenance of the myelin sheath.

With the exception of the outermost surface of the myelin sheath, exposure of the membrane to solutes in the extracellular fluid is limited by a complex series of intra-myelinic junctional complexes. These junctions limit the lateral diffusion of protein along the extracellular apposition of the compacted membrane. Another array of junctional complexes anchor the tips of the paranodal loops to the axonal surface. These myelin–axonal junctions also provide a barrier to the free diffusion of proteins and other large molecules into the periaxonal space which separates the inner surface of the myelin sheath from the axon[27]. Disruption of the paranodal junctions results in the retraction of the myelin sheath from the node of Ranvier (paranodal demyelination) and is an important contributory factor to the pathophysiology of inflammatory diseases of the PNS[28].

The composition of PNS myelin is remarkably simple. It is lipid rich and contains only three major protein components, the PO glycoprotein, myelin basic protein (MBP) and the P2 protein, all of which have some potential to induce EAN[29]. The protein composition of peripheral nerve myelin isolated from several species is illustrated in Figure 5.1. The major protein is the PO glycoprotein which accounts for at least 50% of the total membrane protein in all species studied. The PO protein is a member of the immunoglobulin gene superfamily and its amino acid sequence is compatible with it being a simple transmembrane glycoprotein[30]. Homotropic interactions involving the extracellular, IgG C2-like domain of PO are responsible for compaction of the extracellular apposition of myelin[31]. In addition, the cytoplasmic domain of PO is highly charged and may stabilize the cytoplasmic apposition of peripheral nerve myelin by ionic interactions with membrane lipids[30]. The PO glycoprotein is also one of the few proteins that is specifically expressed in peripheral but not in central nerve myelin. PO-specific antisera therefore provide an ideal immunohistochemical marker for myelinated PNS tissue.

This is not the case for MBP and P2 protein, which together account for a further 15–25% of the PNS myelin membrane protein. The relative concentrations of these proteins in the PNS varies widely between different species (Figure 5.1). In murine PNS myelin, less than 0.1% of the total membrane protein is P2 protein, whereas in bovine PNS myelin P2 protein accounts for almost 20% of the myelin proteins, whereas the converse is true for MBP, which is only a minor component of bovine PNS myelin. In addition neither protein should be considered as PNS specific: MBP is

Figure 5.1 (Opposite) The protein composition of peripheral nerve myelin isolated from several mammalian species. 50 μg samples of peripheral nerve (PNS) myelin protein were separated by SDS–polyacrylamide gel electrophoresis and either stained directly with Coomassie Blue (Panel A), or electroblotted onto cellulose nitrate membranes and P2 protein detected using either a polyclonal rabbit anti-P2 antisera (Panel B), or mouse monoclonal antibodies (mAb) generated using purified bovine P2 protein (Panels C and D). Lane 1, mouse; lane 2, rat; lane 3, human; lane 4, rabbit; lane 5, bovine. In contrast to the P0 glycoprotein, which is the major protein component of PNS myelin in all five species, the concentrations of P2 protein and MBP vary dramatically. The samples have been applied to the gel so that the concentration of MBP in PNS myelin is clearly seen to decrease from mouse to cow, whereas the concentration of P2 protein increases. This is also seen in panels B–D in which the P2 protein is specifically stained. Also note that the two mouse mAbs detect a heterogeneity in the mouse antibody response to bovine P2. The mAb used in C binds to an epitope common to the bovine, rabbit and human proteins, but which is absent in the murine protein. In contrast, the mAb used in D reacts with the P2 protein of all five species. (Illustration by courtesy of Dr T.V. Waehneldt)

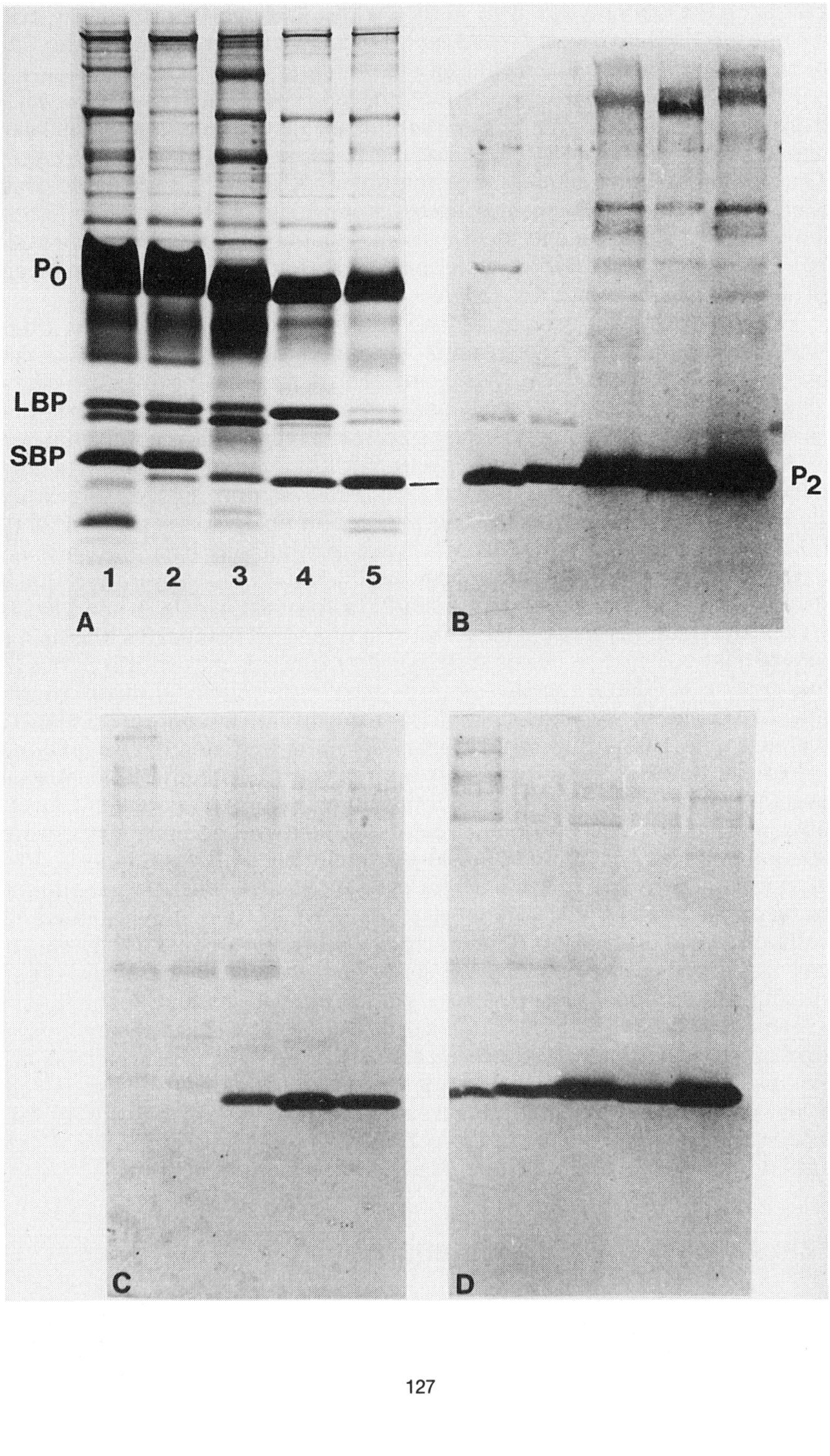
P0
LBP
SBP
1 2 3 4 5
A
B
P2
C
D

present in the CNS myelin of all species, while although P2 protein is specific for murine PNS myelin, it is also present at low concentrations in the CNS of many larger mammals, including man[32,33].

MBP is located at the cytoplasmic surface of compact CNS myelin, where it plays an important role in maintaining the structure of the cytoplasmic apposition[34,35]. However this is not the function of MBP in PNS myelin. This is demonstrated in the dysmyelinating mouse mutant, shiverer, in which exons 3–7 of the MBP gene are deleted, abolishing MBP expression in both the CNS and PNS. This results in a complete absence of CNS myelination, but has no effect on PNS myelination[36], where the structure of the myelin sheath is normal despite the absence of MBP[37].

The function of P2 protein in PNS myelin is also unknown. The amino acid sequence and three-dimensional structure of P2 protein indicates that it is a lipid-binding protein, suggesting that it may have some role related to lipid metabolism[38,39]. A large number of quantitatively minor proteins and glycoproteins, such as 2′,3′-CNPase and the myelin-associated glycoprotein (MAG), are also found in PNS myelin[29,35], but the immunology of these minor components is poorly understood. An exception is MAG which is of clinical interest as it is a target autoantigen in an IgM-associated PAN[40]. Like the PO glycoprotein, MAG is a transmembrane glycoprotein and a member of the immunoglobulin gene superfamily[41], but the localization of the two proteins is different. PO is found in compact myelin, while MAG is localized within membranes adjacent to cytoplasmic compartments, such as the periaxonal and outermost regions of the myelin sheath[42,43]. The localization of MAG, together with its large extracellular domain, suggest that MAG-specific antibodies could disrupt myelin–axonal interactions at the paranodes, in addition to triggering immune-mediated demyelination.

Protein, however, constitutes only a minor part of the myelin membrane: over 70% of the dry weight of PNS myelin is lipid. The major PNS myelin lipids are cholesterol, phospholipids and galactosyl ceramide (GC), whilst plasmalogens and sulphatide are also present in smaller amounts[29]. PNS myelin also contains low concentrations of several different gangliosides and complex glycolipids. These glycolipids have been implicated in the pathogenesis of GBS and antibody-mediated polyneuropathy[44,45]. Unfortunately, it is difficult to explore the pathological significance of glycolipid-specific autoantibody responses in animal models as they exhibit wide interspecies variability in their tissue distribution. Moreover, the epitopes of immunopathological importance are carbohydrate structures, which are also expressed by many glycoproteins. The classical example of this phenomenon is the presence of sulphated glucuronic acid epitopes on both MAG and myelin glycolipids, which are targeted by a pathogenic monoclonal IgM antibody response in a subgroup of patients with an IgM PAN[45–47].

EXPERIMENTAL ALLERGIC NEURITIS

Experimental allergic neuritis (EAN) was first described in rabbits following immunization with peripheral nerve tissue in adjuvant[1]. EAN is characterized clinically by an ascending paraparesis/paralysis which begins 10–14 days after immunization. The onset of clinical disease is associated with the appearance of a perivascular infiltrate of lymphocytes and macrophages in the PNS, together with endoneurial oedema, focal demyelination and varying degrees of axonal degeneration[2]. Macrophages are the major effector cell within the EAN lesion, they not only phagocytose myelin debris, but they also extend processes between the extracellular apposition of compact myelin lamellae and actively strip membrane from the sheath. However, the extent of demyelination in acute models of EAN is dependent on the intensity of the inflammatory response within the nerve. Immunization with low doses of immmunogen results in a mild clinical disease in which the lesions are concentrated in the nerve roots and axonal changes are minimal. High doses of immunogen induce a more severe disease in which the entire PNS is involved, often with a fatal outcome. In this case inflammation of the nerve is intense and axonal degeneration is the major pathological feature of the lesions. The consequence is a massive secondary loss of myelin, but the profound neurophysiological deficit that may persist for many weeks following disease onset in such EAN models is a direct consequence of axonal loss[26].

Modifications of the original immunization protocol for inducing EAN can induce both hyperacute and chronic progressive or relapsing forms of EAN in the appropriate strains of experimental animal. Chronic relapsing EAN (CREAN) can be induced in a number of animal species[3,5,48,49] and provides a useful model of CIDP in man. The histopathology of CREAN is similar to that of acute EAN, with the exception of 'onion bulb' formations of Schwann cells surrounding demyelinated axons. More recently CREAN was induced in Lewis rats either by treatment with cyclosporin[4] or the repetitive transfer of P2 protein-specific T cell lines[6].

The clinical and histopathological features common to both EAN and inflammatory demyelinating diseases of the PNS in man suggest that similar immune effector mechanisms are involved in both situations. EAN has therefore been used to identify PNS autoantigens and to investigate potential therapeutic strategies for the human diseases, GBS and CIDP. Identification of the immune effector mechanisms and autoantigens involved in EAN was initially complicated by the nature of the immunizing antigen. Immunization with either peripheral nerve tissue or PNS myelin triggers a complex autoimmune response involving both T and B cell responses to several PNS autoantigens. It was therefore not surprising that evidence has been obtained implicating both humoral and cellular mechanisms in the immunopathogenesis of the disease. The capacity of EAN serum to induce demyelination both *in vivo* following direct intraneural injection[50], and *in vitro* when added to myelinating organotypic cultures[51] suggested that humoral mechanisms were important in the pathogenesis of EAN. This concept was further supported by the observations that both complement depletion[52] and plasmapheresis[53] also significantly reduce the severity of EAN. However, neither clinical disease nor demyelination can be transferred to naïve recipients by systemic injection of EAN sera. Clinical EAN could only be successfully transferred to syngeneic recipients using lymphocytes obtained from animals immunized with PNS antigens[54,55].

This apparent dichotomy was resolved following the identification of the key autoantigens involved in the pathogenesis of EAN. Both cellular and humoral arms of the immune system are involved in the pathogenesis of EAN induced by active immunization with either PNS tissue or PNS myelin. However these responses are directed against different autoantigens and it is the T cell response that appears to be critical for disease induction. In actively induced EAN the autoaggressive T cell response is directed predominantly against the P2 and P0 proteins[56–59]. The first PNS myelin component to be identified as an autoantigen able to induce EAN was the P2 protein[56,57,60]. The passive transfer of EAN to naïve recipients by P2 protein-specific $CD4^+$ T cell lines in the rat provided the formal proof that EAN is a T cell-mediated autoimmune disease[61–63]. Subsequently, using the same techniques it was demonstrated that P0 protein-specific T cells can also adoptively transfer EAN in the Lewis rat[64]. As the passive transfer of activated T cells specific for either autoantigen induce the same constellation of histopathological and clinical signs as in acutely actively induced EAN[64,65], an autoaggressive $CD4^+$ T cell response is the minimal requirement to initiate EAN.

In contrast to the autoimmune T cell response, autoantibodies to PNS myelin only play a secondary role in the pathogenesis of the disease. Circulating autoantibodies which recognize epitopes exposed at the surface of the myelin sheath can initiate demyelination providing that the permeability of the blood–nerve barrier to serum proteins is enhanced. This was demonstrated in rats which received an intraneural injection of 5-hydroxytryptamine (5-HT) in addition to multiple intraperitoneal injections of serum obtained from rabbits with EAN[66]. The 5-HT induced localized mast cell degranulation, resulting in an increased permeability of the blood–nerve endothelium to antibody in the circulating blood and severe local demyelination. In EAN the local inflammatory response also increases the permeability of the blood–nerve barrier to serum proteins, antibody-dependent complement activation and cell-mediated cytotoxicity responses directed against the myelin sheath can then be expected to enhance demyelination and further amplify the inflammatory response[26].

T cell-mediated autoimmune responses to peripheral nerve myelin

All three major PNS myelin proteins, MBP, P2 protein and the P0 glycoprotein, can induce a T cell-mediated inflammatory response within the peripheral nervous system. However, T cell responses to MBP, which is present in both PNS and CNS myelin[29], induce experimental autoimmune encephalomyelitis (EAE), an inflammatory disease of the CNS in which there is very little peripheral nerve involvement[67]. The reason why the PNS is spared in MBP-induced EAE remains to be determined, but may be related to tissue specific differences in antigen processing and presentation. In the rat, only T cells specific for either the P2 protein or P0 glycoprotein initiate an autoimmune inflammatory response restricted to the PNS[64,65].

Intravenous injection of as few as 5×10^4 P2-specific T cells induces clinical signs of EAN in syngeneic recipients 4–5 days after cell transfer[61]. The pathology of T cell-mediated EAN is dependent on the number of T cells transferred: passive transfer of low numbers of T cells results in the formation of focal perivascular infiltrates of mononuclear cells, predominantly macrophages[65]. The intensity of this inflammatory response increases with the number of cells transferred, as does the extent of demyelination. However, as is also the case in actively induced EAN, demyelination is generally secondary to axonal degeneration, the major pathological feature of EAN induced by the passive transfer of large numbers of P2-specific T cells (Figure 5.2). A similar pathology with extensive axonal degeneration extending into the dorsal columns of the spinal cord is also observed in a chronic relapsing model of EAN induced by the repeated transfer of P2-specific T cells[6].

Active immunization with P0 glycoprotein in adjuvant induces EAN in the Lewis rat with a similar efficiency and time course as the P2 protein[59]. However, as discussed previously, P2 protein is a cytoplasmic component of PNS myelin and is therefore inaccessible to autoantibody. In contrast P0 is a transmembrane glycoprotein with a clearly defined extracellular domain, which can theoretically provide a target for a demyelinating autoantibody response. The successful adoptive transfer of EAN by P0-specific T cell lines[64], however, demonstrates that a common T cell-mediated effector mechanism predominates in the immunopathogenesis of P0-induced EAN.

The autoimmune T cell response to P2 and P0 has been analysed in great detail in the Lewis rat, and disease-inducing T cell epitopes have been identified for both proteins. The P2 protein contains a single immunodominant neuritogenic determinant located within residues 61–70 of the protein's amino acid sequence[68]. In contrast, the P0 glycoprotein contains two neuritogenic T cell epitopes[64]. One epitope is located within the amino acid residues 56–71 of the extracellular IgG-like domain of P0, whilst the second is encompassed by residues 180–199, located within the protein's cytoplasmic, carboxyl-terminal sequence. The immunological properties of these two domains of P0 are very different. The cytoplasmic epitope is immunodominant and EAN-inducing T cell lines specific for this epitope can be selected from the cell repertoire of rats immunized with PNS tissue. This is not the case for the epitope identified within the extracellular domain of P0 which is cryptic, no T cell response being observed following immunization with either PNS tissue, myelin or purified P0 protein[64]. These observations suggest that the proteolytic pathways involved in the processing of P0 protein differ between the PNS and peripheral immune system. This is important with respect to those clinical studies that attempt to identify autoaggressive T cell responses in the peripheral blood, as the autoantigen of interest may not be appropriately processed by the blood APC populations.

The observation that PNS myelin components with such different functions, localization and structure as the P0 glycoprotein and P2 protein initiate T cell-mediated EAN suggests that other neuritogenic PNS autoantigens will be identified. However, regardless of the autoantigen involved it appears that the primary immunopathogenic processes triggered by the autoaggressive T cell response will be the same.

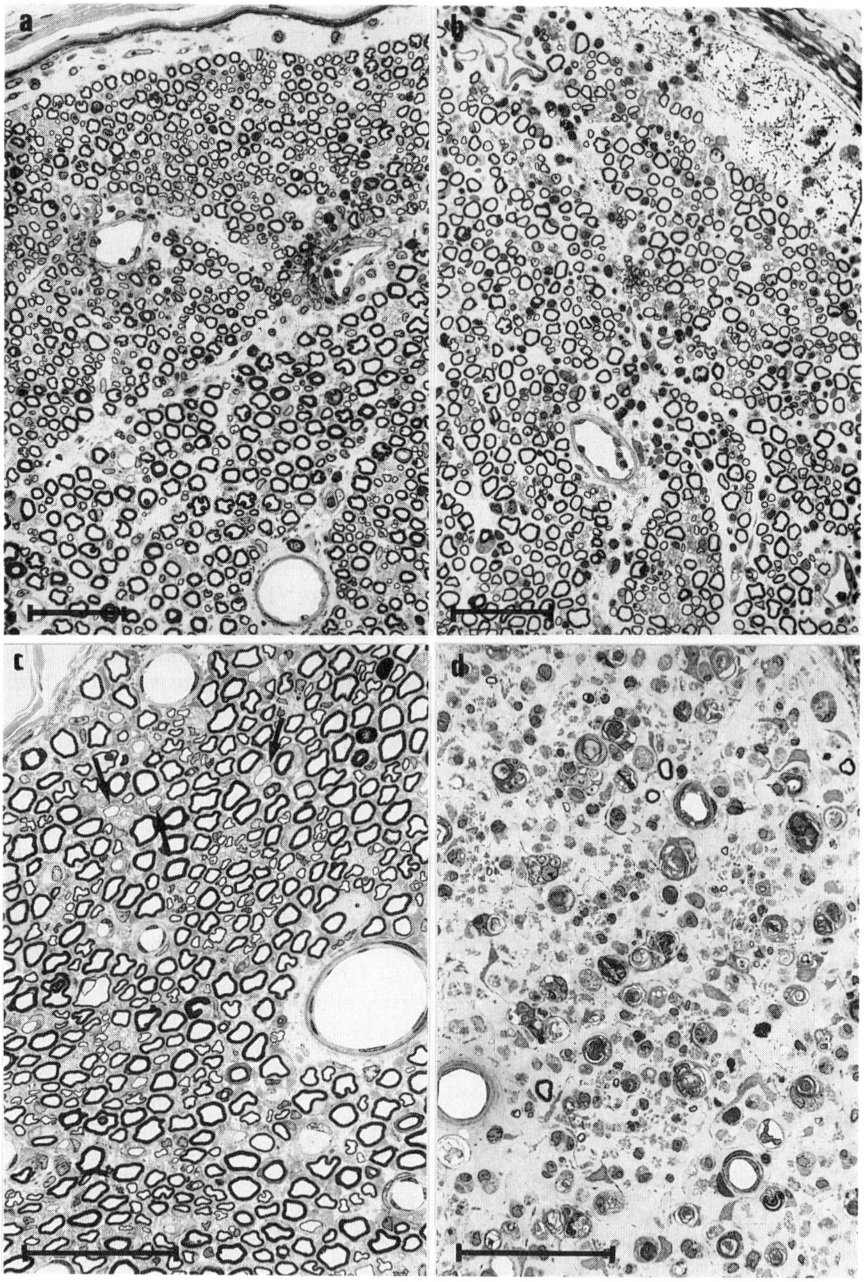
a
b
c
d

Immunopathogenesis of T cell-mediated autoimmune diseases of peripheral nerves

The precise sequence of immunological and cellular events involved in the course of the development of the EAN lesion is still uncertain. However, the initial step in T cell-mediated EAN is the migration of the autoantigen-specific $CD4^+$ T cell into the PNS followed by antigen-specific activation by a local class II MHC-positive APC. In the PNS a population of constitutively class II MHC^+ pericytes probably functions as resident APCs. The antigen-specific interaction of the T cell and APC triggers a variety of cellular functions in both cell types. This may lead to apoptosis of the T cell[69] but, more importantly, the local production of cytokines will be stimulated; this determines the course of the subsequent inflammatory response[26]. One of the earliest effects is on the vascular endothelium, where cytokines act to up-regulate the expression of cell adhesion molecules on the vascular surface of the endothelial cells[70]. Vascular permeability is also increased, both by the direct effects of cytokines on endothelial cells[71], and indirectly via cytokine-induced mast cell degranulation[72]. Although many cytokines are certainly involved in this early response, interferon-γ appears to play a central role, increasing vascular permeability, up-regulating the expression of MHC molecules and cell adhesion molecules on PNS elements and activating infiltrating monocytes. Thus systemic injection of recombinant interferon-γ enhances the clinical and histopathological signs of T cell-mediated EAN, while treatment with antibodies to interferon-γ can suppress disease development[73].

The first detectable pathological changes within the nerve that correspond to this cascade of molecular interactions are an increase in the permeability of the blood–nerve barrier to serum proteins and perivascular infiltration by small numbers of T cells[65,74]. This occurs about 72 h after intravenous injection of activated P2-specific T cells and precedes the onset of clinical disease by 12–24 h[75]. Subsequently there is a rapid migration and accumulation of inflammatory cells, predominantly macrophages, into the peripheral

Figure 5.2 (Opposite) The pathology and extent of tissue damage in P2 protein-specific T cell-mediated experimental allergic neuritis is dependent on the number of T cells transferred. Lewis rats were injected intravenously with either 10^5 (a,c) or 10^7 (b,d) freshly restimulated P2 protein-specific T cell lines and the pathological changes in the sciatic nerves examined 7 (a,b) and 19 days (c,d) later. Animals receiving the lower cell dose exhibited a complete loss of tail tone between 5 and 7 days post-T cell transfer, which had completely resolved by day 10. In contrast animals injected with 10^7 T cells exhibited complete hind limb paralysis by day 5. The clinical severity of the disease decreased after day 7, but severe hind limb paraparesis was still apparent on day 19. Seven days after T cell transfer both groups of animals had infiltrates of inflammatory cells associated with oedema throughout the peripheral nervous system (PNS). However these pathological changes were much more marked in the PNS of rats injected with 10^7 T cells. In these animals demyelination and debris containing macrophages can also be observed (b). Twelve days later the low dose group exhibited minimal pathological changes in the PNS, which included evidence of remyelination (c, arrows). In striking contrast the sciatic nerves of rats injected with 10^7 T cells are almost completely demyelinated and axonal degeneration is the most obvious pathological feature (d). Bar = 50 μm. (Reproduced from reference 130: with permission) nerve, accompanied by a large increase in endoneurial fluid pressure and endoneurial oedema[65,75,76]. These pathological changes within the nerve are associated with a progressive slowing of nerve conduction velocity, and eventually with complete conduction block 4–5 days after T cell transfer[75]. Electrophysiological changes initially reflect paranodal demyelination, but in severe inflammatory lesions conduction failure is due to the overwhelming destruction of axons.

In this subsequent stage of lesion development in T cell-mediated EAN, multiple effector mechanisms are involved, with macrophages playing a central role. Activated macrophages secrete a large number of cytotoxic agents including proteases, lipases, glycosidases, reactive oxygen metabolites and toxic cytokines[77–80]. These have detrimental effects on the blood–nerve barrier, further increasing oedema in the nerve[81], as well as compromising myelin stability and the functional integrity of the axon[26]. Depletion of the macrophage population or inhibition of their biological activities suppresses the development of clinical disease, demonstrating their importance in disease pathogenesis[82,83].

The interaction of macrophages with myelin in EAN lesions appears to be selective. They first attach to apparently normal myelin sheaths and then strip the myelin lamellae from the axon, finally phagocytosing and degrading the membrane (Figure 5.3a,b). The molecular basis of this interaction is unknown, but antibody-independent activation of the alternative complement pathway by the P0 protein on myelin or myelin debris[84] may deposit C3i on the membrane surface, providing a ligand for macrophage CR3 receptor.

Clearly, activation of the complement cascade will be enhanced in the presence of circulating antibody to the myelin surface. Antibody bound to myelin will induce an Fc-dependent ADCC response, whilst opsonization with antibody and complement products will enhance macrophage-mediated phagocytosis. Extrapolating from the pathological consequences of anti-myelin antibodies in T cell-mediated autoimmune CNS disease, the pathology of the lesion will be defined by the balance of T cell- and antibody-mediated effector mechanisms[85]. However, in the absence of an overwhelming antibody response to myelin, the key factors in lesion development are the T cell-mediated increases in the permeability of the blood–nerve barrier to serum proteins, and the recruitment and activation of macrophages in the lesion.

Figure 5.3 (Opposite) Interaction of monocytes with myelinating Schwann cells in P2 protein-specific T cell-mediated experimental allergic neuritis. (A) A mononuclear cell has invaded the myelin sheath and is located between the compact myelin and Schwann cell cytoplasm (asterisks). Although the myelin sheath appears normal at this point in time note that the monocyte is already starting to interact with both the outer surface of the myelin membrane and the contiguous membrane underlying the cytoplasmic compartment of the Schwann cell. (B) At a later stage many debris containing macrophages are seen. In this example several such cells have breached the basal lamina surrounding a demyelinating axon. It should be noted the interactions that target the macrophages to attack a particular Schwann cell/myelin sheath are not understood and it is a common observation that whilst one axon is undergoing active demyelination, other myelin sheaths in the vicinity remain apparently unaffected

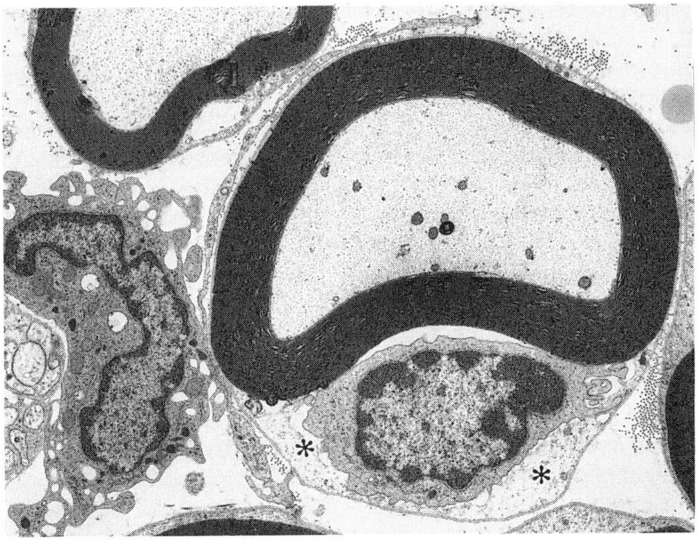

A

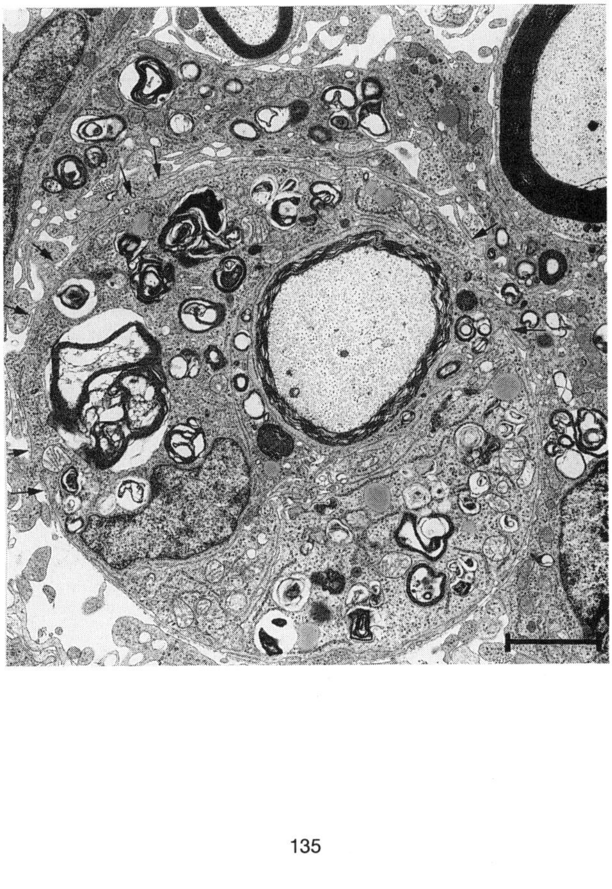

B

THERAPEUTIC STUDIES ON EAN

There are clearly several stages in the development of the EAN lesion that may be amenable to therapeutic intervention. Ideally, one would wish to specifically neutralize the autoaggressive T cell population without compromising general immunological competence[12,13,86]. The strategies investigated have attempted either to render the autoaggressive T cell response anergic/non-reactive, to eliminate the T cell population, or to prevent them from interacting with antigen-presenting cells within the target tissue.

T cell tolerance to the neuritogenic P2 protein can be induced by pretreating rats with soluble P2 in the absence of adjuvant[87,88]. However, the less invasive approach of establishing oral tolerance to PNS autoantigens has yet to be investigated in EAN, although it has proved successful in suppressing EAE[89,90]. In contrast, many studies have investigated the possibility of using monoclonal antibodies (mAb) to $CD4^+$ T cell differentiation antigens to eliminate or functionally inactivate the autoaggressive T cell response. Unfortunately, anti-CD4 mAb treatment is only really effective when the mAb is given prophylactically[91]. Moreover, an anti-CD5 mAb paradoxically enhanced the clinical severity of EAN and caused relapses[92]. A more promising approach uses an antibody recognizing the rat α/β TcR. This antibody not only inhibits the development of T cell-mediated EAN, but also reverses the development of actively induced EAN when given therapeutically[93]. It may also be possible to eliminate specifically the pathogenic T cell population in EAN using TcR V gene-specific mAbs[94,95]. It is, however, uncertain at present whether the neuritogenic T cell responses to P2 or P0 proteins preferentially use specific TcR Vβ genes[96], as has been reported in EAE[97–99]. Interestingly, attempts to prevent EAN induction by vaccination with attenuated P2-specific T cell lines have been unsuccessful[100] suggesting that multiple TcRs may be used in EAN.

In addition to these attempts to inhibit the induction of EAN at the level of the autoaggressive T cell response, a wide range of other less specific therapeutic strategies have been investigated. Intercellular adhesion molecule (ICAM) 1 plays an important role with respect to T cell–endothelial cell interactions, and anti-ICAM 1 antibody can inhibit EAN[101], as can interfering with mast cell degranulation[102] and treatment with cyclosporin A[103]. However, in view of the central role they play in the pathogenesis of the lesion, elimination of macrophages, or the pharmaceutical inhibition of their biological activities are at present the methods of choice with regards treatment of EAN[26,80,82,83,104].

Autoimmune B cell responses to peripheral nerve myelin

Although a myelin-specific autoimmune T cell response is the minimal requirement to induce EAN, it has already been stated that sera from animals with EAN induced using PNS tissue or myelin mediate demyelination, both *in vivo* and *in vitro*. In the rabbit, GC is the immunodominant myelin antigen responsible for this demyelinating autoantibody response[51,105]. Moreover GC-induced EAN in the rabbit appears to be the only paradigm for an autoantibody-mediated neuropathy[7]. A proportion of rabbits injected repeatedly with galactocerebroside and bovine serum albumin develop symptoms of a peripheral neuropathy[7], associated with a multifocal conduction block in the PNS[106] and a demyelinating PNS lesion which has some similarities with classically induced EAN[7]. The pathogenicity of the anti-GC antibody response in this model is not doubted, although anti-GC antibodies do not bind to micellar dispersions of the purified lipid, as the galactose headgroup is tightly hydrogen bonded in the plane of the hydrophobic/hydrophilic interface[107]. The addition of auxiliary lipids, cholesterol and phospholipid, disrupt GC–GC hydrogen bonds and increase the mobility of the galactose headgroup, allowing the antibody to bind to epitopes situated in that region[108]. The ability of anti-GC antibody to mediate demyelination *in vivo* and *in vitro* indicates that a similar conformation is adopted at the surface of the myelin membrane. *In vitro*, anti-GC antibody-mediated demyelination is complement dependent and rapid, whereas in the absence of complement the binding of the anti-GC antibody to the myelin surface induces myelin swelling, i.e. a separation of the extracellular apposition increasing the periodicity of the membrane by about 10–15 nm[109]. Similar changes also occur *in vivo* following injection of the antibody directly into the sciatic nerve[51]. Addition of complement initiates lysis of the Schwann cell and demyelination. In this model the perivascular cuffs of small lymphocytes which are characteristic of T cell-mediated EAN are absent during the early stages, suggesting that GC-induced EAN is primarily antibody-mediated[7].

However, a number of observations suggest that the situation may be more complicated and that, in addition to the GC-specific autoantibody response, other immune effector mechanisms are required to precipitate lesion formation. In particular, not all animals with high titre anti-GC IgG responses develop EAN[170] and remyelination can occur despite a sustained demyelinating, anti-GC antibody response in the serum[7,110,111]. Interestingly, a study of rabbits immunized with only complete Freund's adjuvant revealed the presence of subclinical inflammatory lesions in the PNS[112]. Lymphokines produced in these inflammatory foci may increase the permeability of the vascular endothelium, allowing an initial influx of antibody and complement to initiate demyelination. It should be noted that although GC is also a major component of CNS myelin, no CNS abnormalities have been reported in GC-induced EAN in the rabbit. Although GC-induced EAN is relatively poorly characterized the ability of a glycolipid to initiate a demyelinating neuropathy is of great clinical interest. Autoantibodies to epitopes on sulphated glucuronic acid-containing glycoconjugates, both lipid and protein[45–47], are the pathological entity responsible for a subset of IgM associated PANs. Immunization of rabbits with one of the target antigens, sulphoglucuronyl paragloboside, has also been reported to induce a mild clinical disease, associated with electrophysiological evidence of demyelination[45].

Autoimmune responses to peripheral nerve myelin in human disease

Although the pathology and clinical course of EAN has similarities with both GBS and CIDP, there is no conclusive evidence that these human diseases are autoimmune mediated. Peripheral T cell activation is certainly associated with disease activity in GBS, but the antigen specificity of this response is unknown[113]. Some patients with GBS also exhibit enhanced T cell responses to either P2 protein or the P0 glycoprotein (reviewed in reference 114). However, the data obtained are inconsistent. This may be due in part to differences in the groups of patients studied, the time elapsed between disease onset and sampling, and techniques used to detect the autoimmune T cell response. Studies of the dynamics of autoantigen-specific T cell responses in the blood of animals with EAN indicate that the time at which the patient's peripheral blood lymphocytes are tested is crucial. In EAN induced by active immunization with P2 protein, the P2-specific T cell response in the peripheral blood is transient and can be only detected shortly before and during disease onset[115]. This also appears to be true for GBS. Although a T cell response to P2 protein may be present at disease onset, it is often no longer detectable some days later[116].

It must also be remembered that the presence of an autoimmune T cell response to PNS myelin proteins in the peripheral blood is not restricted to patients with peripheral nerve disease, as P2-specific T cells are present in the immune repertoire of healthy controls[117]. Moreover, a pathogenic T cell response may be restricted to specific epitopes. The Lewis rat mounts a vigorous T cell response to two epitopes in the P2 protein. One epitope involving amino acids 58–72 can induce EAN, whilst the second, amino acids 14–27, is not neuritogenic[118]. The situation is likely to be far more complicated in man than in inbred strains of experimental animal. This has been clearly demonstrated with respect to the human T cell response to MBP, which can utilize multiple MHC class II haplotypes, T cell receptor V and Vβ elements and which recognizes a large number of epitopes[119,120].

Theoretically, it may be easier to detect and demonstrate the presence of a pathogenic autoantibody response. However the significance of autoantibodies and the identity of the putative target autoantigens in GBS and CIDP are still hotly debated. As in EAN, plasmapheresis has a considerable clinical benefit for some patients with GBS or CIDP, indicating that a humoral immune response may be involved in disease pathogenesis[121,122]. The demyelinating activity of immunoglobulins from patients with GBS and CIDP has also been demonstrated, both *in vitro*, following intraneural injection and *in vitro* using myelinating PNS cultures as targets (reviewed in references 114, 123). The titre of anti-peripheral nerve glycolipid antibodies decreases in parallel with clinical improvement in some patients with GBS[124]. Most of the complement fixing anti-myelin antibody response in GBS has been reported to be of the IgM isotype and directed against neutral glycolipids[44], but other investigators implicate autoantibodies recognizing gangliosides and other glycolipids in the pathogenesis of this disease[40,45–47,125–127].

A specific demyelinating autoantibody response has been identified in a large proportion of patients with an IgM PAN. In these patients, the pathogenic entity responsible for their neuropathy is a monoclonal IgM antibody recognizing a carbohydrate determinant expressed by MAG, PO and several acidic, sulphated glucuronyl glycolipids (SGGL) in PNS myelin[40,45–47,125–127]. Injection of this IgM into the cat PNS induced demyelination and associated electrophysiological abnormalities, confirming the pathogenicity of this antibody response[128]. However, the mode of action of the IgM within the patient's PNS is unclear: despite the high circulating concentration of the IgM and the demonstration of IgM and complement in the myelin sheath, complete loss of PNS myelin does not occur. Electron microscopic analysis reveals a selective widening of the extracellular apposition of the myelin sheath, associated with a penetration of IgM along the surface of the membrane. The absence of gross complement-mediated demyelination in these patients may reflect a high expression of CD59 on the surface of the Schwann cell (Lassmann, personal communication). CD59 is a membrane bound inhibitor of complement activation, the function of which is to protect cells from the consequences of autologous complement activation. The electrophysiological deficit in these patients may therefore reflect a decrease in conduction velocity, or conduction block mediated by the disruption of myelin/myelin and myelin/axonal interactions, in addition to myelination *per se*.

Other PAN patients express IgM with specificities other than SGGL or MAG. One group of patients has a monoclonal IgM response to chondroitin sulphate, a component of the extracellular matrix, rather than to PNS myelin. Although the pathogenicity of this IgM response still has to be confirmed it suggests that a peripheral neuropathy can be triggered by antibody-mediated reactions within the nerve that do not directly involve the myelin sheath. This is also the case in patients with lower motor neuron disease and various forms of motor neuropathy[129] in whom IgM autoantibodies to a Gal(β1-3)GalNAc epitope is implicated in the disease pathogenesis. Interestingly, this epitope is expressed by numerous glycoproteins and glycolipids and is widely distributed throughout the nervous system, including peripheral nerve myelin antigens, and other tissues. *In vivo*, however, the autoantibody only appears to be deposited at the nodes of Ranvier, suggesting that molecular microenvironment plays an important role in determining the accessibility of the epitope to antibody.

Analysis of the immunopathogenic mechanisms operating in EAN has identified a number of potential immune effector mechanisms and PNS autoantigens that may be involved in human disease. It is now vital to establish protocols that can differentiate between pathogenic and non-pathogenic autoimmune T cell responses in man. Only when this goal is achieved will it be possible to consider developing antigen-specific immunotherapies for GBS and CIDP. In the meantime it can only be hoped that novel pharmaceutical strategies will be developed for these diseases that will limit the inflammatory response and associated tissue damage in the PNS.

References

1. Waksman BH, Adams RD. Allergic neuritis. An experimental disease of rabbits induced by injection of peripheral nervous tissues and adjuvants. J Exp Med. 1955;102:213–35.
2. Lassmann H, Zimprich F, Rössler K, Vass K. Inflammation in the nervous system. Basic mechanisms and immunological concepts. Rev Neurol. 1991;147:763–81.
3. Adam AM, Atkinson PF, Hall SM, *et al.* Chronic experimental allergic neuritis in Lewis rats. Neuropathol Appl Neurobiol. 1989;15:249–56.
4. McCombe PA, van der Kreek SA, Pender MP. The effects of prophylactic cyclosporin A on experimental allergic neuritis (EAN) in the Lewis rat. Induction of relapsing EAN using low dose cyclosporin A. J Neuroimmunol. 1990;28:131–40.
5. Craggs RI, Brosnan JV, King RH, Thomas PK. Chronic relapsing experimental allergic neuritis in Lewis rats: effects of thymectomy and splenectomy. Acta Neuropathol. 1986;70: 22–7.
6. Lassmann H, Fierz W, Neuchrist C, Meyermann R. Chronic relapsing experimental allergic neuritis induced by repeated transfer of P2-protein reactive T cell lines. Brain. 1991;114: 429–42.
7. Saida T, Saida K, Dorfman SH, *et al.* Experimental allergic neuritis induced by sensitization with galactocerebroside. Science. 1979;204:1103–6.
8. Sadiq SA, Thomas FP, Kilidireas K, *et al.* The spectrum of neurologic disease associated with anti-GM1 antibodies. Neurology. 1990;40:1067.
9. Schönbeck S, Chrestel S, Hohlfeld R. Myasthenia gravis: Prototype of the antireceptor autoimmune diseases. Int Rev Neurobiol. 1990;32:175–200.
10. Ashwell JD, Schwartz RH. T-cell recognition of antigen and the Ia molecule as a ternary complex. Nature. 1986;320:176–9.
11. Berzofsky JA, Brett SJ, Streicher HZ, Takahashi H. Antigen processing for presentation to T lymphocytes: function, mechanisms and implications for the T cell response. Immunol Rev. 1989;106:5–31.
12. Adorini L, Barnaba V, Bona C, *et al.* New perspectives on immunointervention in autoimmune diseases. Immunol Today. 1990;11:383–6.
13. Wekerle H, Hohlfeld R. Principles of therapeutic approaches to autoimmunity. In: Rose NR, Mackay IR, editors. The Autoimmune Diseases, II. Orlando, FL: Academic Press, 1992:387–407.
14. Wekerle H, Linington C, Lassmann H, Meyermann R. Cellular immune reactivity within the CNS. Trends Neurosci. 1986;9:271–7.
15. Hickey WF, Hsu BL, Kimura H. T-lymphocyte entry into the central nervous system. J Neurosci Res. 1991;28:254–60.
16. Hickey WF. Migration of hematogenous cells through the blood–brain barrier and the initiation of CNS inflammation. Brain Pathol. 1991;1:97–105.
17. Butcher EC. Leukocyte-endothelial cell recognition: Three (or more) steps to specificity and diversity. Cell. 1992;67:1033–6.
18. Baron JL, Madri JA, Ruddle NL, Hashim G, Janeway CA. Surface expression of alpha4 integrin by CD4+ is required for their entry into brain parenchyma. J Exp Med. 1993;177:57–68.
19. Naparstek Y, Cohen IR, Fuks Z, Vlodavsky I. Activated T lymphocytes produce a matrix-degrading heparan sulfate endoglycosidase. Nature. 1984;310:241–4.
20. Willenborg DO, Parish CR, Cowden WB. Inhibition of experimental allergic encephalomyelitis by the α-glucosidase inhibitor castanospermine. J Neurol Sci. 1989;90:77–85.
21. Lassmann H, Vass K, Brunner C, Wisniewski HM. Peripheral nervous system lesions in experimental allergic encephalomyelitis. Ultrastructural distribution of T cells and Ia antigen. Acta Neuropathol. 1986;69:193–204.
22. Wekerle H, Schwab M, Linington C, Meyermann R. Antigen presentation in the peripheral nervous system: Schwann cells present endogenous autoantigens to lymphocytes. Eur J Immunol. 1986;16:1551–5.
23. Kingston AE, Bergsteinsdottir K, Jessen KR, Van der Meide PH, Colson MJ, Mirsky R. Schwann cells cocultured with stimulated T cells and antigen express major histocompatibility complex (MHC) class II determinants without interferon-gamma pretreatment:

Synergistic effects of interferon-gamma and tumor necrosis factor on MHC class II induction. Eur J Immunol. 1989;19:177–83.
24. Zhang Y, Porter S, Wekerle H. Schwann cells and myasthenia gravis: Preferential uptake of soluble and membrane bound AChR by normal and immortalized Schwann cells and immunogenic presentation to AChR-specific T line lymphocytes. Am J Pathol. 1990;136: 111–22.
25. Steinhoff U, Kaufmann SHE. Specific lysis by CD8+ T cells of Schwann cells expressing Mycobacterium leprae antigens. Eur J Immunol. 1988;18:969.
26. Hartung H-P, Heininger K, Schaefer B, *et al.* Immune mechanisms in inflammatory polyneuropathy. Ann NY Acad Sci. 1988;540:122–61.
27. Thomas PK, Ochoa J, Berthold C-H, Carlstedt T, Corneliuson. Microscopic anatomy of the peripheral nervous system. In: Dyck PJ, Thomas PK, Griffin JW, Low PA, Poduslo JF, editors. Peripheral Neuropathy. Philadelphia: W.B. Saunders, 1993:28–92.
28. Chiu SY. Channel function in mammalian axons and support cells. In: Dyck PJ, Thomas PK, Griffin JW, Low PA, Poduslo JF, editors. Peripheral Neuropathy. Philadelphia: W.B. Saunders, 1993:94–108.
29. Norton WT, Cammer W. In Morell P, editor. Myelin. New York: Plenum Press; 1984: 147–79.
30. Lemke G, Lamar E, Patterson J. Isolation and analysis of the gene encoding peripheral myelin protein zero. Neuron. 1988;1:73.
31. Filbin MT, Walsh FS, Trapp BD, Pizzey JA, Tennekoon GI. Role of myelin P0 protein as a homophilic adhesion molecule. Nature. 1990;344:871.
32. Deibler GE, Driscoll BF, Kies MW. Immunochemical and biochemical studies demonstrating the identity of a bovine spinal cord protein (SCP) and a basic protein of bovine peripheral nerve myelin (BF). J Neurochem. 1978;30:401.
33. Kadlubowski M, Hughes RAC, Gregson NA. Spontaneous and experimental neuritis and the distribution of the myelin protein P2 in the nervous system. J Neurochem. 1984;42:123–9.
34. Omlin FX, Webster H de F, Palkovitz GG, Cohen SR. Immunocytochemical localization of basic protein in major dense line regions of central and peripheral myelin. J Cell Biol. 1982;95:242.
35. Readhead C, Popko B, Takahashi N, *et al.* Expression of a myelin basic protein gene in transgenic shiverer mice: correction of the dysmyelinating phenotype. Cell. 1987;48:703.
36. Ganser AL, Kirschner PA. Myelin structure in the absence of basic protein in the shiverer mouse. In: Baumann N, editor. Neurological Mutations Affecting Myelination. INSERM Symposium No. 14. Amsterdam: Elsevier/North Holland, 1981:171.
37. Campagnoni AT, Macklin WB. Cellular and molecular aspects of myelin protein gene expression. Mol Neurobiol. 1988;2:41–89.
38. Jones TA, Bergfors T, Sedzik J, Unge T. The three-dimensional structure of P2 myelin protein. EMBO J. 1988;7:1597–604.
39. Sundelin J, Das SR, Eriksson U, *et al.* The primary structure of bovine cellular retinoic acid-binding protein. J Biol Chem. 1985;260:6494.
40. Latov N, Hays AP, Sherman WH. Peripheral neuropathy and anti-MAG antibodies. Crit Rev Neurobiol. 1988;3:301.
41. Salzer JL, Holmes WP, Colman DR. The amino acid sequences of the myelin-associated glycoproteins: homology to the immunoglobulin gene superfamily. J Cell Biol. 1987;104:957.
42. Trapp BD. Distribution of the myelin-associated glycoprotein during myelin compaction in quaking mouse peripheral nerve. J Cell Biol. 1988;107:675.
43. Trapp BD, Quarles RH, Suzuki K. Immunochemical studies of quaking mice support a role for the myelin-associated glycoprotein in forming and maintaining the periaxonal space and periaxonal cytoplasmic collar of myelinating Schwann cells. J Cell Biol. 1984;99:594.
44. Koski CL, Chou DHK, Jungalwala FB. Anti-peripheral nerve myelin antibodies in Guillain–Barré syndrome bind to a neutral glycolipid of peripheral myelin and cross-react with Forssman antigen. J Clin Res. 1989;84:280.
45. Yu RK, Ariga T, Kohriyama T, *et al.* Autoimmune mechanisms in peripheral neuropathies. Ann Neurol. 1990;27:S30.
46. Ariga T, Kohriyama T, Freddo L, *et al.* Characterization of sulfated glucuronic acid containing glycolipids reacting with IgM M-proteins in patients with neuropathy. J Biol Chem. 1987;262:848.

47. Burger D, Simon M, Perruisseau G, Steck AJ. The epitope(s) recognized by HNK-1 antibody and IgM paraprotein in neuropathy is present on several N-linked oligosaccharide structures on human P0 and myelin-associated glycoprotein. J Neurochem. 1990;54:1569.
48. Wisniewski HM, Brostoff SW, Carter H, Eylar EH. Recurrent experimental allergic polyganglioradiculoneuritis. Multiple demyelinating episodes in rhesus monkeys sensitized with rabbit sciatic nerve myelin. Arch Neurol. 1974;30:347–58.
49. Suzumura A, Sobue G, Sugimura K, Matsuoka Y, Sobue I. Chronic experimental allergic neuritis (EAN) in juvenile guinea pigs: Immunological comparison with acute EAN in adult guinea pigs. Acta Neurol Scand. 1985;71:364–72.
50. Saida T, Saida K, Silberberg DH, Brown MJ. Transfer of demyelination by intraneural injection of experimental allergic neuritis serum. Nature. 1978;272:639–41.
51. Saida T, Saida K, Silberberg DH. Demyelination produced by experimental allergic neuritis serum and antigalactocerebroside antiserum in CNS cultures. An ultrastructural study. Acta Neuropathol. 1979;48:19–25.
52. Feasby TE, Filbert JJ, Hahn AF, Neilson M. Complement depletion suppresses Lewis rat experimental allergic neuritis. Brain Res. 1987;419:97.
53. Harvey GK, Schindhelm K, Anthony JH, Pollard JD. Membrane plasma exchange in experimental allergic neuritis: Effect on antibody levels and clinical course. J Neurol Sci. 1988;88:207–18.
54. Aström K-E, Waksman BH. The passive transfer of experimental allergic encephalomyelitis and neuritis with living lymphoid cells. J Pathol Bacteriol. 1962;83:89–107.
55. Szymanska I, Ramvani J, Eylar EH. The passive transfer of severe allergic neuritis in the Lewis rat with lymphoid cells preincubated with P2 protein. Cell Immunol. 1983;82:422.
56. Brostoff SW, Burnett P, Lampert PW, Eylar EH. Isolation and characterization of the protein from sciatic nerve myelin responsible for allergic neuritis. Nature. 1972;235:210–12.
57. Kadlubowski M, Hughes RAC. Identification of the neuritogen for experimental allergic neuritis. Nature. 1979;277:140–1.
58. Carlo DJ, Karkhanis YD, Bailey PJ, Wisniewski HM, Brostoff SW. Experimental allergic neuritis: Evidence for involvement of the P0 and P2 proteins. Brain Res. 1975;88:580–4.
59. Milner P, Lovelidge CA, Taylor WA, Hughes RAC. P0 myelin protein produces experimental allergic neuritis in Lewis rats. J Neurol Sci. 1987;79:275–85.
60. Kadlubowski M, Hughes RAC, Gregson NA. Experimental allergic neuritis in the Lewis rat: characterization of the activity of peripheral myelin and its major basic protein, P2. Brain Res. 1980;184:439–54.
61. Linington C, Izumo S, Suzuki M, Uyemura K, Meyermann R, Wekerle H. A permanent rat T cell line that mediates experimental allergic neuritis in the Lewis rat *in vivo*. J Immunol. 1984;133:1946–50.
62. Rostami A, Burns J, Brown MJ, *et al.* Transfer of experimental allergic neuritis with P2-reactive T cell lines. Cell Immunol. 1985;91:354–61.
63. Linington C, Mann A, Izumo S, *et al.* Induction of experimental allergic neuritis in the BN rat: P2 protein specific T cells overcome resistance to actively induced disease. J Immunol. 1986;137:3826–31.
64. Linington C, Lassmann H, Ozawa K, Kosin S, Mongan L. Cell adhesion molecules of the immunoglobulin supergene family as tissue-specific autoantigens: Induction of experimental allergic neuritis (EAN) by P0 protein-specific T cell lines. Eur J Immunol. 1992;22:1813–17.
65. Izumo S, Linington C, Wekerle H, Meyermann R. Morphologic study of experimental allergic neuritis mediated by T cell line specific for bovine P2 protein in Lewis rats. Lab Invest. 1985;53:209–18.
66. Harvey GK, Pollard JD. Peripheral nervous system demyelination from systemic transfer of experimental allergic neuritis serum. J Neuroimmunol. 1992;41:159–66.
67. Lassmann H, Vass K, Brunner C, Wisniewski HM. Peripheral nervous system lesions in experimental allergic encephalomyelitis. Ultrastructural distribution of T cells and Ia antigen. Acta Neuropathol. 1986;69:193–204.
68. Olee T, Powers JM, Brostoff SW. A T cell epitope for experimental allergic neuritis. J Neuroimmunol. 1988;19:167–74.
69. Schmied M, Breitschopf H, Gold R, *et al.* Apoptosis of T lymphocytes in experimental autoimmune encephalomyelitis. Evidence for programmed cell death as a mechanism to control inflammation in the brain. Am J Pathol. 1993;143:446–52.

70. Shimizu Y, Newman W, Tanaka Y, Shaw S. Lymphocyte interactions with endothelial cells. Immunol Today. 1992;13:106–13.
71. Brett J, Gerlach H, Nawroth P, Steinberg S, Godman G, Stern DM. Tumor necrosis factor cachectin increases permeability of endothelial cell monolayers by a mechanism involving regulatory G-proteins. J Exp Med. 1989;169:1977–91.
72. Brosnan CF, Lyman WD, Tansey FA, Carter TH. Quantitation of mast cells in experimental allergic neuritis. J Neuropathol Exp Neurol. 1985;44:196–203.
73. Hartung H-P, Schäfer B, Van der Meide PH, Fierz W, Heininger K, Toyka KV. The role of interferon-gamma in the pathogenesis of experimental autoimmune disease of the peripheral nervous system. Ann Neurol. 1990;27:247–57.
74. Powell HC, Braheny SL, Myers RR, Rodriguez M, Lampert PW. Early changes in experimental allergic neuritis. Lab Invest. 1983;47:332–8.
75. Heininger K, Stoll G, Linington C, Toyka KV, Wekerle H. Conduction failure and nerve conduction slowing in experimental autoimune neuritis induced by P2-specific T cell lines. Ann Neurol. 1986;19:44–9.
76. Powell HC, Olee T, Brostoff SW, Mizisin AP. Comparative histology of experimental allergic neuritis induced with minimum length neuritogenic peptides by adoptive transfer with sensitized cells or direct sensitization. J Neuropathol Exp Neurol. 1991;50:658–74.
77. Brosnan CS, Selmaj K, Raine CS. Hypothesis: a role for tumor necrosis factor in immune-mediated demyelination and its relevance to multiple sclerosis. J Neuroimmunol. 1988;18: 87–94.
78. Hartung H-P, Schäfer B, Heininger K, Toyka KV. Suppression of experimental autoimmune neuritis by the oxygen radical scavengers superoxide dismutase and catalase. Ann Neurol. 1988;23:453–60.
79. Schabet M, Whitaker JN, Schott K, *et al.* The use of protease inhibitors in experimental allergic neuritis. J Neuroimmunol. 1991;31:265–72.
80. Hartung H-P, Schäfer B, Heininger K, Stoll G, Toyka KV. The role of macrophages and eicosanoids in the pathogenesis of experimental allergic neuritis. Brain. 1988;111:1039–59.
81. Claudio L, Kress Y, Factor J, Brosnan CF. Mechanisms of edema formation in experimental autoimmune encephalomyelitis. Am J Pathol. 1990;137:1033–45.
82. Heininger K, Schäfer B, Hartung H-P, Fierz W, Linington C, Toyka KV. The role of macrophages in experimental autoimmune neuritis induced by a P2-specific T-cell line. Ann Neurol. 1988;23:326–31.
83. Tansey FA, Brosnan CF. Protection against experimental allergic neuritis with silica quartz dust. J Neuroimmunol. 1983;3:169–79.
84. Koski CL, Vanguri P, Shin ML. Activation of the alternative pathway of complement by human peripheral nerve myelin. J Immunol. 1985;134:1810–14.
85. Lassmann H, Brunner C, Bradl M, Linington C. Experimental allergic encephalomyelitis: The balance between encephalitogenic T lymphocytes and demyelinating antibodies determines size and structure of demyelinated lesions. Acta Neuropathol. 1988;75:566–76.
86. Hohlfeld R. Neurological autoimmune disease and the trimolecular complex of T-lymphocytes. Ann Neurol. 1989;25:531–8.
87. Brosnan CF, Craggs RI, King RHM, Thomas PK. Attempts to suppress experimental allergic neuritis in the rat by pretreatment with antigen. Acta Neuropathol. 1984;64: 153–60.
88. Cunningham JM, Powers JM, Brostoff SW. Prevention of experimental allergic neuritis in the Lewis rat with bovine P2 protein. Brain Res. 1983;258:285–9.
89. Bitar D, Whitacre CC. Suppression of experimental autoimmune encephalomyelitis by the oral administration of myelin basic protein. Cell Immunol. 1988;112:364–70.
90. Higgins PJ, Weiner HL. Suppression of experimental autoimmune encephalomyelitis by oral administration of myelin basic protein and its fragments. J Immunol. 1988;140:440–5.
91. Holmdahl R, Olsson T, Moran T, Klareskog L. *In vivo* treatment of rats with monoclonal anti-T-cell antibodies. Immunohistochemical and functional analysis in normal rats and in experimental allergic neuritis. Scand J Immunol. 1985;22:257–69.
92. Strigard K, Larsson P, Holmdahl R, Klareskog L, Olsson T. *In vivo* monoclonal antibody treatment with OX19 (anti-rat CD5) causes relapse and terminates P2-induced immunospecific tolerance in experimental allergic neuritis. J Neuroimmunol. 1989;23:11–18.
93. Jung S, Krämer S, Schluesener HJ, Jünig T, Toyka KV, Hartung H-P. Prevention of

experimental autoimmune neuritis by an antibody against T cell receptor-α/β. J Immunol. 1992;148:3768–75.

94. Acha-Orbea H, Mitchell DJ, Timmermann L, *et al.* Limited heterogeneity of T cell receptors from T lymphocytes mediating autoimmune encephalomyelitis allows specific immune intervention. Cell. 1988;54:263–73.
95. Torres-Nagel NE, Gold DP, Hünig T. Identification of rat TCR Vβ8.2, 8.5, and 10 gene products by monoclonal antibodies. Immunogenetics. 1993;37:305–8.
96. Clark L, Heber-Katz E, Rostami A. Shared T-cell receptor gene usage in experimental allergic neuritis and encephalomyelitis. Ann Neurol. 1992;31:587–92.
97. Urban JL, Kumar V, Kono DH, *et al.* Restricted use of T cell receptor V genes in murine autoimmune encephalomyelitis raises possibilities for antibody therapy. Cell. 1992;54: 577–92.
98. Chluba J, Steeg C, Becker A, Wekerle H, Epplen JT. T cell receptor β chain usage in myelin basic protein-specific rat T lymphocytes. Eur J Immunol. 1989;19:279–84.
99. Burns FR, Li X, Shen H, *et al.* Both rat and mouse T cell receptors specific for the encephalitogenic determinant of myelin basic protein use similar Vα and Vβ chain genes even though the major histocompatibility complex and encephalitogenic determinants being recognized are different. J Exp Med. 1989;169:27–40.
100. Jung S, Schluesener HJ, Toyka KV, Hartung H-P. T cell vaccination does not induce resistance to experimental autoimmune neuritis. J Neuroimmunol. 1991;35:1–11.
101. Archelos J, Mäurer M, Jung S, Toyka KV, Hartung HP. Suppression of experimental allergic neuritis by an antibody to the intercellular adhesion molecule ICAM-1. Brain. 1993;116:1043–58.
102. Brosnan CF, Tansey FA. Delayed onset of experimental allergic neuritis in rats treated with reserpine. J Neuropathol Exp Neurol. 1984;43:84–93.
103. King RHM, Craggs RI, Gross MLP, Tompkins C, Thomas PK. Suppression of experimental allergic neuritis by cyclosporin A. Acta Neuropathol. 1983;59:262–8.
104. Craggs RI, King RHM, Thomas PK. The effect of suppression of macrophage activity on the development of experimental allergic neuritis. Acta Neuropathol. 1984;62:316–23.
105. Raine CS, Johnson AB, Marcus DM, Suzuki A, Bornstein MB. Demyelination *in vitro*. Absorption studies demonstrate that galactocerebroside is a major target. J Neurol Sci. 1981;52:117–31.
106. Niedieck B, Kuwert E, Palacios O, Crees O. Immunochemical and serological studies on the lipid hapten of myelin with relationship to experimental allergic encephalomyelitis (EAE). Ann NY Acad Sci. 1965;122:266–76.
107. Pascher I, Sundell S. Molecular arrangements in sphingolipids: the crystal structure of cerebroside. Chem Phys Lipids. 1977;20:175.
108. Raine CS, Bornstein MB. Experimental allergic neuritis. Ultrastructure of serum-induced myelin aberrations in peripheral nervous system cultures. Lab Invest. 1979;40:423–32.
109. Sumner AJ, Saida K, Saida T, Silberberg DH, Asbury AK. Acute conduction block associated with experimental antiserum-mediated demyelination of peripheral nerve. Ann Neurol. 1982;11:469.
110. Stoll G, Schwendemann G, Heininger K, *et al.* Relationship of clinical, serological, morphological, and electrophysiological findings in galactocerebroside-induced experimental allergic neuritis. J Neurol Neurosurg Psychiatry. 1986;49:258.
111. Stoll G, Reiners K, Schwendemann G, *et al.* Normal myelination of regenerating peripheral nerve sprouts despite circulating antibodies to galactocerebroside in rabbits. Ann Neurol. 1986;19:189.
112. Powell HC, Mizisin AP, Wiley CA, *et al.* Relationship of adjuvants and swine influenza vaccine to experimental neuropathy in rabbits. Acta Neuropathol. 1987;73:12–17.
113. Hartung HP, Hughes RAC, Taylor WA, Heininger K, Reiners K, Toyka KV. T cell activation in Guillain–Barré syndrome and in MS: Elevated serum levels of soluble IL-2 receptors. Neurology. 1990;40:215–18.
114. Linington C, Brostoff SW. Peripheral nerve antigens. In: Dyck PJ, Thomas PK, Griffin JW, Low PA, Poduslo JF, editors. Peripheral Neuropathy. Philadelphia: W.B. Saunders. 1992:410.
115. Taylor WA, Hughes RAC. Responsiveness to P2 of blood- and cauda equina-derived lymphocytes in experimental allergic neuritis in the Lewis rat: preliminary characterization

of a P2-specific cauda equina-derived T cell line. J Neuroimmunol. 1988;19:279.
116. Khalili-Shirazi A, Hughes RAC, Brostoff SW, Linington C, Gregson N. T cell responses to myelin proteins in Guillain–Barrè syndrome. J Neurol Sci. 1992;111:200–3.
117. Burns J, Krasner LJ, Rostami A, Pleasure D. Isolation of P2 protein-reactive T-cell lines from human blood. Ann Neurol. 1986;19:391.
118. Olee T, Weise M, Powers J, Brostoff SW. A T cell epitope for experimental allergic neuritis is an amphipathic alpha-helical structure. J Neuroimmunol. 1989;21:235.
119. Giegerich G, Pette M, Meinl E, Epplen JT, Wekerle H, Hinkkanen A. Diversity of T cell receptor α and β chain genes expressed by human T cells specific for similar myelin basic protein peptide/major histocompatibility complexes. Eur J Immunol. 1992;22:753–8.
120. Wekerle H. Myelin-specific, autoaggressive T cell clones in the normal immune repertoire: Their nature and their regulation. Int Rev Immunol. 1992;9:231–41.
121. Tharakan J, Ferner RE, Hughes RAC, *et al.* Plasma exchange for Guillain–Barré syndrome. J Roy Soc Med. 1989;82:458.
122. Dyck PJ, Daube J, O'Brian PC, *et al.* Plasma exchange in chronic inflammatory demyelinating polyradiculoneuropathy. N Engl J Med. 1986;314:461.
123. Hartung HP, Stoll G, Toyka KV. Immune reactions in the peripheral nervous system. In: Dyck PJ, Thomas PK, Griffin JW, Low PA, Poduslo JF, editors. Peripheral Neuropathy, Philadelphia: W.B. Saunders, 1992:431.
124. Koski CL, Gratz E, Sutherland J, Mayer RF. Clinical correlation with anti-peripheral nerve myelin antibodies in Guillain–Barré syndrome. Ann Neurol. 1986;19:573.
125. Ilyas AA, Willison HJ, Quarles RH, *et al.* Serum antibodies to gangliosides in Guillain–Barré syndrome. Ann Neurol. 1988;23:440.
126. Latov N, Gross RB, Kastelman J, *et al.* Complement-fixing antiperipheral nerve myelin antibodies in patients with inflammatory polyneuritis and with polyneuropathy and paraproteinemia. Neurology. 1981;31:1530.
127. Quarles RH, Ilyas AA, Willison HJ. Antibodies to glycolipids in demyelinating diseases of the human peripheral nervous system. Chem Phys Lipids. 1984;42:235.
128. Trojaborg W, Galassi G, Hays AP, *et al.* Electrophysiological study of experimental demyelination induced by serum of patients with IgM M proteins and neuropathy. Neurology. 1989;39:1581.
129. Latov N. Neuropathy and anti-GM1 antibodies. Ann Neurol. 1990;27:S41.
130. Linington C, Wekerle H, Meyermann R. T lymphocyte autoimmunity in peripheral nervous system autoimmune disease. Agents Actions. 1986;19:256–65.

6
Immunology of the motor nerve terminal

A. VINCENT and J. NEWSOM-DAVIS

INTRODUCTION

The approaches that have so successfully established the autoimmune basis of myasthenia gravis (MG; see Chapter 7, this volume) have lent themselves to the study of other putative autoimmune disorders. Development of an animal model of MG by immunization against purified acetylcholine receptors (AChR) from the electric ray, and identification of the reduced numbers of muscle AChRs using the specific neurotoxin [^{125}I]α-bungarotoxin (α-BuTx), predated the observations that confirmed the role of antibodies in this disease, i.e. the detection of anti-AChR antibodies, the clinical response to plasma exchange, and passive transfer of MG to experimental animals. By contrast, in the Lambert–Eaton myasthenic syndrome (LEMS) and acquired neuromyotonia (Isaacs' syndrome, NMT) the autoimmune nature of the human disorder was evident before the target antigens could be identified. It is now thought that the target in LEMS is the voltage-gated calcium channel (VGCC), and in NMT may be the voltage-gated potassium channel (VGKC). When the relevant human channels have been better characterized, and their genes cloned and expressed, it should be possible to identify directly the target(s) of the autoantibodies, and to establish experimental disease in animals. The success of the experimental approaches described in this review has begun to influence treatment of these conditions, and further investigation into their immune aetiologies may lead eventually to specific immunotherapy.

LEMS

LEMS, first characterized electrophysiologically by Lambert *et al.*[1], is one of a group of disorders that can arise as a 'remote effect' of a neoplasm.

Table 6.1 Paraneoplastic neurological disorders

Site	*Disorder*	*Neoplasm*	*Target of antibodies*
Cerebrum	Limbic encephalitis	Small cell lung	Neurones
Brain stem	Opsoclonus–myoclonus	Neuroblastoma, gynaecological	Neuronal nuclei
	Encephalitis	Small cell lung	Neurones
Cerebellum	Subacute degeneration	Ovarian, lymphoma, small cell lung	Purkinje cells
Retina	Retinitis	Small cell lung	Retinal cells
Spinal cord	Myelopathy	Small cell lung	Spinal cord protein
Peripheral nerve	Subacute sensory neuropathy	Small cell lung	Neuronal nuclei of dorsal root ganglia
	Neuromyotonia	Lung cancer, thymoma	Peripheral nerve, ? K^+ channels
Neuromuscular junction	LEMS	Small cell lung	Presynaptic Ca^{2+} channels
	Myasthenia gravis	Thymoma	Postsynaptic acetylcholine receptors

These paraneoplastic disorders can involve the cerebrum, brainstem, retina, cerebellum, dorsal root ganglia and spinal cord as well as peripheral nerve and the neuromuscular junction (for review, see reference 2). Table 6.1 lists the principal diseases and their associated neoplasms. It should be noted that some of the conditions can occur in the absence of an associated tumour (e.g. opsoclonus–myoclonus, LEMS, NMT, MG). As the table shows, the range of associated neoplasms is small. Small cell lung cancer (SCLC) is the most common, perhaps because it is probably of neuroectodermal origin and may therefore share cross-reactive determinants with the nervous system[3].

Incidence

A prospective survey of 150 patients with SCLC[4], taken together with other retrospective studies, suggests a LEMS incidence of 3% (and an overall incidence in the general population of about 4 per million). LEMS was the most common paraneoplastic syndrome encountered in this series. However, not all patients with LEMS have an associated cancer. In the series of 50 patients reported by O'Neill *et al.*[5], about one-third had no detectable cancer, and most of these were non-smokers (i.e. low risk for SCLC) with a clinical history of LEMS of longer than 5 years.

Clinical features

The syndrome is characterized by proximal muscle weakness, most marked in the lower limbs, and autonomic dysfunction, including dry mouth, sexual impotence and constipation. Ptosis and bulbar symptoms may also occur,

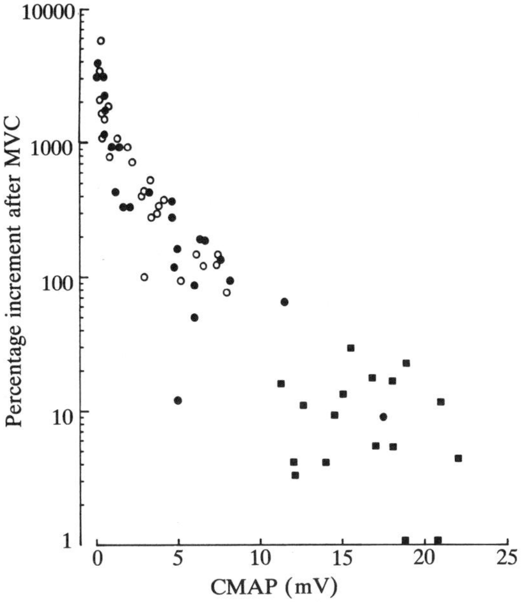

Figure 6.1 Relationship between increment in the compound muscle action potential (CMAP) after maximal voluntary contraction (MVC) and initial CMAP amplitude. Electrophysiological findings in LEMS patients (●, cancer detected; ○, no cancer detected). Filled squares are values from control subjects, the lowest of which was 8.4 mV. Only two LEMS patients had values within the control range. The percentage increment after maximal voluntary contraction for 10–15 s, MVC, shown on a logarithmic scale, shows an inverse correlation with the compound muscle action potential (CMAP) amplitude. Taken with permission from reference 5

and there may be respiratory involvement. On examination, muscle weakness is typically accompanied by augmentation of strength and recovery of reflexes during the first few seconds of sustained maximum effort (in contrast to MG), and the initially depressed tendon reflexes often show post-tetanic potentiation. A complete list of symptoms and signs is given in reference 5.

The edrophonium ('Tensilon') test may be positive, as it is in MG, and there may be increased jitter on single-fibre EMG. The definitive diagnosis is made by demonstrating a reduced compound muscle action potential amplitude in a resting muscle that increases more than 2-fold following 15 s maximal voluntary contraction of the muscle (see Figure 6.1). LEMS has to be distinguished from MG, from the congenital myasthenias, and from poisoning by *Botulinum* toxin (BoTx). Anti-AChR antibodies are usually detectable in MG, and reflexes are typically brisk. Most of the congenital myasthenic syndromes begin in infancy or early childhood (for a review see reference 6). BoTx poisoning could be difficult to exclude, although it is rare. The presence of anti-VGCC antibodies would confirm LEMS, but raised titres are only clearly detected in a proportion of patients using the current method with $[^{125}I]\omega$-conotoxin from *Conus geographus*.

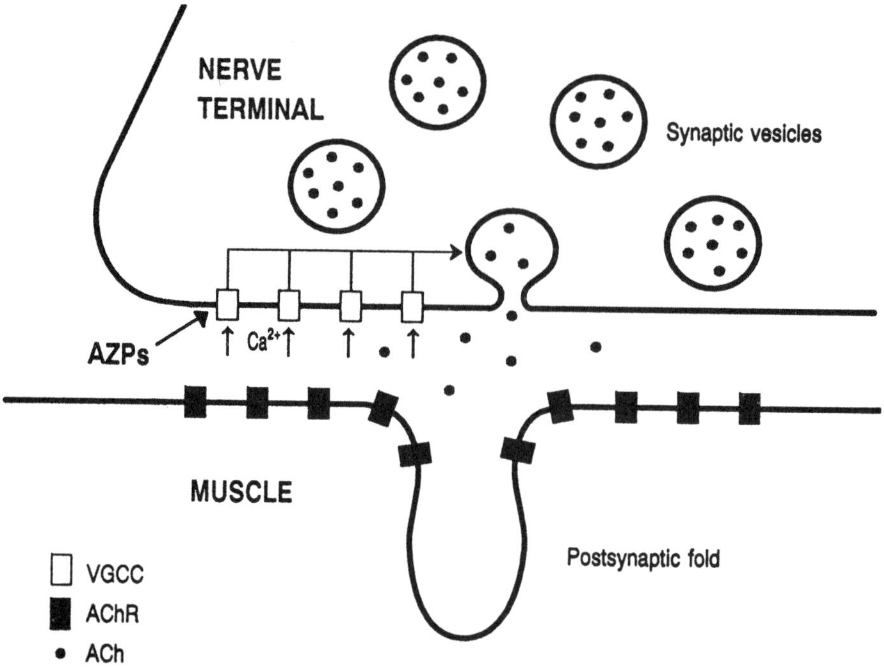

Figure 6.2 Ca^{2+} dependency of ACh release at the neuromuscular junction. Schematic diagram showing position of active zone particles (AZP), thought to be the voltage-gated calcium channels (VGCC), in the 'active zones' on the nerve terminal membrane opposite the postsynaptic folds. Release of ACh takes place when nerve terminal depolarization causes the VGCCs to open allowing a rapid local increase in Ca^{2+} concentration. This leads to the fusion of the synaptic vesicles with the nerve terminal, and ACh release. The intraterminal mechanisms are unknown

Experimental studies on LEMS muscle

Electrophysiology of neuromuscular transmission in LEMS

Neuromuscular transmission depends on the release of acetylcholine (ACh) from the nerve terminal and its interaction with postsynaptic AChRs (Figure 6.2; for reviews see reference 7). ACh is released in packets, or quanta, each of which contains 5000–10 000 molecules of the neurotransmitter. It diffuses across the synaptic cleft, binds to the AChRs and causes opening of the AChR-associated ion channel, allowing cations (mainly Na^{+}) to enter the muscle fibre. When individual packets of ACh are released the resulting depolarization (the miniature endplate potential, MEPP) can be recorded by a microelectrode inserted into the muscle fibre close to the endplate.

When a nerve impulse invades the nerve terminal, the action potential causes the opening of VGCC, which allows the rapid local influx of Ca^{2+} ions into the cytoplasm. Ca^{2+} acts on a presynaptic mechanism to cause the almost simultaneous release of about 50 packets of ACh. The combined effect of all the ACh results in the endplate potential (EPP) which, in normal muscle, triggers a muscle action potential (MAP) and muscle contraction. The quantal content (*m*), that is the number of packets of ACh released per impulse, can be measured by various methods (see reference 7). The use of μ-conotoxin, a neurotoxin that predominantly blocks the muscle action potential[8], leaving the nerve action potential intact, makes it possible to record MEPPs and EPPs from the same muscle fibres in the absence of muscle contraction. *m* can then be calculated from the ratio between the MEPP and EPP after the appropriate corrections.

In LEMS the number of quanta released is substantially reduced, and the EPP may be too small to trigger the muscle action potential[9]. During repetitive nerve stimulation the size of the EPP increases with restoration of muscle fibre activation. The abnormality of quantal release, overcome by repetitive stimulation, can be reproduced by treating normal human muscle with high levels of Mg^{2+}. Mg^{2+} competitively blocks the entry of Ca^{2+} into the nerve terminal, and thus these observations are consistent with a defect in Ca^{2+} influx underlying the abnormality of quantal release in LEMS[9]. The recovery of muscle contraction during repetitive stimulation is thought to be due to build-up of Ca^{2+} within nerve termini.

These conclusions were reinforced by the studies of Engel and his associates[10] who applied freeze-fracture electron microscopy to muscle biopsies from LEMS patients. They found that the active zone particles (AZP), thought to represent the transmembrane VGCC, were reduced in number and lacked their usual orderly arrangement in double parallel arrays (Figure 6.3). Biochemical measurements made in muscle biopsies from LEMS patients showed that ACh release was reduced even though the storage and synthesis of the neurotransmitter were normal[11].

Autoimmune basis for LEMS

Several observations suggested an autoimmune basis. Organ-specific autoantibodies and an increased incidence of other autoimmune disorders are frequently found[12,13]. Substantial clinical improvement, sustained for several weeks, followed plasma exchange, implying the existence of a humoral factor[14]. This improvement could be maintained by administration of the immunosuppressive drugs prednisolone and/or azathioprine[15]. The association of LEMS with an increased incidence of the HLA haplotype A1, B8, DR3, and with certain immunoglobulin heavy chain markers also indicated the importance of immunogenetic factors in susceptibility[16].

In order to investigate the presence of a causative antibody, mice were injected intraperitoneally with IgG prepared from LEMS plasma, at a dose of 10 mg/day, for periods ranging from 2 to 80 days[14,17,18]. Although the animals did not generally show clinical weakness (probably because the safety factor for neuromuscular transmission is high in rodents), there was a significant reduction in *m* measured at diaphragm endplates *in vitro*[17,18]. This made it possible to investigate in greater detail the underlying basis for the defect in quantal release.

First, the reduction in *m* was not due to an effect on the propagation of

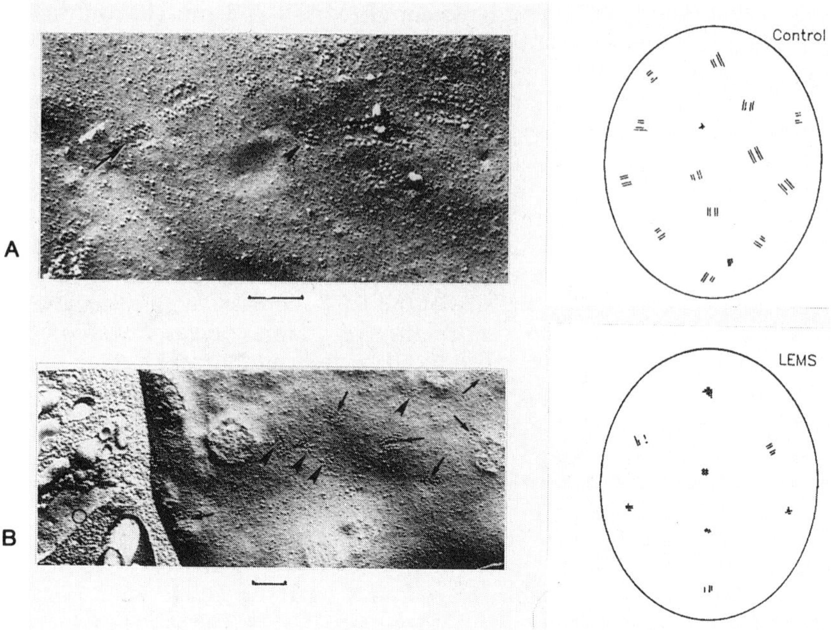

Figure 6.3 Active zones in LEMS. Active zones in the presynaptic membrane face of nerve terminals from human muscle biopsies. **A**. Healthy control muscle: active zones consist of double parallel rows of AZPs (arrows) and a few smaller parallel rows or clusters (arrow-heads). **B**. LEMS muscle: there are fewer parallel rows, and more clusters of AZPs. However, the total number of particles in rows or clusters is reduced overall. The schematic reconstructions are based on the mean results of nine patients and 14 controls. Scale 1 μm. Taken with permission from reference 10. Courtesy of Dr A Engel

the action potential into the nerve terminal, since both MEPP frequency and ACh release were reduced in LEMS IgG-treated diaphragms when release was stimulated directly by incubating the muscle in high concentrations of K^{+} [19]. Neither was the effect at the intraterminal site of Ca^{2+} activation of the release mechanism; the Ca^{2+}-independent K^{+}-stimulated increase in MEPP frequency which occurs in Ca^{2+}-free solutions, or in the presence of the pharmacological agents ouabain and lithium, was not affected by LEMS IgG[20]. These observations indicate that release which is not dependent on Ca^{2+} entry is normal. On the other hand there was clearly a reduced sensitivity to external Ca^{2+}. The quantal content, *m*, (Figure 6.4), and Ca^{2+}-dependent K^{+}-stimulated increase in MEPP frequency, both responded to increases in external Ca^{2+}. These observations are consistent with a reduced number of functional VGCC[21,22] limiting the amount of Ca^{2+} entry into the nerve terminal following depolarization.

LEMS IgG usually had no short-term effect on the mouse diaphragm *in vitro*, and appeared to require several hours to achieve any reduction in *m*[19,22]. This is probably not due to a problem with accessibility of the IgG to the neuromuscular junction, since some MG IgG preparations have reduced AChR function within 3 h[23], and similar results are found with

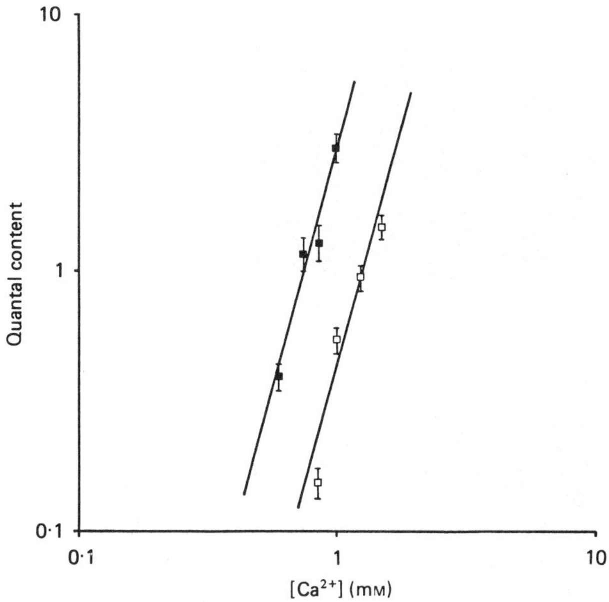

Figure 6.4 Ca^{2+} dependency of quantal content in LEMS. *m* was measured in mouse diaphragms after injection with control (■) or LEMS (□) IgG. The preparation was kept in a high Mg^{2+} concentration (7.2 mM) to reduce the quantal content to levels which could be easily measured. At each Ca^{2+} concentration the quantal content is reduced in LEMS IgG-treated mice (shifted to the right), but it responds normally to increases in Ca^{2+} in the bathing fluid (slope of line is not changed). Log-log plot. Taken with permission from reference 21

application of the LEMS preparations to cultured cells (see below). The electrophysiological studies on passively-transferred LEMS are further reviewed by Wray[24].

Antibody binding in the passive transfer model

Fukunaga *et al.*[25] found that passively transferred LEMS produced changes in the number and orderly arrangement of AZPs, very similar to those previously observed in biopsies from patients with LEMS[10]. In further studies, the early events were investigated in mice after 2 days of injections. The earliest sign was a decrease in the distance between the active zone particles in the outside rows, followed by clustering of the particles, finally resulting in a reduced number of active zones and of particles that were identified as AZPs by careful stereoscopic measurements[26]. In parallel with these observations, Fukuoka *et al.*[27] demonstrated IgG binding to the nerve terminal membrane by immunoperoxidase and immunoferritin staining (Figure 6.5). These studies not only suggested that the LEMS antibodies were directed against the active zone particles, but also suggested that their mechanism of action involved cross-linking of the AZPs on the surface of the nerve terminal, followed by internalization. This was confirmed by

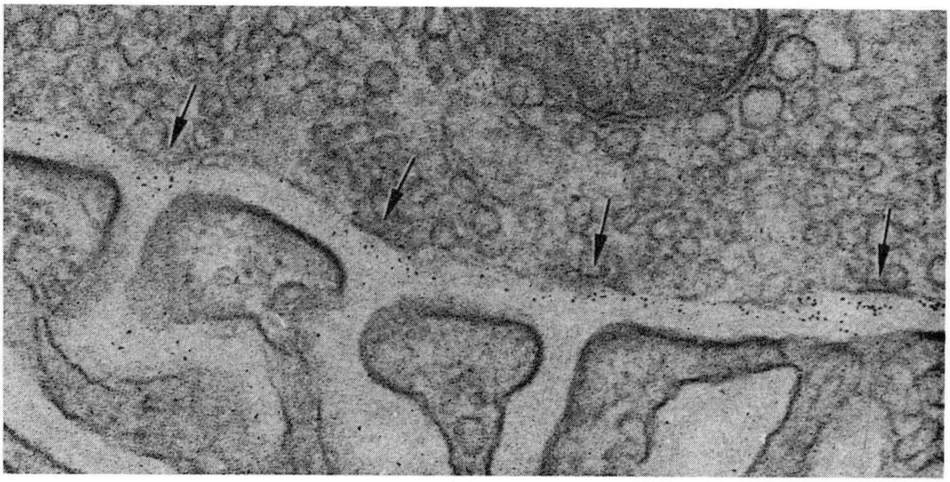

Figure 6.5 Immunoferritin localization of human IgG after injection with LEMS IgG. The ferritin particles are concentrated near the active zones (arrows). Magnification ×81 900. Taken from reference 27, courtesy of Dr A Engel

showing, in organ culture that, whereas Fab monomers derived from LEMS IgG by papain digestion were ineffective, divalent $F(ab')_2$ generated by pepsin digestion produced results which were similar to those with whole IgG[28]. None of the morphological studies on muscles from either LEMS patients or mice with passively transferred disease have suggested complement-mediated damage to the nerve terminal; indeed the physiological evidence suggests that the nerve terminal function is normal except with respect to the number of functioning VGCCs. These findings have been reviewed by Engel[29].

Role of small cell lung cancer in LEMS

Before the autoimmune basis for LEMS was established it had been suggested that a peptide secreted by SCLC tumours was responsible for the neurological syndrome. This theory did not receive support from the studies of Lambert and Lennon[30], who successfully transplanted SCLC tumours into athymic nude mice but found no neuromuscular dysfunction in the recipients. It is now clear that, in SCLC-associated LEMS, tumour cells trigger autoantibodies to surface determinants that cross-react with similar determinants at the neuromuscular junction.

SCLC expresses various neurone-specific markers, including neurone-specific enolase and UJ13A, and can secrete neuroactive peptides such as ACTH and bombesin[31]. It can generate short-duration action potentials which are similar to those found in cultured neurones[3], inhibited by VGCC antagonists. Thus it is not surprising that individuals in whom particular immune response genes appear to be markers for increased susceptibility[16] develop antibodies against cell surface components of the tumours, including VGCCs, and that these autoantibodies have the potential to cross-react with CNS determinants. Interestingly, tumour biopsies from patients with SCLC and LEMS show more macrophage infiltration but lower levels of expression of HLA class I than SCLCs from patients without LEMS[32]. One explanation for these features would be that an active immune response to the tumour could have triggered destruction of the more highly differentiated, HLA-expressing cells.

Effect of LEMS sera on cultured cells

In order to investigate the nature of the target antigen in LEMS and to help establish a source of the antigen for diagnostic assay, various neuronal and small cell lung cancer cells have been investigated for expression of functional VGCC. Depolarization of the SCLC line, MAR 10, with high K^+ resulted in influx of $^{45}Ca^{2+}$ which could be inhibited by incubation in the presence of known VGCC blockers such as dihydropyridines, phenylalkylamines and large divalent cations[33]. This K^+-stimulated Ca^{2+} flux was reduced when the SCLC cells were cultured in the presence of LEMS IgG, but unaffected by control IgG, including that from patients with other neurological diseases. LEMS IgG inhibits Ca^{2+} flux, though to a varying extent, in a number of different neuronal and SCLC lines[34] (Figure 6.6). A similar effect could be demonstrated by electrophysiological experiments using whole-cell patch clamp recordings from the neuronal cell line, NG108, adrenal chromaffin and rat pituitary cells[35–37]. In most cases the effects depended on exposure of the cells for a minimum of several hours, consistent with the evidence cited above that the autoantibodies act by cross-linking the VGCCs leading to their internalization, rather than by direct blocking of the Ca^{2+} channel itself. However, occasional LEMS IgG preparations have demonstrated a more direct effect.

The relevance of these observations to the aetiology of LEMS is indicated by a close correlation between the inhibition of Ca^{2+} flux by an individual patient's IgG and the CMAP measured in the patient's muscle at the time of serum sampling[38] (Figure 6.6).

Immunoprecipitation assay using [^{125}I]ω-conotoxin

The Ca^{2+} flux studies suggested that the cell lines might be a good source of the antigen to use in immunoprecipitation assays for diagnosis and monitoring the disease. Calcium channels are heterogeneous and several different subtypes have been described based on their inactivation kinetics and pharmacological properties (Table 6.2). Cells of neuronal origin were thought to express N type VGCC as well as L and T types. N type are poorly blocked by dihydropyridines but susceptible to inhibition by ω-conotoxin, another neurotoxin (distinct from the μ-conotoxin that inhibits Na^+ channels, see above) from *Conus geographus*, the fish-eating snail. For this reason several groups have extracted VGCCs from neuronal cell lines, labelled them with

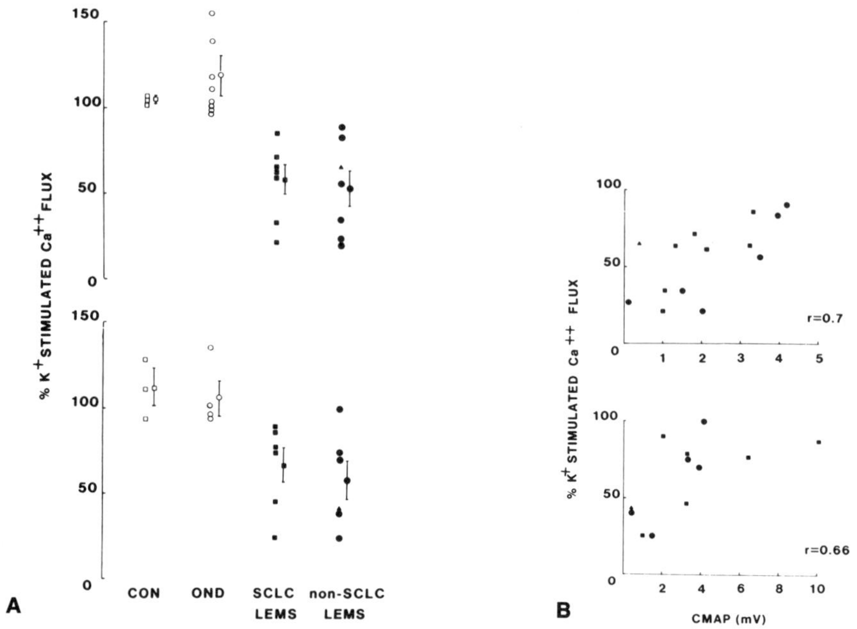

Figure 6.6 LEMS IgG reduces VGCC function. **A**. Effect of IgG on K^+-stimulated Ca^{2+} flux in a small cell cancer line (top) and the PC12 phaeochromocytoma cell line (bottom). Cells were incubated for 7 or 3 days, respectively, with IgG from healthy controls (CON), other neurological disorders (OND) and LEMS patients with or without small cell lung cancer (SCLC). Results are expressed as a percentage of values in cells grown in medium without IgG. **B**. Correlations between inhibition of K^+-stimulated Ca^{2+} flux and amplitude of the CMAP in individual LEMS patients. Results from both cell lines as in A. Taken with permission from reference 38

Table 6.2 Neuronal calcium channel subtypes

	Sensitivity of Ca^{2+} flux to antagonists		
Type	*Dihydropyridines*	*ω-conotoxin*	*ω-aga-toxin*
L	+	+	–
N	–	++	–
P	–	–	++

+, Relatively weak inhibition or reversible binding
++, Strong inhibition or binding

[^{125}I]ω-conotoxin, and showed that LEMS sera can immunoprecipitate the radioactivity (Figure 6.7). However, the proportion of LEMS patients in whom this assay is positive varies[39–41].

Recently, immunoprecipitation asays have been performed using as antigen VGCCs extracted from a SCLC tumour cell line derived from a LEMS patient[42]. Interestingly, sera from only four of 13 LEMS patients immunoprecipitated [^{125}I]ω-conotoxin-labelled VGCCs, whereas all 13 inhibited K^+-dependent Ca^{2+} flux in the line. This was consistent with the relative lack of effect of w-conotoxin on the K^+-dependent Ca^{2+} flux, suggesting that in

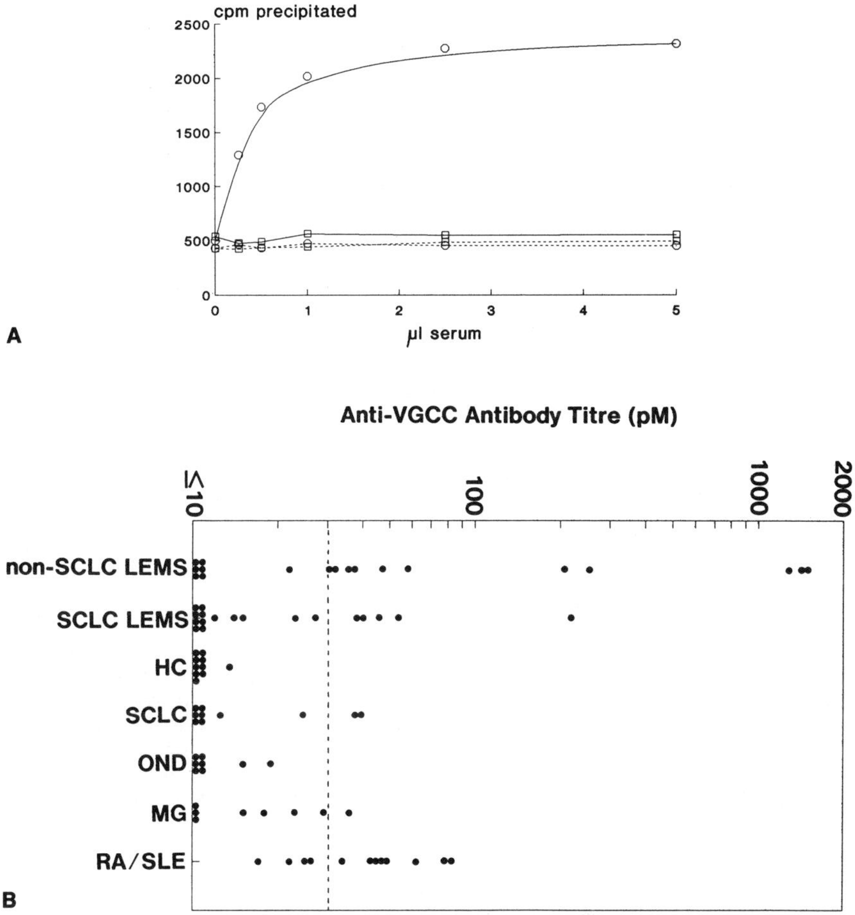

Figure 6.7 Radioimmunoassay for LEMS. **A.** Immunoprecipitation of [^{125}I]ω-conotoxin-labelled VGCCs, extracted from a human neuroblastoma cell line, by serum from a LEMS patient (○). Serum from a healthy control (□) did not precipitate any radioactivity. Dotted lines show precipitation when the cell line was presaturated with non-radioactive ω-conotoxin. **B.** Serum antibody titres against [^{125}I]ω-conotoxin-labelled VGCCs, measured as in A, in LEMS and control groups (HC, healthy; SCLC, small cell lung cancer without LEMS; OND, other neurological controls; MG, myasthenia gravis; RA/SLE; rheumatoid arthritis and systemic lupus erythematosus). Taken with permission from reference 41

this line, and possibly in the neuronal cell lines mentioned above, ω-conotoxin binds to a subpopulation of VGCCs which are not the main target for LEMS antibodies. There is still considerable debate about the importance of different VGCC types in neuronal function and recent work suggests that the P type channel, first described in Purkinje cells[43], might be most important functionally at the neuromuscular junction[44]. This channel is not susceptible to µ-conotoxin but is inhibited by FTX and ω-aga-toxin fractions of the American funnel web spider, *Agelenopsis aperta*[45]. Studies in progress aim to use this and other P-type toxins to label VGCCs for diagnostic assays.

Other antigens in LEMS

There has been some interest in the possible involvement of antigens other than the VGCC in the aetiology of LEMS. Chapman *et al.*[46] reported electromyographic evidence of LEMS in rats immunized with purified *Torpedo* cholinergic nerve terminals. About 50% of animals showed a small initial MAP with an increment of the second of paired stimuli. The antigen has not been identified, but recently a 56 kDa polypeptide, possibly synaptotagmin, a synaptic vesicle protein, has been shown to bind some LEMS antibodies on Western blots[47]. It appears, therefore, that either VGCCs are not the only target antigens in LEMS, or VGCCs are associated with synaptic vesicle proteins and co-purify with them. It was interesting that the sera positive for binding to synaptotagmin were also positive for immunoprecipitation of ω-conotoxin-binding[47]. A possible interaction between VGCC and synaptotagmin is suggested.

Treatment of LEMS

Both groups of patients may benefit symptomatically from 3,4 diaminopyridine (3,4DAP) that increases ACh release by blocking nerve K^+ channels[48]. In SCLC-associated LEMS, specific tumour therapy often leads to improvement in or even recovery from neurological symptoms[49]. This implies that removal of the antigenic stimulus leads to reduced levels of anti-VGCC antibodies though this has not yet been reported. In patients without SCLC for whom 3,4DAP is insufficient treatment, immunosuppressive drugs (prednisolone and azathioprine) can be valuable[15]. Patients who are apparently cancer-free at presentation should be followed carefully to ensure early detection of the appearance of SCLC if they are in a high-risk group.

ACQUIRED NEUROMYOTONIA

Acquired neuromyotonia (NMT) (Isaacs' syndrome[50]) is a syndrome of continuous, spontaneous muscle fibre activity that causes muscle stiffness, painful muscle cramps and in most cases visible undulating myokymia. Excessive sweating and hypertrophy of the muscles may occur as a result of the hyperactivity, and creatine kinase levels may be raised. It may arise in isolation, but has also been reported in association with peripheral neuropathies, thymoma, myasthenia gravis and occasionally with lung cancer (for review see reference 51). The characteristic electromyographic findings are spontaneous doublet, triplet or multiplet motor unit discharges with high instantaneous frequencies, that occur as irregular bursts or immediately following nerve activation (Figure 6.8), and may be associated with fasciculations and fibrillation potentials[50,52]. Its abolition by *d*-tubocurarine and its typical persistence after proximal peripheral nerve block indicated its origin in the terminal portion of the motor nerves[50]. It also continues during sleep or general anaesthesia. It should be distinguished from other causes of

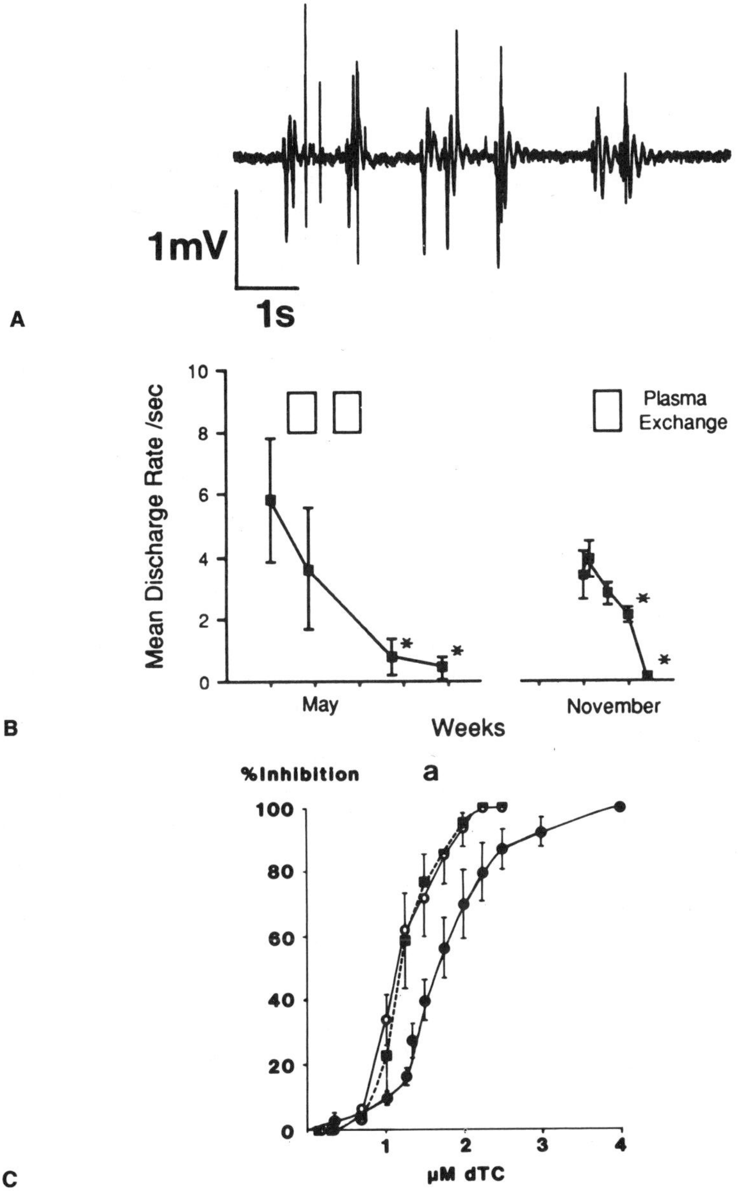

Figure 6.8 Evidence for an autoimmune basis for neuromyotonia (NMT) in a 17-year-old male. **A**. Spontaneous motor unit discharges recorded with a concentric needle electrode from the resting gastrocnemius muscle. **B**. Mean discharge rate/s of motor units in medial gastrocnemius showing marked improvement following two treatments with plasma exchange with a 6-month interval. **C**. Curare sensitivity of neuromuscular transmission in mice injected with patient's IgG (●), compared with control IgG (○) or untreated (■). NMT IgG treatment resulted in resistance to curare with a shift of the dose–response curve to the right. Taken from reference 54 with permission

visible myokymia, which tend to be more focal and rhythmical in distribution, and from the stiff man syndrome which is of central origin.

Aetiology of neuromyotonia

The nature of this rare condition was unknown until recently. However, in the last few years it has become apparent that in some patients the aetiology is autoimmune. Several cases have been reported in association with thymoma, and/or with MG and also occasionally with lung cancer (Table 6.1). Penicillamine, a drug which is known to induce a variety of autoimmune diseases, has been reported to induce neuromyotonia which improved after withdrawal of treatment[53]. These clinical features thus raised the possibility of an autoimmune aetiology. This was supported by the report of a clear response to plasma exchange[54] (Figure 6.8), confirmed in other cases[55], that implicates a humoral factor. Moreover, passive transfer of NMT IgG into mice resulted in increased efficacy of neuromuscular transmission[54], as shown by enhanced resistance to *d*-turbocurarine (Figure 6.8). These experiments indicate that the IgG had an effect on the neuromuscular junction, though the mice did not show any overt hyperactivity, and there was no evidence of spontaneous nerve activity.

An interpretation proposed for these observations was the presence of antibodies to voltage-gated K^+ channels that normally control nerve excitability and transmitter release. This was supported by recent experiments which have shown an increase in the number of quanta of ACh released per nerve impulse in mice receiving IgG from two patients with NMT[56]. The increase was similar to that found when normal mouse muscle was incubated with the K^+ channel blocker 3,4DAP. Thus anti-K^+ channel antibodies, by reducing the number of functional channels, may underlie the increase in nerve terminal excitability that characterizes NMT. Whether similar or related antibodies affect targets within the blood–nerve barrier in the human condition remains to be seen, but it is of interest in this context that oligoclonal bands were detected in the cerebrospinal fluid of three NMT patients[51], consistent with the production of IgG within the CNS.

Voltage-gated K^+ channels, like their calcium counterparts, are known to be heterogeneous, in this case deriving from alternate splicing of several different, but related, genes. Defining the exact nature of the antigen, and finding a suitable antigen source for an immunoassay will not be easy, but an approach based on the use of specific neurotoxins, similar to that being used in LEMS, appears to be promising.

CONCLUSIONS

The approaches described in this review have proved successful in establishing an autoimmune basis for LEMS. In particular the passive transfer of IgG to mice has allowed more detailed investigations of antibody-mediated physiological effects than can be performed on human muscle biopsies, and the study of inhibitory effects on ion fluxes in human neuronal cell lines has made it possible to begin to identify and characterize the target antigen in LEMS. Similar approaches are now being used to investigate the aetiology of NMT. Appropriate cell lines will, in the future, provide the starting material for purification and cDNA cloning of the antigens for both LEMS and NMT. These in turn will enable further investigation of the underlying immune mechanisms involved in the aetiology of the diseases, and should lead eventually to attempts to provide specific immunotherapy.

ACKNOWLEDGEMENTS

We are grateful to Dr Bethan Lang for her helpful comments on the manuscript and to Dr Kerry Mills for providing the electrophysiological data.

References

1. Lambert EH, Rooke ED, Eaton LM, Hodgson Ch. Myasthenic syndrome occasionally associated with bronchial neoplasm: neurophysiologic studies. In: Viets H, editor. Myasthenia gravis. Springfield: Charles C Thomas, 1961:362–410.
2. Posner JB. Paraneoplastic syndromes. Curr Neurol. 1989;9:245–8.
3. Tischler AS, Dichter MA, Biales B. Electrical excitability of oat cell carcinoma. J Pathol. 1977;122:153–6.
4. Elrington GM, Murray NMF, Spiro SG, Newsom-Davis J. Neurological paraneoplastic syndromes in patients with small cell lung cancer: a prospective survey of 150 patients. J Neurol Neurosurg Psychiatry. 1991;54:764–7.
5. O'Neill JH, Murray NM, Newsom-Davis J. The Lambert–Eaton myasthenic syndrome. A review of 50 cases. Brain. 1988;111:577–96.
6. Engel A. Congenital myasthenic syndromes. In: Vincent A, Wray D, editors. Neuromuscular Transmission. Oxford: Pergamon Press, 1992.
7. Vincent A, Wray D, editors. Neuromuscular Transmission. Oxford: Pergamon Press, 1992: 1–288.
8. Hong SJ, Chang CC. Use of geographutoxin II (μ-conotoxin) for the study of neuromuscular transmission in mice. Br J Pharmacol. 1989;97:934–40.
9. Lambert EH, Elmqvist D. Quantal components of endplate potentials in myasthenic syndrome. Ann NY Acad Sci. 1971;183:183–99.
10. Fukunaga H, Engel AG, Osame M, Lambert EH. Paucity and disorganisation of presynaptic membrane active zones in the Lambert–Eaton myasthenic syndrome. Muscle Nerve. 1982;5:686–97.
11. Molenaar PC, Newsom-Davis J, Polak RL, Vincent A. Eaton–Lambert syndrome: acetylcholine and choline acetyltransferase in skeletal muscle. Neurology. 1982;32:1062–5.
12. Gutmann L, Crosby TW, Takamori M, Martin JD. The Lambert Eaton syndrome and autoimmune disorders. Am J Med. 1972;53:354–6.
13. Lennon VA, Lambert EH, Whittingham S, Fairbanks V. Autoimmunity in the Lambert–Eaton myasthenic syndrome. Muscle Nerve. 1982;5:S21–5.
14. Lang B, Newsom-Davis J, Wray D, Vincent A, Murray NMF. Autoimmune aetiology for myasthenic (Eaton–Lambert) syndrome. Lancet. 1981;ii:224–6.
15. Newsom-Davis J, Murray NM. Plasma exchange and immunosuppressive drug treatment in the Lambert–Eaton myasthenic syndrome. Neurology. 1984;34:480–5.
16. Willcox N, Demaine AG, Newsom-Davis J, Welsh KI, Robb SA, Spiro SG. Increased frequency of IgG heavy chain marker Glm(2) and of HLA-B8 in Lambert–Eaton myasthenic syndrome with and without associated lung carcinoma. Human Immunol. 1985;14:29–36.
17. Lang B, Newsom-Davis J, Prior C, Wray D. Antibodies to motor nerve terminals: an electrophysiological study of a human myasthenic syndrome transferred to mouse. J Physiol Lond. 1983;344:335–45.

18. Kim Y. Passive transfer of the Lambert–Eaton myasthenic syndrome: neuromuscular transmission in mice injected with plasma. Muscle Nerve. 1985;8:162–72.
19. Prior C, Lang B, Wray D, Newsom-Davis J. Action of Lambert-Eaton myasthenic syndrome IgG at mouse motor nerve terminals. Ann Neurol. 1985;17:587–92.
20. Lande S, Lang B, Newsom-Davis J, Wray D. Site of action of Lambert–Eaton myasthenic syndrome antibodies at mouse motor nerve terminals. J Physiol. 1985;371:61p.
21. Lang B, Newsom-Davis J, Peers C, Prior C, Wray DW. The effect of myasthenic syndrome antibody on presynaptic calcium channels in the mouse. J Physiol Lond. 1987;390:257–70.
22. Wray DW, Lang B, Newsom-Davis J, Peers C. Antibodies against calcium channels in the Lambert–Eaton myasthenic syndrome. Ann NY Acad Sci. 1989;560:269–77.
23. Burges J, Wray DW, Pizzighella S, Hall Z, Vincent A. A myasthenia gravis plasma immunoglobulin reduces miniature endplate potentials at human endplates *in vitro*. Muscle Nerve. 1990;13:407–13.
24. Wray D. The Lambert–Eaton myasthenic syndrome. In: Vincent A, Wray D, editors. Neuromuscular Transmission. Oxford: Pergamon Press. 1992:249–67.
25. Fukunaga H, Engel AG, Lang B, Newsom-Davis J, Vincent A. Passive transfer of Lambert–Eaton myasthenic syndrome with IgG from man to mouse depletes the presynaptic membrane active zones. Proc Natl Acad Sci USA. 1983;80:7636–40.
26. Fukuoka T, Engel AG, Lang B, Newsom-Davis J, Prior C, Wray DW. Lambert–Eaton myasthenic syndrome: I. Early morphological effects of IgG on the presynaptic membrane active zones. Ann Neurol. 1987;22:193–9.
27. Fukuoka T, Engel AG, Lang B, Newsom-Davis J, Vincent A. Lambert–Eaton myasthenic syndrome: II. Immunoelectron microscopy localization of IgG at the mouse motor endplate. Ann Neurol. 1987;22:200–11.
28. Nagel A, Engel AG, Lang B, Newsom-Davis J, Fukuoka T. Lambert–Eaton myasthenic syndrome IgG depletes presynaptic membrane active zone particles by antigenic modulation. Ann Neurol. 1988;24:552–8.
29. Engel AG, Nagel A, Fukuoka T, *et al.* Motor nerve terminal calcium channels in Lambert–Eaton myasthenic syndrome. Morphologic evidence for depletion and that the depletion is mediated by autoantibodies. Ann NY Acad Sci. 1989;560:278–90.
30. Lambert EH, Lennon VA. Neuromuscular transmission in nude mice bearing oat cell tumors from Lambert–Eaton myasthenic syndrome. Muscle Nerve. 1982;5:S39–45.
31. Allan PM, Garson JA, Harper EI, *et al.* Biological characterization and clinical applications of a monoclonal antibody recognizing an antigen restricted to neuroectodermal tissues. Int J Cancer. 1983;31:591–8.
32. Morris CS, Esiri MN, Marx A, Newsom-Davis J. Immunocytochemical characteristics of small cell lung carcinoma associated with the Lambert–Eaton myasthenic syndrome. Am J Pathol. 1992;140:839–45.
33. Roberts A, Perera S, Lang B, Vincent A, Newsom-Davis J. Paraneoplastic myasthenic syndrome IgG inhibits $^{45}Ca^{2+}$ flux in a human cell carcinoma line. Nature. 1985;317: 737–9.
34. Lang B, Leys K, Vincent A, Newsom-Davis J. K^+-stimulated Ca^{2+} influx in cell lines derived from small cell lung cancer and neuronal tumors. Ann NY Acad Sci. 1989;560: 294–6.
35. Kim YI, Neher E. IgG from patients with Lambert–Eaton syndrome blocks voltage dependent calcium channels. Science. 1988;239:405.
36. Login IS, Kim YI, Judd AM, Spangelo BL, MacLeod RM. Immunoglobulins of Lambert–Eaton myasthen: syndrome inhibit rat pituitary hormone release. Ann Neurol. 1987;22: 610–14.
37. Peers C, Lang B, Newsom-Davis J, Wray DW. Selective action of myasthenic syndrome antibodies on calcium channels in a rodent neuroblastoma x glioma cell line. J Physiol Lond. 1990;421:293–308.
38. Lang B, Vincent A, Murray NM, Newsom-Davis J. Lambert–Eaton myasthenic syndrome: immunoglobulin G inhibition of Ca^{2+} flux in tumor cells correlates with disease severity. Ann Neurol. 1989;25:265–71.
39. Sher E, Canal N, Piccolo G, *et al.* Specificity of calcium channel autoantibodies in Lambert–Eaton myasthenic syndrome. Lancet. 1989;ii:640–3.
40. Lennon VA, Lambert EH. Autoantibodies bind solubilised calcium channel-omega-

conotoxin complexes from small cell lung carcinoma: a diagnostic aid for Lambert–Eaton myasthenic syndrome. Mayo Clin Proc. 1989;64:1498–504.
41. Leys K, Lang B, Johnston I, Newsom-Davis J. Calcium channel autoantibodies in the Lambert–Eaton myasthenic syndrome. Ann Neurol. 1991;29:307–14.
42. Johnston I, Lang B, Leys K, Newsom-Davis J. Heterogeneity of calcium channel antibodies detected using a small cell lung cancer line derived from a Lambert–Eaton syndrome patient. Neurology. 1994;44:334–8.
43. Llinas R, Sugimori M, Hillman DE, Cherksey B. Distribution and functional significance of the P-type voltage-dependent Ca^{2+} channels in the mammalian central nervous system. TINS. 1992;15:351–5.
44. Uchitel OD, Protti DA, Sanchez V, Cherskey BD, Sugimori M, Llinas R. P-type voltage-dependent calcium channel mediates presynaptic calcium influx and transmitter release in mammalian synapses. Proc Natl Acad Sci USA. 1992;89:3330–3.
45. Mintz I, Venema CJ, Swiderek KM, Lee TD, Bean BP, Adams ME. P-type calcium channels blocked by the spider toxin w-Aga IVA. Nature. 1992;355:827–9.
46. Chapman J, Rabinowitz R, Kroczyn A, Michaelson D. Rats immunized with cholinergic synaptosomes: a model for Lambert Eaton syndrome. Muscle Nerve. 1990;13:726–33.
47. Leveque C, Hoshino T, David P, *et al.* The synaptic vesicle protein synaptotagmin associates with calcium channels and is a putative Lambert–Eaton myasthenic syndrome antigen. Proc Natl Acad Sci USA. 1992;89:3625–9.
48. Murray NMF, Newsom-Davis J, Karni Y, Wiles CM. Oral 3,4-diaminopyridine in the treatment of the Lambert–Eaton myasthenic syndrome (LEMS). J Neurol Neurosurg Psychiatry. 1984;47:1052–3.
49. Chalk CH, Murray NM, Newsom-Davis J, O'Neill JH, Spiro SG. Response of the Lambert–Eaton myasthenic syndrome to treatment of associated small-cell lung carcinoma. Neurology. 1990;40:1552–6.
50. Isaacs H. A syndrome of continuous muscle-fibre activity. J Neurol Neurosurg Psychiatry. 1961;24:319–25.
51. Newsom-Davis J, Mills KR. Immunological associations of acquired neuromyotonia (Isaacs' syndrome): report of five cases and literature review. Brain. 1993;116:453–69.
52. Denny-Brown D, Foley JM. Myokymia and the benign fasciculation of muscular cramps. Trans Assoc Am Physicians. 1948;61:88–96.
53. Raeback J, Benton S, Swash M, Schwartz MS. Penicillamine-induced neuromyotonia. Br Med J. 1979;279:1464–5.
54. Sinha S, Newsom-Davis J, Mills K, *et al.* Autoimmune etiology for acquired neuromyotonia (Isaacs' syndrome). Lancet. 1991;ii:75–7.
55. Bady B, Chauplannaz G, Vial C, Savet J-F. Autoimmune aetiology for acquired neuromyotonia. Lancet. 1991;338:1330.
56. Shillito P, Lang B, Newsom-Davis J. Evidence for an autoantibody-mediated mechanism in acquired neuromyotonia. J Neurol Neuropathol Psychiatry. 1993;55:1214.

7
Myasthenia gravis

D. B. DRACHMAN and R. W. KUNCL

INTRODUCTION

Myasthenia gravis (MG) is undoubtedly the most thoroughly understood neuromuscular autoimmune disease, and is perhaps the best understood of all human autoimmune disorders. The clinical features of muscle weakness and fatigue were first recognized in the seventeenth century[1], and were well described by 1900[2,3]. The neuromuscular junction was identified as the general site of abnormality because of the resemblance of MG to curare poisoning, and the favourable clinical response to treatment with anticholinesterase drugs[4]. The development and application of neurotoxins from elapid snake venoms[5], that bind specifically to acetylcholine receptors (AChRs), led to the precise identification of the deficit of available AChRs at neuromuscular junctions[6]. These highly specific neurotoxins permitted purification and characterization of the AChR molecule, initially from the richest sources – the electric organs of electric eels and rays[7] – and subsequently from a wide variety of sources, including human muscle. At present, genes for all subunits of the AChR have been sequenced and cloned[8–10], and AChR subunits have been produced by recombinant technology[11,12]. An experimental model (EAMG) induced by immunization of animals with purified AChR[13] has greatly facilitated studies of the pathogenesis and treatment of MG. The key role of AChR-specific antibodies in the pathogenesis of MG[14], and the mechanisms by which they interact with AChRs[15], have now been clearly elucidated.

From the clinical point of view, both diagnosis and treatment of MG have advanced remarkably. Formerly a fatal or disabling disease in the majority of cases[16], MG no longer carries a 'grave' prognosis. With the use of modern immunotherapy, most myasthenic patients can be restored to fully productive lives[17].

Despite these important advances, significant gaps in our knowledge remain, and are the focus of current research. The factors that initiate and maintain the pathological autoimmune response in MG are not yet known, as is also true for all other spontaneously occurring autoimmune diseases. The cellular immunology of MG is currently the subject of intensive study. Based on detailed knowledge of the molecular structure of the AChR, efforts to map the epitopes with which B cells and T cells interact are underway. As will be discussed further, the heterogeneity of the immune responses at both B cell and T cell levels makes this a formidable task.

In view of the extensive knowledge of the pathogenesis and immunology of MG, it should be possible to devise specific methods of immunotherapy, and ultimately, to cure the underlying disorder. However, this goal has as yet remained elusive.

In this chapter, we will attempt to summarize current knowledge about the pathogenesis, immunology, clinical features, diagnosis, and present and future treatment of MG.

THE NEUROMUSCULAR JUNCTION IN MG

It is now thoroughly established that the basic abnormality in MG is a deficit of available AChRs at neuromuscular junctions. This was first demonstrated by the use of ^{125}I-labelled α-bungarotoxin (α-BuTx), which binds specifically and virtually irreversibly to nicotinic AChRs of skeletal muscles[5]. The number of AChRs can be determined by saturation of a muscle biopsy specimen with [^{125}I]α-BuTx, and measurement of the amount of radioactivity bound to neuromuscular junctions[6,18]. Comparison of the number of AChR binding sites per neuromuscular junction in deltoid muscles from large groups of healthy individuals and myasthenic patients showed a highly significant difference: the myasthenic patients' junctions had only one-third as many AChRs on the average ($0.7 \pm 0.1 \times 10^7$, compared with $2.1 \pm 0.2 \times 10^7$ for normal individuals), and there was only 5% overlap between the two groups[6,19]. Indeed, measurement of junctional AChRs in muscle biopsies, when available, is one of the most sensitive and reliable diagnostic tests for MG. In addition to the reduction of AChRs, neuromuscular junctions from myasthenic patients show morphological changes of simplification of the postsynaptic membrane folds, and an increase in the gap between pre- and postsynaptic membranes[20].

The reduction in junctional AChRs accounts for most, if not all, of the clinical and physiological abnormalities in MG. No additional defects of pre- or postsynaptic function that might further impair neuromuscular transmission have been reported in MG. Neither resting nor stimulation-evoked release of ACh is reduced[21,22]. Channel properties of the remaining AChRs at myasthenic junctions were reportedly normal, in terms of open times and current flow[23]. Moreover, an experimental animal model in which the number of available AChRs in rats was reduced by specific blockade with α-cobratoxin, reproduced the characteristic features of human MG. The animals were weak, and showed decremental responses on repetitive nerve stimulation, typical of the pattern in MG[24]. The decremental responses were markedly improved by administration of anticholinesterase agents. Post-tetanic responses, thought to be particularly characteristic of MG, were also reproduced by the AChR blockade model.

Both the clinical and the electrophysiological features of MG are well explained by the reduction of available AChRs. The basic principle is that the amplitude of endplate potentials (epps) depends on the number of interactions between presynaptically released ACh molecules and postsynaptic AChR molecules. A reduction of either the amount of ACh released, or the number of AChRs, would result in a reduction of the epp amplitude. At the normal junction, the interactions are more than sufficient to produce epps large enough to trigger muscle potentials without failures. The excess above threshold has been termed the 'safety margin' of neuromuscular transmission[25]. In MG, the decreased number of AChRs limits the number of interactions, giving rise to epps of diminished amplitude. Therefore, epps at some neuromuscular junctions are below the threshold necessary to trigger muscle action potentials. This results in failure of neuromuscular transmission, which has been demonstrated both by intracellular recording[26,27] and by the method of single fibre electromyography (SFEMG)[28] (see section on diagnosis). When transmission fails at many junctions, the power of the whole muscle is reduced, which is manifested clinically as weakness. Neuromuscular fatigue is the single most characteristic feature of MG. The patient cannot sustain or repeat forceful muscular contractions. Electrophysiologically, fatigue is recognized as a progressive decrement in the amplitude of muscle responses evoked by repetitive stimulation of motor nerves. These fatigue phenomena result from the reduced safety margin at myasthenic junctions, superimposed on the normal decline of evoked ACh release, which is termed 'presynaptic rundown'. During repeated stimulation of normal motor nerves, the amount of ACh released per impulse decreases after the first few impulses, since the nerve is unable to sustain its original release rate[29]. In the myasthenic patient, this results in progressive failure of transmission because of the reduced numbers of AChRs (low safety factor) at neuromuscular junctions. In healthy individuals, the safety margin is sufficiently great so that transmission failure and fatigue do not occur except at high stimulation rates of 40–50 Hz.

THE ACETYLCHOLINE RECEPTOR

The nicotinic AChR of skeletal muscle is the target of the autoimmune response in MG. The AChR is a ligand-gated channel, composed of five subunits arranged around a central pore. It extends through the muscle membrane, with about half the total height of the molecule (55 Å) projecting outside the membrane, and about 15 Å within the cytoplasm[30]. As seen from above, it has been compared to a doughnut; the arrangement of subunits is like that of barrel staves around a central cavity[31]. Each AChR molecule consists of two α-subunits, and one each of β, δ, and either γ or ε (see below). The different subunits have considerable homology to each other[8], suggesting a common ancestral origin. Each of the subunits has four hydrophobic domains, implying that it traverses the membrane four times[32]. The amino terminus is located extracellularly, but it is not yet certain whether the carboxyl terminus is external or internal[33,34]. Each of the two α-subunits bears an ACh binding site, which is located extracellularly, and is centred around amino acids 192–193. Functionally, the ion channel is closed in the resting state. It is activated to open when both α-subunit binding sites are occupied by the agonist, ACh, or by closely related analogues. Blocking agents such as α-BuTx or curare bind at or near the same site, preventing access to ACh.

AChRs are closely regulated by motor nerves[35–39]. There are important differences between the AChRs of innervated mature muscles and those of denervated or immature muscles. In normally innervated mature muscle cells, AChRs are localized almost exclusively at the neuromuscular junction. Following denervation, or in immature skeletal muscle cells, AChRs are distributed over the entire surface of the muscle membrane, due to increased synthesis and insertion of extrajunctional-type AChRs. The junctional AChRs of innervated muscles have an ε subunit in place of a γ subunit[40,41], have channel properties of high conductance and short open times[42], and the majority of the AChRs turn over relatively slowly (half-life in mice, about 12 days)[42]. By contrast, the extrajunctional type AChRs of denervated or immature muscles have a γ subunit rather than an ε subunit, have low conductance and long open time channel properties[42], and turn over rapidly (half-life in mice <1 day). The motor nerves regulate the synthesis, subunit composition, distribution, and stabilization of AChRs[35–45]. There is substantial evidence that ACh transmission plays a key role in the regulation of these properties[36,39,44,45].

The richest natural source of AChR is the electric organ of the electric ray (*Torpedo*) or eel (*Electrophorus*), which consists of arrays of neuromuscular junction-like structures capable of producing powerful electrical discharges[46]. Fetal bovine muscle has been used for the production of relatively large amounts of mammalian AChR[47]. Human AChR extracted from amputated limbs is commonly used for diagnostic radioimmunoassay (RIA) of anti-AChR antibodies[48]. Relatively small amounts of AChR can be purified from this source by affinity chromatography. The human cell line TE671, derived from a rhabdomyosarcoma, was found to express AChR of the extrajunctional type, and has been used as a source of human AChR[49,50]. One of the most important advances in this area has been the cloning and sequencing of genes for all the AChR subunits of many species, including *Torpedo* and man[8–10]. It is now possible to produce fusion proteins consisting of large stretches, or even entire subunits, of AChR by genetic engineering[11,12]. Although these proteins lack the conformational attributes of natural AChR, they are useful for studies of T cell recognition in MG. Structurally and functionally intact AChRs have also been produced in frog oocytes[51]. Eventually, AChR generated by modern biotechnology may play a key role in future therapeutic strategies.

Table 7.1 Antibody-mediated autoimmune disease: criteria

1.	Antibody is present in patients with the disease.
2.	Antibody interacts with the target antigen.
3.	Passive transfer of the antibody reproduces the disease features.
4.	Immunization with the antigen produces a model disease.
5.	Reduction of the antibody ameliorates the disease.

HUMORAL PATHOGENESIS OF MG: INTERACTION OF ANTIBODIES WITH AChR

It is now widely accepted that the neuromuscular abnormalities in MG are brought about by antibody-mediated processes. The evidence for this satisfies a set of five criteria recently proposed to define the relationship between a putative autoantibody and a disease presumed to be autoimmune (Table 7.1)[52]. It is instructive to apply these criteria to MG, as well as to the other neuromuscular diseases described in this volume.

(1) Antibody is present. Overall, 80–90% of patients with MG have detectable serum antibodies to AChR, as measured by the standard RIA[53–55]. The high proportion of antibody-positive patients supports the concept of antibody-mediated pathogenesis of MG. However, the absence of detectable circulating antibodies in more than 10% of myasthenic sera, including some from patients with severe generalized disease, provides an intriguing exception. Moreover, the serum antibody concentration does not correspond well with the clinical severity of weakness in MG[53,56,57]. These disparities initially led to questions about the relationship of anti-AChR antibodies to the pathogenesis of MG (see below).

(2) Interaction with target antigen. One of the seminal developments in MG was the identification of the AChR at the neuromuscular junction as the molecular target of the disease process[6,13]. Despite knowledge of the target, demonstration of antibody at the site of junctional AChRs proved technically difficult. However, electron microscopic immunochemistry identified IgG at the postsynaptic membranes of myasthenic patients' neuromuscular junctions, localized appropriately so as to affect AChRs[58].

(3) Passive transfer experiments provided the most direct evidence of the pathogenic role of autoantibodies. IgG from myasthenic patients was repeatedly injected into mice, reproducing the characteristic features of MG, including reduced amplitudes of miniature endplate potentials, and a reduction of AChRs at neuromuscular junctions, as well as weakness and decremental responses to repetitive nerve stimulation[15,59]. The success of these studies depended on adequate cross-species reactivity between the human antibody and the mouse AChR; and reliable methods for detecting the key features of MG in the mice.

(4) Model disease (EAMG). The availability of purified AChR permitted the immunization of experimental animals to produce EAMG[13,60–62]. This model, which is discussed in detail in Chapter 8, clearly demonstrated that an immune response directed against AChRs is capable of producing

key features of MG. However, the model does not reproduce the spontaneous human disease exactly, since the immunizing event (injection of relatively large amounts of AChR in adjuvant) is highly artificial. Further, the cellular effector mechanisms and the rapid course of the response in EAMG differ from those of spontaneous human MG.

(5) Reduction of serum anti-AChR antibodies by immunosuppression or plasmapheresis results in marked clinical improvement in the great majority of patients[63,64].

In summary, the criteria linking the autoantibody and the disease process have been amply satisfied in MG, and the principle of antibody-mediated pathogenesis is widely accepted.

Mechanisms of action of AChR antibodies

How do anti-AChR antibodies effect a reduction in the number of junctional AChRs? At least three mechanisms are thought to participate in this effect: (1) accelerated endocytosis and degradation of AChRs; (2) functional blockade of ACh binding sites; and (3) damage to AChRs, in conjunction with complement and/or cellular elements.

Accelerated degradation of AChRs

The ability of myasthenic patients' IgG to accelerate the degradation of AChRs was first demonstrated in a rat skeletal muscle cell culture system, using [^{125}I]α-BuTx as a probe to follow receptor degradation[65–67]. The rate of appearance of the breakdown product [^{125}I]tyrosine in the medium reflects degradation of AChRs[68]. When immunoglobulin from myasthenic patients is added to the cultures, the AChR degradation rate increases by up to 2–3 fold. Sera from approximately 90% of myasthenic patients produce significant acceleration of AChR degradation in muscle culture systems[55,57]. This accelerated loss or 'modulation' of AChRs is the basis for a commercially available diagnostic test for MG. The ability of myasthenic patients' IgG to induce accelerated degradation of AChRs depends on its capacity to cross-link the receptors[69,70]. Cross-linking can be produced by IgG molecules because they are divalent, and are therefore capable of binding to identical antigenic sites on different AChR molecules. Monovalent Fab fragments, prepared by enzymatic cleavage of IgG from myasthenic patients, do not cause accelerated degradation, although they retain their ability to bind to single AChRs. However, if a second 'piggyback' antibody against the Fab fragments is added, to cross-link AChR–Fab complexes in the culture system, AChR degradation is accelerated. Morphological studies using freeze-fracture electron microscopy show that antibody-linked AChRs are drawn together in tightly packed clusters within the muscle membrane[71]. The clustered AChRs are rapidly endocytosed by way of clathrin-coated pits that are known to transport a variety of other surface components to the interior of cells. The internalized AChRs then undergo enzymatic degradation within lysosomes. The critical step that is accelerated by anti-AChR antibodies is endocytosis of the AChRs.

Antibody-accelerated degradation of AChRs has also been shown to occur at intact neuromuscular junctions *in vivo*[72]. This is not a trivial point, since junctional AChRs differ from the extrajunctional type AChRs of cultured skeletal muscles in their subunit composition, immunological reactivity, and turnover rates.

Blockade of AChRs

Antibodies from many myasthenic patients are capable of blocking the ligand-binding site of AChRs. Depending on the method used, the proportion of myasthenic patients' sera that block the ligand binding site has been reported to vary from 7% to nearly 90% under optimal conditions[57,73–75]. Because of the small size of the ACh-binding site (see above), it is unlikely that blockade is due to attachment of the antibody directly to the site itself. The blocking antibodies are thought to bind near the site, producing steric hindrance.

Damage to neuromuscular junctions

Several lines of evidence suggest that complement-mediated damage contributes to the effect of anti-AChR antibodies. Electron microscopy of neuromuscular junctions from myasthenic patients revealed simplification of postsynaptic folds, which has been attributed to complement-mediated damage[20]. Immunocytochemical methods have demonstrated the presence of the 'membrane attack complex' of complement at most neuromuscular junctions[76]. In the passive transfer model, the pathogenic effect of myasthenic IgG is enhanced by the presence of complement in recipient animals[59].

Anti-AChR antibodies and the severity of MG

It has been repeatedly noted that there is a poor correlation between the clinical severity of MG and the absolute concentration of circulating anti-AChR antibody[53,56,57]. However, a relative change in the serum anti-AChR antibody concentration in a given patient generally correlates with a change in clinical status[63,64,77–79]. This suggested that different subsets of antibodies may have different capacities to alter the neuromuscular junction, and thereby produce the clinical manifestations of MG. There is evidence that the functional ability of the antibodies to reduce the available junctional AChRs by the mechanisms outlined above, might reflect their role in the disease process more accurately than the absolute antibody concentration. Using a rat skeletal muscle culture system, the ability of immunoglobulin from MG patients to induce accelerated degradation and/or blockade of AChRs was measured[57]. Interestingly, immunoglobulin from some patients had a predominant effect on degradation, while others predominantly produced blockade. The potential of different antibodies for producing these differential effects may relate to the specific AChR epitopes to which they bind. When these two functional effects produced by each serum were mathematically combined, the result corresponded most closely with the clinical status of the patient[57]. Others have argued that the ability to induce loss of AChRs in culture may merely correlate with anti-AChR antibody titres, but differences in experimental conditions make comparisons difficult[80,81]. In any case, it is clear that these two functional activities of the autoantibodies represent at least some of their clinically relevant properties. Undoubtedly, other factors, such as the ability of the antibodies to bind complement, or intrinsic properties of the patient's neuromuscular junctions such as the safety factor of neuromuscular transmission, can also influence the degree of muscle weakness in individual patients.

Binding sites of anti-AChR antibodies

The large size and complex structure of the AChR molecule make it highly likely that the specific epitopes to which anti-AChR antibodies bind play an important role in the antibodies' ability to alter neuromuscular function. First, pathologically relevant antibodies probably bind to the extracellular domains of the AChR molecule, to which they would have access[82]. Second, the ability of antibodies to cross-link AChR molecules, and thus induce accelerated degradation, must be critically dependent on spatial considerations. In order to permit cross-linking of AChRs, the epitope must be located at a site close enough to its outer rim to permit the arms of the IgG molecule to span adjacent AChR molecules. On the other hand, there must not be two identical sites available for internal cross-linking within a single AChR molecule. Third, blocking antibodies must bind at or near the ACh binding site, close to amino acids 192–193 of the α-subunit. Finally, other spatial constraints could influence the ability to achieve a high enough antibody density to induce activation of complement.

In order to study the binding sites of anti-AChR antibodies, competition studies have been carried out[82–85]. Monoclonal antibodies (Mabs) with known binding sites were used to 'protect' the particular region of AChR to which they bind. The binding of individual patients' sera to Mab-protected AChR, or to unprotected AChR, was measured by RIA. Competition between the Mab and the patient's serum antibodies was indicated by a reduction in the amount of serum antibody bound to the protected AChR. Competition studies give only an approximation of the antibody specificity, since the large size of the antibody relative to the small size of the epitope to which it binds may sterically hinder access to the competing antibodies. Nevertheless, using this type of analysis, it is clear that the majority of anti-AChR antibodies bind to the α-subunit. Lindstrom *et al.* have emphasized that a relatively large proportion of anti-AChR antibodies from human MG patients bind to a restricted portion of the α-subunit[82,83], which they have designated the 'main immunogenic region' (MIR)[82,83,85]. In nearly 80% of patients, more than half of the anti-AChR antibody was found to bind the MIR[83]. However, the remainder of the antibodies bound to other sites, both on the α-subunit and on each of the other AChR subunits. The MIR is conformationally determined, and its antigenic properties are greatly altered by denaturation[82]. Initial studies located the MIR in the region of amino acids 46–127 of the α-subunit[86]. More recent studies using site-directed mutagenesis have suggested a critical core extending over 10 amino acids, 67–76 of the α-subunit, in both human and *Torpedo* AChR[85]. It should be emphasized that the MIR does not constitute a single epitope, since antibodies of differing fine specificity can bind to it[82–85]. Its role in human MG is still controversial[87].

Heterogeneity of antibodies

Extensive evidence indicates the existence of heterogeneous populations of anti-AChR antibodies in individual myasthenic patients, with only limited sharing of specificities among different patients[84,88]. Anti-AChR antibody heterogeneity has been analysed in several ways. First, as described above, antibodies from different patients have varied patterns of functional effects on blocking and degradation of AChRs, that reflect differences in their sites of binding[57]. Second, competition studies, including those described above, have revealed that the great majority of patients have antibodies that bind both to different subunits, and to different sites on each subunit[82–85]. Despite the fact that competition studies give only a coarse-grained approximation of the binding sites of the anti-AChR antibodies, they were able to demonstrate significant heterogeneity of binding sites of the antibodies. Third, antibodies from different myasthenic patients differ in their ability to cross-react with AChR from non-human species, indicative of antibody heterogeneity[89]. Fourth, differences in light chains and in subclass composition of anti-AChR antibodies have been reported[83,90,91]. Lastly, anti-idiotypic antibodies raised against anti-AChR antibodies were used to test for idiotype sharing between patients. The cross-reactivity between patients was extremely limited, suggesting very little sharing of idiotypes between myasthenic patients[84,92,93]. Taken together, these findings indicate that there is extensive heterogeneity of antibodies, and therefore of the B cells that produce them, in patients with myasthenia gravis.

Antibody-negative MG

About 10–20% of patients with acquired MG lack circulating anti-AChR antibodies detectable by the standard RIA[53–55]. Although some of these patients have mild, localized MG, some 'antibody-negative' patients have generalized MG whose disease corresponds to conventional MG in other clinical respects[88,94–97]. These patients have decremental responses on repetitive nerve stimulation, respond favourably to anti-cholinesterase agents, and improve in response to plasmapheresis or immunosuppressive treatment. Motor point biopsies obtained in seven antibody-negative patients revealed significantly reduced numbers of AChRs per neuromuscular junction, consistent with findings in patients with RIA-detectable antibodies[95]. Passive transfer of IgG from six of seven antibody-negative patients to mice resulted in reduced numbers of junctional AChRs and reduced amplitudes of miniature endplate potentials[88,95]. Moreover, sera from 8 of 11 patients was shown to bind significantly to a mammalian skeletal muscle line that expressed AChRs[98], and 11 of 12 sera induced significantly increased 'modulation' of AChRs in human myotube cultures. The Oxford group has recently reported that serum immunoglobulin from antibody-negative patients can interfere acutely with AChR channel function in the TE671 (rhabdomyosarcoma) cell model, without inducing loss of AChRs themselves[99]. The pathogenic factor copurified with IgM in their studies, although IgM binding to AChRs was not observed. Histologically, thymus glands from antibody-negative patients showed abnormal cellular infiltration (thymitis), as did patients with positive antibody titres, but most had significantly fewer germinal centres[100].

Taken together, these studies lead to the conclusion that antibody-negative MG is autoimmune, and that its pathogenesis involves circulating antibodies not detected by RIA. The differing antibody-mediated mechanisms reported suggest that the rubric 'antibody-negative MG' may include a heterogeneous group of autoimmune myasthenic disorders. The inability to detect AChR-binding antibodies by the conventional RIA indicates that the antibodies must differ in some way from those of the majority of MG patients. One possibility is that the antibodies may be directed at epitopes that are not present in the soluble AChR extract, either because the AChR molecule is altered in the process of extraction, or because the epitopes are associated with, but not intrinsic components of, the AChR. Alternatively, the affinity of the antibodies for AChR may be too low for detection in the RIA, which uses soluble AChR as the target antigen. Either of these hypotheses is consistent with the demonstrated activity of serum immunoglobulin from antibody negative patients when applied to solid phase test systems.

ROLE OF T CELLS IN MG

Thus far, the discussion has focused on antibodies, and their direct involvement in the pathogenesis of the fundamental AChR deficit in MG. It is now abundantly clear that T cells play a pivotal role in the immune response to AChR. The AChR antibody response is T cell-dependent: the requirement for T cells has been formally demonstrated in EAMG in rats[101]. In the human immune response, AChR-specific $CD4^+$ T cells have been shown to augment the production of AChR antibodies by B cells *in vitro*[102].

Many studies have shown that T cells from myasthenic patients respond to stimulation with AChR, in the presence of appropriate antigen-presenting cells (APCs)[103–111]. Early studies used AChR purified from *Torpedo* as the source of stimulating antigen[103–105]. Although *Torpedo* AChR stimulated proliferation of T cells from some patients, the responses were relatively weak, and the differences between *Torpedo* and human AChR led to selective stimulation of a narrow range of T cells capable of reacting with the *Torpedo* receptor. More recently, the human antigen, in the form of purified AChR, recombinant human AChR subunits or polypeptide sequences, and synthetic peptides of up to 20 amino acids in length, have been used to stimulate T cells, with more robust and more relevant responses[105–111]. AChR-reactive T cell lines or clones have been isolated from peripheral blood lymphocytes, or more efficiently from thymuses, of myasthenic patients[112], and have been propagated *in vitro*. These T cells are $CD4^+$ $CD8^-$ (helpers), and MHC restricted (see reference 113). Depletion of $CD8^+$ (cytotoxic/suppressor) T cells has been reported to enhance the responsiveness of peripheral blood lymphocytes[108]. Although proliferation responses to AChR are more readily obtained from myasthenic patients' T cells, it is important to note that lymphocytes from normal individuals can also respond to AChR[111]. This observation supports the concept that potentially autoreactive T cells can exist in the normal immune system.

Much work has been done to determine the response patterns of T cells in MG. In general, $CD4^+$ T cells respond to enzymatically degraded, or 'processed' antigens, in the context of self MHC class II antigens[114]. MHC class II molecules contain a groove that accommodates linear peptides approximately 15–20 amino acids in length[115]. The specific MHC molecule plays an important part in determining which peptides can be bound, and therefore presented. The T cell receptor (TCR) 'sees' the peptide only in the context of the appropriate self MHC class II molecule. Analysis of T cells from myasthenic patients has revealed striking heterogeneity in their patterns of responsiveness. Not only do each individual's cells respond to multiple epitopes, but there are significant differences in the epitopes to which different individuals respond[105–110,116–118]. Although the majority of T cell recognition sites are on the α-subunit, T cells also recognize epitopes on the other subunits. Moiola *et al.* identified more than 30 AChR-derived peptides to which myasthenic patients' T cells respond[119]. The over-representation of α-subunit recognition is not yet explained, but may be due to the presence of two α-subunits per AChR molecule. The T cells do not appear to recognize most B cell epitopes, including the MIR. This is consistent with the concept of 'complementarity', i.e. B cells and T cells recognize non-overlapping epitopes[120]. Attempts to identify increased use of specific T cell receptors, by Southern blot analysis of TCR genes or using TCR-specific Mabs, has thus far yielded conflicting results[121,122].

In summary, the present evidence strongly suggests that the T cell response to AChR is highly heterogeneous. This heterogeneity may greatly complicate efforts to design specific immunotherapeutic approaches aimed at AChR-responsive T cells, unless only restricted subpopulations of the T cells are found to be clinically important.

ORIGIN OF THE AUTOIMMUNE RESPONSE IN MG: POSSIBLE ROLE OF THE THYMUS

One of the unsolved problems in MG, as in other spontaneously occurring autoimmune diseases of man, concerns the origin of the autoimmune response. The pathological changes in the thymus glands of patients with MG and the favourable results of thymectomy first suggested the possibility that the thymus may play a role in initiating the autoimmune response. Approximately 75% of myasthenic patients have thymic abnormalities. Of these, 85% show germinal centre formation ('hyperplasia'), and thymomas are found in approximately 15%[123]. Surgical thymectomy results in clinical remission in approximately 35% of patients, with improvement in another 50%[124] (reviewed in reference 125).

Several other features of the myasthenic thymus support its possible role in the immune pathogenesis of MG. T cells obtained from thymus glands of myasthenic patients are more responsive to AChR than are T cells derived from peripheral blood[112]. Myasthenic thymus glands contain an increased proportion of B cells, and exhibit increased production of antibodies, especially those directed against AChR[126–128]. In addition to lymphocytes, the thymus gland contains cells of other types, including muscle-like, or 'myoid' cells[129]. Typical muscle cells, presumably derived from the myoid cell population, have been cultured from thymus glands of myasthenic patients and from thymuses of normal rats[130,131]. They are striated and multinucleated, and express surface AChRs[131]. The myoid cells are thought to be the source of AChR and of mRNA for the α-subunit of AChR found in thymic extracts[131,132]. *In situ*, myoid cells may be located in association with $CD4^+$ T cells and interdigitating cells[133]. Because of their strategic location within the thymus, in apposition to immunocompetent cells, the AChR-bearing myoid cells may be particularly vulnerable to immune attack. Some alteration of the muscle cells or the lymphocytes, or a breach of immunoregulation, may serve to break tolerance, and thereby lead to an immune attack directed against AChRs, as well as other components of skeletal muscles. The fact that 'anti-striational' antibodies are also present in sera of a majority of MG patients further suggests that the myoid cells or other intact skeletal muscle cells may serve as the antigenic stimulus in MG, rather than some alternative source of isolated AChR or even AChR-like epitopes. On the other hand, thymomas have not been found to contain either myoid cells or AChR[134]. The discovery that thymomas in myasthenic patients contain a single 10 amino acid epitope of the AChR α-subunit, located on an unrelated polypeptide, has led to the suggestion that it might trigger an autoimmune response in these individuals[134,135], eventually generalizing to involve the AChR. The possibility that a viral infection of the thymus could trigger the autoimmune response has been suggested[136], but detailed studies of the thymus glands of patients with recent onset MG failed to yield evidence of viral infection[137].

The hypothesis that the autoimmune response to AChR may be initiated as a result of 'molecular mimicry' has acquired some support[138–140]. According to this concept, the immune response to an infectious agent with an epitope that mimics an epitope of AChR may set in motion the autoimmune response to AChR. A sequence of the α-subunit of human AChR[139] has significant homology with a sequence of the herpes simplex virus (HSV). Sera from six of 40 MG patients tested recognized this α-subunit sequence, and cross-reacted with the HSV sequence[139]. Bacterial cross-reactivity with AChR has also been noted: monoclonal antibodies raised to AChR have been shown to cross-react with epitopes of various bacteria[140]. Whether these findings provide a link between an apparently unrelated infection and an autoimmune disease, or merely reflect non-uniqueness of the epitopes, or promiscuity of the antibodies, remains to be determined.

Abnormalities of immune regulation may play a role in the development and maintenance of MG. A wide variety of other autoimmune diseases have been reported in association with MG, including Hashimoto's thyroiditis, Graves' disease, pernicious anaemia, rheumatoid arthritis, polymyositis, lupus erythematosus, pemphigus, Lambert–Eaton myasthenic syndrome, idiopathic thrombocytopenic purpura, vitiligo and alopecia areata[141–143]. The association of MG with these autoimmune diseases in some patients, and in some of their family members, supports the concept of a defect in immune regulation, and further suggests that there may be a heritable component to this defect.

Other genetic factors may also predispose to MG. There is a consistent, but only moderate, association of MG with the HLA antigens B8 and DR3, particularly in young females with thymic hyperplasia[144,145], while a stronger association with DQW2 is somewhat controversial[145,146].

Certain intriguing clues that may eventually help to understand the origin of MG have been reported. In some cases, the use of penicillamine to treat other diseases results in the development of MG. Unlike spontaneous MG, the clinical, serological, and neuromuscular abnormalities recover after discontinuation of the drug[147,148]. It has been suggested that penicillamine binds to AChR, and may thereby render it immunogenic[149]. In addition, a proportion of patients who receive bone marrow transplants subsequently develop MG in association with graft versus host disease[150].

In summary, many gaps remain in the present understanding of the origin of the autoimmune response and the complex role of the thymus gland in MG.

CLINICAL FEATURES AND DIAGNOSIS OF MG

The prevalence of MG is approximately 4–6/100 000 population[151]. The incidence is age- and sex-related, with two peaks: one in the second and third decade, mostly women, and one in the sixth and seventh decade, mostly men. Because it is a disease of the nicotinic AChR, only the motor system is impaired. The cardinal features are weakness and fatigability of skeletal muscles. Sensation, reflexes, cognition, and other neural functions remain normal. The clinical severity is usually graded functionally and regionally according to modifications of the Osserman[57,77,152] scale: grade I (focal, e.g. ocular), grade II (mild, generalized), grade III (severe, generalized), and grade IV (crisis, i.e. life-endangering impairment of respiration and swallowing).

Since treatment of MG often involves a lifetime commitment between patient and neurologist, it is essential to establish the diagnosis unequivocally. The history includes weakness, usually in a characteristic distribution involving the elevators of the eyelids and extraocular muscles (ptosis and diplopia), and frequently affecting the neck extensors (head drooping) and proximal limb muscles. When the muscles of expression, phonation, articulation, and chewing are affected, there may be a characteristic facial 'snarl', nasal dysarthric speech, and the need to prop the jaw closed. There is usually a history of fluctuation and fatigability (worse with repeated activity, improved by rest). If the weakness occurs in a vague and variable pattern, it may be misinterpreted as having a psychogenic origin.

In women, weakness may worsen in relation to the menstrual cycle. Transient weakness of infants born to myasthenic mothers may be reported. The effects of previous treatment attempts may be revealing.

On physical examination, the findings are limited exclusively to the motor system, without loss of reflexes or alteration of sensation or coordination. A survey of motor power should document the patient's baseline strength quantitatively, to allow later evaluation of the results of treatment. The deltoids, triceps, and iliopsoas are the most frequently involved limb muscles. The most useful quantitative measures include timed forward arm abduction, vital capacity, and dynamometry of selected muscles and grip.

Diagnostic testing

Confirmatory laboratory testing is essential prior to immunotherapy, and may be approached in the following order.

(1) Anti-cholinesterase test. Drugs that inhibit the enzyme acetylcholinesterase (AChE) allow ACh to interact repeatedly with the limited number of AChRs, producing improvement in the strength of myasthenic muscles. Edrophonium (Tensilon®) is commonly used because of the rapid onset (30 s) and short duration (about 5 min) of its effect. The strength of objectively weak muscles should be used to evaluate the effects of edrophonium. An initial dose of 2 mg is given intravenously. If definite improvement occurs, the test is considered positive and terminated. If there is no change, the patient is given an additional 8 mg. As an alternative, 1 mg of neostigmine can be given by intramuscular injection, which allows for about 30 min of observation.

(2) Repetitive nerve stimulation. It is best to test weak muscles, or proximal muscle groups. Electric shocks are delivered at a rate of 3–5/s to the appropriate nerves, and action potentials are recorded from the muscles. A rapid reduction in the amplitude of evoked muscle action potentials (decremental response of 10–15%) is considered positive[153].

(3) Anti-AChR antibody assay. The raioimmunoassay using human AChR labelled with $[^{125}I]\alpha$-BuTx is the standard test[48].

(4) Single-fibre EMG. Increased 'jitter' and 'blocking' with normal fibre density is considered positive[154,155].

The edrophonium test and repetitive nerve stimulation are the least sensitive and specific of the tests. The presence of anti-AChR binding antibodies is specific for MG, but antibodies are detectable in only about 85% of all MG patients, and in approximately 50% of patients with weakness confined to the ocular muscles[156]. Special assays are also available to measure antibodies that produce AChR blocking of the ACh binding site of the receptor and modulation (accelerated degradation) of the AChR[55,57,65–67]. Single fibre EMG is a highly sensitive test, positive in 88–99% of patients[155], but is limited in its specificity for MG.

CT or MRI scan of the mediastinum should be obtained to search for a tumour or enlargement of the thymus. Other laboratory tests should include evaluation of thyroid function, spirometry, and fasting blood glucose. Conditions that may exacerbate MG include hyperthyroidism, hypothyroidism, occult infection, and certain medications (including but not limited to anti-arrhythmic agents and aminoglycoside antibiotics). Penicillamine[147–149], used for the treatment of scleroderma, rheumatoid arthritis and Wilson's disease, may result in true autoimmune MG, but recovery occurs within weeks or months after discontinuing its use[147–149]. Disorders that may interfere with immunosuppressive therapy include tuberculosis (a skin test should always precede any proposed immunotherapy), other chronic infections, diabetes, peptic ulcer, occult GI bleeding, and hypertension.

It is important to screen for other autoimmune disorders often linked with MG (see above): these may add to the diagnostic picture of immune dysregulation and may complicate therapy.

TREATMENT

The prognosis for myasthenic patients has improved strikingly as a result of advances in treatment; most myasthenic patients can be returned to full productive lives with proper therapy. The most important methods used currently in the treatment of MG include anti-cholinesterase agents, thymectomy, immunosuppressive drugs, and plasmapheresis.

Anti-cholinesterase agents

Anti-cholinesterase agents continue to be used as the first line of treatment for most patients with MG. They prolong the action of acetylcholine released at the neuromuscular junction, thereby enhancing neuromuscular transmission. Pyridostigmine bromide is the most widely used drug. Its action begins within 10–30 min, reaches a peak at about 2 h, and declines gradually thereafter. The initial dose is usually 60 mg every 4 h during the day. The dosage schedule is then readjusted on the basis of the patient's recorded evaluations. A sustained release preparation containing 180 mg of pyridostigmine is available, but should be used only at bedtime, and only if the patient otherwise experiences weakness at night or in the early morning. The maximum useful dosage of pyridostigmine rarely exceeds 120 mg every 3 h.

Anti-cholineserase treatment is generally safe, though it should be used with care in patients with asthma or cardiac conduction defects. The most common side-effect is diarrhoea, which can be controlled with such agents as diphenoxylate hydrochloride, atropine or glycopyrrolate taken once or twice a day. Excessive amounts of anti-cholinesterases may cause increased weakness that is reversible after decreasing or discontinuing treatment.

Although anti-cholinesterases benefit most patients, the improvement is often incomplete. Most patients will therefore require further therapeutic measures.

Thymectomy

Thymectomy has been advocated empirically for more than half a century[157], even before the key role of the thymus in the origin and perpetuation of immune dysregulation in MG was appreciated. Thymoma is a universally accepted indication for surgery, since these tumours may spread locally and become invasive, though they rarely metastasize. If complete removal of the tumour is not possible, postoperative radiation should be carried out. Some patients become weaker after thymomectomy and require immunosuppressive therapy.

Regardless of whether the thymus gland is enlarged, thymectomy is indicated in all patients with generalized MG between puberty and about age 50, in whom a satisfactory response has not been obtained with anti-cholinesterase medication alone[158,159]. The available evidence suggests that up to 85% of patients improve after thymectomy, and of these, about 35% may achieve drug-free remission[124]. However, benefit from thymectomy is delayed, rarely occurring within 6 months and requiring up to 2–5 years for demonstrated efficacy[124,160,161]. The risks of surgery include injury to the phrenic or recurrent laryngeal nerves, atelectasis, pleural effusion, pneumonia, myasthenic crisis, intercurrent pulmonary embolism, impaired wound healing, and later sternal instability[162]. Thymectomy should, therefore, always be carried out in an institution where this procedure is performed regularly, and where the staff is experienced in the pre- and postoperative management, anaesthesia, and surgical techniques of thymectomy. Preoperative preparation should optimize the patient's strength, but immunosuppressive agents should be avoided if possible because of the risks of infection, and corticosteroids should be avoided because of the additional impairment of wound healing. In patients with significant respiratory impairment or bulbar muscle dysfunction, plasmapheresis before surgery provides temporary improvement.

The optimal surgical technique is a 'maximal' trans-sternal approach designed to remove as much thymus tissue as possible[163]. The anterior mediastinum and the adjacent space extending up to the neck should be explored, and all the thymic tissue and related fat removed. Postoperatively, the patient should be cared for in an intensive care unit, where intravenous anti-cholinesterase medication can be given as necessary, and respiratory care can be optimized.

Table 7.2 Standard immunotherapy in myasthenia gravis

Drug	*Usual adult dose*	*Time to onset of improvement*	*Time to maximal improvement*	*Toxicity monitoring*
Prednisone	Gradually ascending to 60 mg q.d. orally followed by q.o.d. regimen	2–3 weeks	3–6 months	Weight Blood pressure Fasting blood glucose Electrolytes Ophthalmic examination Bone density 24 h urine Ca 25-OH vitamin D (especially in postmenopausal women)
Cyclosporin (Sandimmune)	5 mg/kg/day orally, divided b.i.d. (125–200 mg b.i.d.)	2–12 weeks	3–6 months	BP Serum creatinine Blood urea nitrogen Cyclosporin level, 12 h trough by RIA Amylase Cholesterol
Azathioprine (Imuran)	2–3 mg/kg/day orally (100–250 mg daily)	3–12 months	1–2 years	WBC (> 3500) and Differential (< 1000 lymphocytes) MCV Platelets Liver function tests Amylase

Immunosuppressive agents

Prednisone, azathioprine, and cyclosporin are now considered first line drugs for chronic immunosuppressive therapy in MG. A comparison of these drugs is outlined in Table 7.2.

Corticosteroids in MG

Mechanisms

Corticosteroids have been a mainstay of therapy in MG for more than 20 years. Though their effects are legion, the details of their mechanisms of action in MG are not fully known. The immunosuppressive effects of corticosteroids in MG could occur through several of the various known effects on immunocompetent cells[164].

(1) Corticosteroids induce lymphocytopenia by redistributing lymphocytes out of circulation into other compartments less accessible to sites of immunoreactivity.
(2) Corticosteroids reduce differentiation and proliferation of lymphocytes (reviewed in reference 165). Both mechanisms 1 and 2 affect T lymphocytes more than B lymphocytes and plasma cells[166].
(3) Perhaps most important in an autoimmune disease such as MG,

corticosteroids disrupt the intercellular communication among leukocytes through interference with the production or function of numerous lymphokines, especially interleukin-1 (IL-1), interleukin-2 (IL-2), tumour necrosis factor, and migration-inhibitory factor (MIF)[164,167–169]. These actions inhibit the recruitment of leukocytes and macrophages in an immune response.

(4) Corticosteroids inhibit many functions of macrophages, including elaboration of IL-1 (hence all the downstream effects of IL-1 on lymphocytes)[170], the action of MIF (hence promoting the egress of macrophages)[168], and phagocytosis, and the presentation of antigen that is facilitated by interferon-γ[171,172]. Thus, in all these ways, not only cell number but phagocytosis, migration, antigen processing presentation, and all aspects of the inflammatory response are affected.

Besides having immunosuppressive effects, corticosteroids may have other direct beneficial effects in MG. Experimentally, certain direct actions on muscle and neuromuscular transmission have been reported, including an increase in the synthesis of AChR in cell culture[173,174] and enhancement of neuromuscular transmission[175,176].

Pharmacokinetics

Many of the immunosuppressive effects of corticosteroids may last far longer than their suppression of ACTH secretion by the pituitary. This allows the use of alternate-day therapy in MG. If the drug is administered in a single dose in the morning at a time when the normal endogenous cortisol level would peak, it would no longer be present in the circulation by evening, and the hypothalamus–pituitary–adrenal axis would secrete ACTH. This, in turn, will stimulate secretion of endogenous cortisol the next morning, when the patient depends not on exogenous hormone but on homeostatic maintenance on the 'off' day. The longer immunosuppressive effect maintains disease control, while the single alternate-morning dose schedule mimics the normal diurnal cortisol cycle, reduces side-effects, and facilitates eventual tapering of the total dose.

Indications for corticosteroids

Corticosteroids are indicated when either generalized MG or ocular symptoms are not adequately controlled by cholinesterase inhibitors, and are sufficiently disabling to the patient that they outweigh the risks of possible side-effects of these drugs. Corticosteroids can produce improvement in patients with all degrees of weakness, from localized ocular involvement to severe respiratory insufficiency. Diplopia, which is rarely corrected by anticholinesterase agents alone, usually responds well to steroid treatment. Older men with MG seem to respond particularly well to steroid therapy[177].

Relative contraindications to steroid treatment include severe obesity, poorly controlled diabetes mellitus, uncontrolled hypertension, ulcer disease, osteoporosis, or ongoing infection. These problems can usually be circumvented by appropriate medical measures. Long-term treatment with steroids requires medical attention by an experienced physician; patients who are unable or unwilling to be followed medically should never be treated with steroids.

Induction

Prior to initiation of steroid therapy, anti-cholinesterase medication should be adjusted optimally. Patients with moderate to severe generalized weakness should be admitted to hospital for initiation of prednisone therapy because of the risk of transient steroid-induced exacerbation, which occurs during the first week of treatment in up to 48% of patients[178]. The cause of this initial steroid-induced deterioration is not clear.

In order to minimize the risk of exacerbation, we recommend a gradually increasing dosage schedule[179], beginning with 15–20 mg/day and increasing gradually by about 5 mg every 2 or 3 days, until the patient attains a satisfactory clinical response or reaches the level of 50–60 mg/day. The rate of increase must not be decided in advance, but should be guided by the patient's clinical response. Only if the patient is already on a ventilator is a high dose appropriate initially. Several other induction schemes have been advocated, although we find none of them satisfactory from the point of view of safety or speed of induction[180–187].

More than 80% of myasthenic patients can be expected to improve with steroid treatment alone[178]; the clinical effect usually begins within 2–4 weeks, occasionally longer, though maximal benefit may not be realized until 6–12 months or more.

Maintenance

The goal of maintenance steroid therapy is to achieve optimal control of myasthenic weakness, while minimizing the toxic side-effects of steroids. The high daily dose of prednisone is maintained for about 3 months, and is then gradually modified to an alternate-day regimen, so as to minimize side-effects. Eventually, an alternate-day regimen is established in most patients; occasionally a small dose of prednisone must be given on the 'off' day to prevent fluctuations in strength. When the patient reaches a plateau of improvement on an alternate-day regimen, the total dose is tapered gradually, but months or years may be needed to determine the minimum effective dose, and close monitoring is required by patient and doctor. Few patients are able to do without prednisone entirely.

Patients on long-term glucocorticoid therapy must be carefully followed to prevent or treat adverse side-effects. The list of side-effects of chronic steroid therapy is unfortunately long (Table 7.3). While not every patient develops every symptom, most patients will have some side-effects. Fortunately, many of these problems can be prevented or treated effectively with the use of alternate-day therapy and with scrupulous attention to follow-up. Close monitoring of chronically treated patients is therefore mandatory.

Table 7.3 Side effects of corticosteroid treatment

Obesity
Abnormal truncal fat distribution with moon facies, buffalo hump, and thinning of extremities
Impaired glucose tolerance; frank diabetes mellitus
Hypertension
Hypokalaemia
Sodium retention with oedema
Adrenal suppression
Growth retardation in children
Osteoporosis and vertebral compression fractures, especially in postmenopausal women
Avascular necrosis of bone, especially femoral head
Steroid 'myopathy' (atrophy)
Behavioural and affective changes; nervousness, irritability, moodiness, insomnia, depression: steroid psychosis
Pseudotumour cerebri
Peptic ulcer
Skin striae, friability, and ecchymoses
Impaired wound healing
Acne
Facial hirsutism
Posterior subcapsular cataracts
Glaucoma
Herpes zoster and other opportunistic infections

Use of azathioprine in MG

Pharmacology

Since a completely intact immune response requires antigen processing and presentation (dependent in part on RNA synthesis) as well as proliferation and differentiation of immunocompetent cells (dependent on DNA and RNA synthesis), purine analogues such as azathioprine and mercaptopurine can interrupt the immune response potently at multiple sites[165]. A tight relationship exists between azathioprine dose and its biological effects on dividing cells such as lymphoid and erythroid cells. Leukopenia and macrocytosis occur predictably and are monitored as guides to azathioprine dosage[188].

Pharmacokinetics

Azathioprine is actually a precursor that is cleaved *in vivo* to active 6-mercaptopurine. Blood levels are of no predictive value for therapy since the magnitude of clinical effects correlates with thioprine nucleotide levels in tissues rather than with plasma drug levels. The drug is extensively oxidized and methylated in red blood cells and liver. Concurrent administration of allopurinol (for treatment of gout) can increase the toxicity of azathioprine by interfering with its metabolism by xanthine oxidase, an important degradative pathway. Azathioprine dosage must be reduced by as much as 75% in patients who take allopurinol.

Indications

The manner in which azathioprine is used often derives from its chief disadvantage – beneficial effects may take 6 months or more to appear. It therefore tends to be used as additional therapy in patients whose myasthenia has not been adequately controlled by thymectomy and corticosteroids. However, based on European experience, azathioprine may be used effectively as initial therapy in MG, either alone or in combination with corticosteroids[189,190]. The combination affords the relatively rapid onset of immunosuppression produced by the steroids, and allows prompt tapering of corticosteroids once the azathioprine has had time to take effect[189,191]. The addition of azathioprine also allows a reduction of steroid dosage in patients with otherwise well-controlled disease who show excessive toxic effects of prednisone, or who require a chronic maintenance dose of prednisone of more than about 50 mg on alternate days.

Contraindications

Patients who are unable or unwilling to be followed medically should never be treated with azathioprine. Approximately 10% of patients are unable to tolerate azathioprine because of an idiosyncratic reaction consisting of flu-like symptoms of fever and myalgia, bone marrow depression, or abnormalities of liver function. The question of a slightly increased risk of malignancy in azathioprine-treated patients has not been resolved; experience with azathioprine in organ transplantation suggests an increased risk of malignancy. However, patients with myasthenia or rheumatoid arthritis have been treated for years with the drug, and no increase in the incidence of malignancies has been found[190,192,193].

Induction

The usual target dose of azathioprine is 2–3 mg/kg/day. A test dose of approximately 50 mg/day should be given for the first week. If this is well tolerated, the dose should be gradually raised by 50 mg each week, while the white blood cell count (WBC), differential count, platelets, and liver function tests are monitored closely. To establish the optimum dose, several end-points may be used. A total WBC of 3000–4000/mm^3 is a safe end-point. Azathioprine should be briefly discontinued if the WBC falls below 2500/mm^3 or the absolute neutrophil count is less than 1000/mm^3, then reintroduced at a lower dose. This measure cannot be used in patients receiving prednisone, because of steroid-induced leukocytosis. In that situation, an absolute lymphocyte count of <1000 is the appropriate target. A rise in the RBC mean corpuscular volume to above 100 also provides a useful gauge of biological activity, and in MG usually correlates with clinical improvement[188], but macrocytosis does not require discontinuation of therapy.

It is important to realize that in obese patients, the optimum dose of azathioprine depends on the total body weight, not on lean body weight.

Maintenance

An adequate therapeutic trial of azathioprine as sole therapy must last at least 1–2 years, since the lag to onset of effect may range from 3 to 12 months, and the point of maximum benefit may be delayed until 1–3 years. While azathioprine is decidedly slow to act, it is well tolerated by most patients. Close monitoring for toxicity should continue indefinitely, and patients should be seen at a minimum of every 3 months after a stable, non-toxic dose is reached. Although most myasthenic patients require life-long immunosuppression, it is worth attempting to taper azathioprine to establish a minimum effective dose. Because of the slow onset of the drug's effect, tapering of azathioprine must also be carried out gradually, with close monitoring of both neurological status and anti-AChR antibody titre. A doubling of the titre (optimally sera from two different dates measured in simultaneous assay) may predict clinical relapse[194].

Based on European experience with the drug as sole therapy[195], only a minority of myasthenic patients remain in remission after discontinuation of azathioprine[189,194]: close and continued follow-up is necessary after therapy is stopped.

Toxicity[196,197]

As with other immunosuppressive agents, azathioprine increases susceptibility to opportunistic infections, which should be treated promptly and vigorously. The haematological toxicity discussed above – leukopenia, anaemia, and thrombocytopenia – are all reversible upon reduction of the dose of azathioprine. Hepatic toxicity, with mild elevation of transaminases, is common, and responds to lowering the dose. A rise in transaminase levels up to 2-fold is usually well tolerated by patients. Gastrointestinal discomfort, with nausea and anorexia, is usually mild, and responds to the use of divided doses taken after meals.

Cyclosporin in MG

Mechanisms

Cyclosporin, a fungus-derived cyclic peptide with potent immunosuppressive activity, found its first major role in preventing transplant rejection. The drug inhibits the activation of helper inducer ($CD4^+$) T cells[198,199], and their production of IL-2[200,201]. It was first shown to be applicable to myasthenia in an experimental model[202], and has been used increasingly in the treatment of myasthenic patients[203–206]. Its therapeutic effect in MG may be explained by interference with helper T cells, which are necessary for the activation of B cells and production of anti-AChR antibodies. This relatively selective immunomodulatory action contrasts with the broad-spectrum effects of corticosteroids, azathioprine, and cyclophosphamide. Unlike cytotoxic immunosuppressants, cyclosporin does not cause generalized myelosuppression, thereby limiting the risk of opportunistic infections.

Pharmacokinetics and drug interactions

Cyclosporin reaches peak plasma concentrations within 3–4 h after ingestion. The drug has a large volume of distribution and is sequestered in tissues. It is cleared from blood with a half-time of about 19 h. Most of the drug is metabolized in the liver and excreted in the bile. This accounts for its ability to potentiate greatly the risk of necrotizing myopathy or myoglobinuria due to lovastatin, which also depends on biliary excretion. Because cytochrome P_{450}-mediated oxidation of the drug is extensive, hepatic dysfunction or concomitant administration of agents that affect the cytochrome P_{450} system can cause dramatic changes in the elimination of cyclosporin. Cyclosporin's independent mechanism of action produces an effect that is additive to that of corticosteroids. Because of evidence that the combination of cyclosporin with azathioprine and prednisone for suppression of organ rejection increases the risk of malignancies and infectious complications[207], most centres prefer to use only prednisone in combination with cyclosporin. It should be noted that corticosteroids increase plasma cyclosporin levels.

Indications

Cyclosporin is the only drug that has been shown to be effective for the treatment of MG in a prospective double-blinded, randomized, placebo-controlled trial[206]. Improvement began at about 2 weeks, with maximal improvement by 4 months, correlating with a reduction in anti-AChR antibody levels. Although that original trial was small and limited, reported experience with the drug in open trials for MG has also been generally positive[203,204], and a large multicentre controlled trial has been completed and awaits publication. The efficacy of cyclosporin is similar to that of azathioprine[205] but it has the advantage of a more prompt effect, usually occurring within weeks[203–206].

The most prominent side-effects of cyclosporin are nephrotoxicity[208] and hypertension. It should therefore only be used with great caution in patients with pre-existing uncontrolled hypertension or significant renal disease. There is an increased risk of nephrotoxicity in elderly patients. Other side-effects include facial hirsutism, gastrointestinal disturbance, headache, tremor, convulsions, and rarely hepatotoxicity. As with other immunosuppressive agents, there is a possible increase in the long-term risk of malignancy.

Induction

The efficacy of cyclosporin relates to the lowest ('trough') plasma levels, while toxicity depends on peak concentrations. Therefore, the drug is given in a divided dosage schedule, twice a day. Because it is lipid soluble and variably absorbed, cyclosporin should be taken with a fat-containing meal or snack. The initial dose is 2.5 mg/kg twice a day.

Maintenance

Although the dose is eventually guided by clinical efficacy, it is initially adjusted by monitoring plasma cyclosporin levels and side-effects. Plasma levels should be measured every 2 weeks until stable, and then approximately monthly. Trough levels are measured in the morning, 12–14 h after the last dose. The reported levels depend on the method of assay; using the RIA, with a specific monoclonal antibody, the trough level should be maintained between 100 and 200 ng/ml. The blood pressure, serum creatinine and blood urea nitrogen levels are monitored, and the dose of cyclosporin is decreased if the creatinine level rises above 1.4 times the baseline level.

With close attention to management, cyclosporin can be used safely in nearly 90% of patients[209].

Cyclophosphamide in MG

Because of its potential toxicity, cyclophosphamide is reserved for rare patients with severe myasthenia unresponsive to or intolerant of other therapies. Published experience with its use in MG is limited[210–212]. Cyclophosphamide is an alkylating agent and therefore selectively interferes with rapidly proliferating cells, including B and T cells. Synthesis of pathogenic antibodies is decreased. The drug may be given orally or intravenously as monthly pulses for rapid induction or as a daily dose regimen[210]. The reported response rates of up to 80–90% are difficult to evaluate, because in most series the patients were unusually difficult to treat and were receiving multiple concomitant immunotherapies. Most authorities recommend a dose of 2.5–3.0 mg/kg/day, adjusted to maintain a WBC of 2500–4000/mm^3 and a relative lymphocyte count of $<10\%$.

Toxicity is substantial. Myelosuppression may result in leukopenia, anaemia and thrombocytopenia. Anorexia, nausea and vomiting are frequent, probably due to direct effects on the brainstem of the metabolite, phosphoramide mustard. Infertility, diarrhoea, stomatitis, and alopecia result from the alkylation effects in rapidly turning over tissues. The drug is also teratogenic.

Haemorrhagic cystitis is a side-effect unique to cyclophosphamide which can usually be prevented by ensuring adequate urinary output. It should be monitored by frequent urinalysis. As with all immunosuppressive drugs, the risk of cancer is increased (haematological, skin, bladder); in the case of cyclophosphamide the risk appears to increase significantly with duration of treatment, and with cumulative doses over 85 g[213].

Short-term immunotherapies: plasma exchange and human immune globulin

Plasma exchange

Plasma exchange, which depletes circulating antibodies, can produce short-term improvement in patients with symptomatic MG. Several uncontrolled trials, as well as long experience, have proved its effectiveness[214–218]. Plasma exchange is now used primarily to stabilize patients in myasthenic crisis or for short-term management of patients undergoing thymectomy, in order to avoid use of corticosteroids and immunosuppressants. Less commonly, it is used as adjuvant therapy in severely ill patients who are slow to respond to immunosuppressants. Repeated plasma exchange as a chronic form of therapy, because the patient is either intolerant or unresponsive to conventional immunosuppressant treatment, is rarely indicated. Plasma exchange works rapidly, with objective improvement measurable within days of treatment. Improvement (in the individual patient) correlates roughly with reduction in anti-AChR antibody titres[215]. The beneficial effects of plasma exchange are temporary, lasting only days to weeks, unless concomitant immunosuppressive agents are used[219]. Even patients with initially undetectable anti-AChR binding antibody may improve after plasma exchange[94,97,220,221].

Many protocols for plasma exchange have been advocated[215,218,222,223]. Five exchange treatments of 3–4 l each, over a 2-week period, is a typical programme at our institution. In centres with adequate experience, plasma exchange is safe. The vital signs as well as serum concentration of potassium, calcium and magnesium should be monitored. The major risks are due to problems of vascular access: blood flow from peripheral veins is frequently insufficient for processing by modern high-volume haemapheresis machines, and indwelling catheters in large veins are used. This can cause infection, thrombosis, perforation and even pneumothorax[224]. Sepsis, arrhythmia, anaphylactic shock, pulmonary embolism, and systemic haemorrhage from disseminated intravascular coagulation, among other hazards, have also been reported. The benefit of plasma exchange must be weighed against problems of vascular access, the risks of pheresis, and the high cost of the procedure.

Intravenous human immune globulin

The indications for use of intravenous human immune globulin (HIG) are the same as those for plasma exchange, i.e. to produce rapid improvement in a patient suffering a difficult period of myasthenic weakness. The largest review of the efficacy of HIG[225] summarized eight independent studies of 60 patients and reported overall improvement in 73%, but this figure is likely to be biased by the selective reporting of positive uncontrolled trials. The usual dose is 400 mg/kg/day on each of 5 consecutive days. When patients respond, the onset of improvement is within 4–5 days and the maximal response occurs within 1–2 weeks of initiation of HIG. The effect is transient but may be sustained for weeks to months, allowing intermittent chronic therapy. The mechanism of action of HIG in MG is not known, but it has no consistent effect on the measurable amount of AChR antibody *in vivo* or *in vitro*. Possible mechanisms that have been suggested to explain the immunomodulatory action of HIG include blockade of Fc receptors on macrophages and other cells and inhibition of the immune response to AChR by specific anti-idiotypic antibodies in the HIG pool[226].

Adverse reactions occur in fewer than 10% of patients and are generally mild; they include allergy, headache, fluid overload, various gastrointestinal symptoms and, rarely, renal shutdown. The process of preparation of HIG has been shown to inactivate human immunodeficiency virus and hepatitis B. HIG is very expensive, and this factor as well as the possible risks should be carefully weighed against the potential of rapid benefit[227].

Comparisons and current immunotherapy

Each of the available treatment options has its own advantages and disadvantages. Prednisone generally acts rapidly, is tried and true, but is beset by the problems of prevention and treatment of side-effects. Azathioprine is safe and moderately effective, but slow. Cyclosporin is about equal to azathioprine in effectiveness; it is rapid in onset, but expensive to use. Cyclophosphamide is potent but highly toxic, and is therefore reserved for special cases. Plasmapheresis or intravenous immunoglobulin are often useful for the short-term management of acute problems, or as pre- or postoperative therapy. However, the effects of both are transient, and their costs are extremely high. The therapeutic armamentarium now available provides a broad spectrum of effective treatment modalities. However, more specific and long-lasting treatments are still needed.

SPECIFIC IMMUNOTHERAPY: EXPERIMENTAL APPROACHES

Ideally, the goal of therapy in MG should be to eliminate the autoimmune response to AChR specifically, without otherwise interfering with the immune system. The treatment should be non-toxic, and long-lasting or permanent. Indeed, the goal of achieving discrete control of a specific immune response has been considered the 'holy grail' of immunology. Given the detailed knowledge now available, it should be possible to design rational and specific therapy for MG: this could lead the way to treatment for a wide variety of other immune disorders.

Certain of the features of MG outlined above present important considerations in the design of therapeutic strategies, and are therefore recapitulated here:

(1) The pathogenesis of MG depends on antibody-dependent mechanisms. In this respect, MG differs from several cell-mediated autoimmune conditions for which novel therapeutic methods have recently been described, including thyroiditis, experimental allergic encephalomyelitis, and adjuvant arthritis. Approaches that specifically inhibit cellular responses do not necessarily inhibit antibody responses.
(2) The antibody response to AChR is T cell-dependent, as discussed above. This affords an important avenue for therapy.
(3) AChR is a highly immunogenic antigen. Perhaps because of this, immune responses to AChR may not be as amenable to certain therapeutic manoeuvres that are successful for less powerful antigens.
(4) Immune responses to AChR are highly heterogeneous. Therapeutic

strategies must take into account the broad range of specificities of both T cells and B cells.

In considering the entire arc of pathogenesis of MG, from antigen presentation to impairment of neuromuscular transmission, there is an astonishingly large number of sites at which therapeutic intervention can be applied. Table 7.4 outlines many possible approaches, arranged in more or less reverse order, starting at the neuromuscular junction and working backwards. Each of these approaches has either been used clinically or tested experimentally in EAMG or other autoimmune conditions, as referenced. The very length of the list attests to the fact that an ideal therapeutic strategy has yet to be devised. A few representative approaches will be summarized in this section.

Targeting B cells

Since B cells produce the pathogenic antibodies in MG, it seems logical to attempt to interrupt the disease process at this penultimate step. To do so requires targeting all the B cells that produce antibodies specific for AChR. As discussed above, both the AChR antibodies and the relevant B cells are highly heterogeneous. Since these B cells bear antibodies that act as surface receptors for various epitopes of AChR, they are therefore capable of binding AChR. If the AChR molecule is armed with a lethal 'warhead', the relevant B cells will bind and take up the lethal antigen, and be killed. Experimentally, immunotoxins composed of AChR and either the toxic A chain of ricin[228] or radioactive iodine[229] have been used successfully *in vitro* or in naïve animals. However, there are serious potential problems in applying this method to ongoing autoimmune diseases. In ongoing MG, precisely the same antibodies that serve as B cell receptors are present in the circulation. The AChR immunotoxin must therefore escape circulating antibodies. The immunotoxic molecules may be complexed by the antibodies, and the complexes precipitated in the lungs, liver or kidneys, without ever reaching their goal, but with the risk of producing damage to these organs. Further, even if the AChR-specific B cells were eliminated, the ability of B cell genes to mutate and rearrange allows for the appearance of new AChR-specific B cells, which can be up-regulated in response to antigenic stimulation, resulting in recurrence of MG. These problems would apply to virtually any strategy designed to target antigen-specific B cells in ongoing disease.

T cell-directed approaches

As noted above, T cells play a key role in the autoimmune response in MG, and T cells have certain characteristics that make them more favourable for therapeutic approaches. Their receptors recognize linear epitopes (in association with MHC class II)[114]; as a rule, T cell epitopes generally differ from B cell epitopes[120], permitting targeting of the relevant T cells, while minimizing the possibility of interception by circulating antibodies. Unlike

Table 7.4 Outline of current and future therapeutic interventions in myasthenia gravis

Neuromuscular junction	
Anti-cholinesterases	Prolong ACh–AChR interaction
3,4-Diaminopyridine	Increase ACh release[257]
3-Deazaadenosine (3DZA)	Decrease AChR turnover[258,259]
Antibody depletion	
Plasmapheresis	Semiselective pheresis; Preferential removal of AChR Ab; (polyvinyl alcohol with tryptophane)[260]
General immune treatment	
Thymectomy	
Adrenal corticosteroids	
Azathioprine	
Cyclosporin A[202–206]	
Cyclophosphamide	
Total lymphoid irradiation[261]	
Intravenous IG	
Unusual immunosuppressive agents tried	
Dimethylsulphoxide	Suppressive in EAMG[262]
Thalidomide	Used in bone marrow transplantation No benefit in EAMG[263]
Pristine immune system	
Cyclophosphamide + total body irradiation; bone marrow 'rescue'	Abolishes immune response to AChR, in EAMG[264]
Deplete AChR-specific B cells	
'Hot antigen suicide'	Effective in naïve animals, culture
*a) AChR + ricin A[228]	See text
*b) AChR + ^{125}I[265]	
Deplete T helper cells	
*Anti-CD4 Ab[230]	
*IL-2 toxin[236]	See text
Target antigen-specific T cells	
*T cell vaccination[240–246]	Effective in EAE; not EAMG; See text
*Immunize with TCR peptide(s)[248,249]	EAE; See text
*APCs used to target AChR-specific T cells[254]	
Specific suppression	
T suppressor cells[266,267]	
Large suppressor cells	Antigen-specific macrophages[268–270]
Antigen presenting cells	
Ab vs. MHC Class II[271]	
Ab vs. MHC Class II + peptide	EAE[272]
MHC-blocking peptide[273]	
Anti-idiotypic approach	Mixed results in EAMG[274–277]
Tolerance induction	
Deaggregated antigen[278]	
Route of administration	Oral, inhalation[279]
TLI + antigen	Effective for some antigens; not AChR[280]
Anti-CD4 + antigen	Effective for some antigens[281]
Antigen-coupled cells	Effective in EAMG[282]
?Tolerogenic fragment[283]	

*Discussed in text

B cells, T cell receptor genes do not undergo mutation, which obviates a potential source of resupply of pathogenic cells. Moreover, various surface markers on T cells can serve as semispecific 'addresses' for targeting. Finally, methods are now available for inactivating antigen-specific T cells (rendering them 'anergic'), which provides a powerful mechanism for silencing them.

Depletion of T helper cells

T helper (T_h) cells can be depleted or inactivated by injection of antibodies specific for the CD4 surface antigen[230,231], or the T cell receptor (CD3 antigen)[232]. These antibodies interfere with T_h cells indiscriminately, producing a general immunosuppressive effect. Further, an immune response to the injected antibodies may develop, precluding repeated treatment. Efforts to produce 'humanized' monoclonal antibodies to these epitopes should mitigate or eliminate this problem for clinical use.

Targeting activated T cells: IL-2 toxin

T cells involved in an active immune response express receptors for IL-2, while resting and memory T cells do not[233,234]. This property can be used to target activated T cells, including those involved in the immune response to AChR. A recently developed IL-2 toxin, produced by recombinant technology[235], has been used for this purpose[236]. This consists of the receptor-binding moiety of IL-2 and the cytotoxic portion of diphtheria toxin; it binds to cells bearing IL-2 receptors, is internalized by endocytosis, and irreversibly inhibits protein synthesis, resulting in death of the target T cell[237]. Experimentally, IL-2 toxin is extremely effective *in vitro* in inhibiting both AChR-driven T cell proliferation and anti-AChR antibody production[236]. However, treatment in live rats with IL-2 toxin is only moderately effective in preventing cellular and humoral immune responses to AChR; this is attributable to the fact that it is rapidly inactivated in the intact animal[238]. These findings suggest that a strategy aimed at IL-2 receptors of T cells can provide semiselective (although not antigen-specific) suppression of an active autoimmune response, but its effectiveness may depend on the use of an IL-2 toxin with more prolonged bioavailability *in vivo*[239].

Targeting antigen-specific T cell receptors

The principle underlying these strategies is that elimination or inactivation of T cells specific for the autoantigen should effectively treat the autoimmune disease. One approach, termed 'T cell vaccination', involves immunization with T cells activated to the particular antigen, in order to induce specific immunological unresponsiveness[240]. The inhibitory effect is believed to result from an immune response directed against the specific antigen receptors of the T cells used in the vaccination procedure[241]. This method has been used successfully to suppress immune responses to several cell-mediated experimental autoimmune disorders, including experimental allergic encephalomyelitis (EAE)[242], thyroiditis[243], adjuvant arthritis[244], and interstitial nephritis[245]. However, this approach was not successful in treating EAMG, an antibody-mediated disease[246]. Vaccination of Lewis rats with T cells sensitized to AChR produced an interesting dichotomous immune effect. The vaccination itself actually primed the rats, resulting in increased antibody production in response to a challenge with AChR. On the other hand, splenic lymphocytes from the vaccinated rats produced antigen-specific suppression *in vitro*. These observations indicate that vaccination with antigen-specific T cells can elicit both a positive antibody response and a suppressive cellular response in the same animal. These findings in EAMG are consistent with the results of T cell vaccination in autoimmune thyroiditis in mice[243]. Vaccination with T cell lines specific for thyroglobulin inhibited the development of thyroiditis, which is a cell-mediated condition, but did not inhibit the anti-thyroglobulin antibody response.

A more narrowly focused approach to targeting T cell receptors has been used in studies of EAE, where the antigen used to produce the disease is myelin basic protein (MBP). The logic is that if immunization with whole T cells can induce an inhibitory response against T cell receptors, then immunization with the relevant T cell receptors in pure form might also be effective. The key question is: how many T cell receptors, and which ones are relevant in a given autoimmune disease? In certain strains of rodents, the number of T cell receptors used in acute EAE appears to be relatively restricted[247,248]. Active immunization with the peptide moieties of the relevant T cell receptors has had a therapeutic effect in preventing or modifying experimental EAE in rats[248,249]. However, it must be emphasized that such an approach directed against identified T cell receptors requires that the receptor usage in the particular autoimmune disease must be markedly restricted. This requirement applies not only to the T cell repertoire of each individual, but also to the potential variation between individuals. In contrast to the restricted pattern of T cell responses in acute experimental autoimmune diseases in inbred strains of rodents, it appears that T cell responses are highly heterogeneous in chronic autoimmune diseases both in animals and in humans[250,251]. In particular, there is now abundant evidence in MG in humans and EAMG in rats that the epitopes of AChR to which T cells respond are highly heterogeneous[105–111,116–118,252] (see above). Since T cells recognize epitopes only in association with the appropriate self MHC class II antigens, this produces yet another level of heterogeneity[253]. Thus, targeting the repertoire of AChR-specific T cells of any individual patient, requires presentation of the entire spectrum of processed AChR peptides appropriate to that individual, in association with the proper MHC class II antigen. Unless some restrictive principle limits the spectrum of pathogenic peptides and MHC antigens, this is likely to be an extremely complex undertaking.

We have recently developed a method by which the individual's own antigen presenting cells (APCs) can be used for this purpose[254], since they process and present the antigen appropriately, and express the correct MHC class II antigen. A novel method of binding AChR to surface immunoglobulin with a heterobifunctional antibody conjugate[255] allows all B cells, regardless of their inherent specificity, to be used as ACPs for AChR[254]. If these APCs are 'fixed' with cross-linking reagents, they induce long-lasting or permanent anergy of the specific T cells with which they interact[254,256]. Experimentally, culture of these fixed AChR-presenting cells with AChR-specific T cells induced anergy. When restimulated with fresh APCs and AChR, the T cells showed markedly reduced proliferative responses and IL-2 production, compared with controls. This strategy represents an attempt to deal with the critical issue of heterogeneity of T cell responses, in designing specific therapy for MG.

CONCLUSIONS

Much has been learned during the past two decades about the pathogenesis, immunology and molecular biology of MG. The diagnosis and practical treatment are well defined and usually successful. Despite these impressive advances, there are still important gaps in our understanding of the origin of MG, the factors that contribute to its chronic maintenance, and how to 'cure' it. If progress continues at the present pace, MG should continue to lead in the field of autoimmunity, with the ultimate goal of specific therapy for the underlying disorder.

ACKNOWLEDGEMENTS

The original work in the manuscript was carried out with partial support from the National Institutes of Health #1RO1 NS23719, the Muscular Dystrophy Association and the Myashenia Gravis Foundation. We are grateful to Christine Fackler Salemi for her help in the preparation of the manuscript.

References

1. Willis T. De Anima Brutorum. Oxford: Theatro Sheldoniano, 1672:404–6.
2. Erb W. Zur casuistik der bulbaren lahmungen. Uber einen neuen wahrscheinlich bulbaren symptom-complex. Arch Psychiatr Nervenkr. 1879:336–50.
3. Campbell H, Bramwell E. Myasthenia gravis. Brain. 1900:277–336.
4. Walker MB. Treatment of myasthenia gravis with physostigmine. Lancet. 1934;1:1200–1.
5. Chang CE, Lee CY. Isolation of neurotoxins from the venom of *Bungarus multicinctus* and their modes of neuromuscular blocking action. Arch Pharmacodyn Ther. 1962;144:241–57.
6. Fambrough DM, Drachman DB, Satyamurti S. Neuromuscular junction in myasthenia gravis: Decreased acetylcholine receptors. Science. 1973;182:293–5.
7. Lindstrom J, Patrick J. Purification of the acetylcholine receptor by affinity. In: Bennett MVI, editor. Synaptic Transmission and Neuronal Interaction. New York: Raven Press, 1974:191–215.
8. Noda M, Furutani Y, Takahashi H, *et al.* Cloning and sequence analysis of calf cDNA and human genomic DNA encoding α-subunit precursor of muscle acetylcholine receptor. Nature. 1983;305:818–23.
9. Changeux J-P, Devillers-Thiery A, Chemouilli P. Acetylcholine receptor: An allosteric protein. Science. 1984;225:1335–45.

10. Mishina M, Kurosaki T, Tobimatsu T, *et al.* Expression of functional acetylcholine receptor from cloned cDNAs. Nature. 1984;307:604–8.
11. Beeson D, Brydwon M, Wood H, Vincent A, Newsom-Davis J. Human muscle acetylcholine receptor: cloning and expression in *Escherichia coli* of cDNA for the alpha-subunit. Biochem Soc Trans. 1989;17:219–20.
12. Barkas T, Gabriel JM, Mauron A, *et al.* Monoclonal antibodies to the main immunogenic region of the nicotinic acetylcholine receptor bind to residues 61–76 of the α subunit. J Biol Chem. 1988;263:5916–20.
13. Patrick J, Lindstrom J. Autoimmune response to acetylcholine receptor. Science. 1973;180:871–2.
14. Drachman DB, Adams RN, Stanley EF, Pestronk A. Mechanisms of acetylcholine receptor loss in myasthenia gravis. J Neurol Neurosurg Psychiatry. 1980;43:601.
15. Toyka KV, Drachman DB, Pestronk A, Kao I. Myasthenia gravis: passive transfer from man to mouse. Science. 1975;190:397–9.
16. Grob D, Brunner NG, Namba T. The natural course of myasthenia gravis and effect of therapeutic measures. Ann NY Acad Sci. 1981;377:652–69.
17. Drachman DB. Treatment of myasthenia gravis. In: Fauci A, editor. Current Therapy in Rheumatology and Immunology, 4th edn. Pennsylvania: BC Decker, 1992:347–52.
18. Devreotes PN, Fambrough DM. Turnover of acetylcholine receptors in skeletal muscle. Cold Spring Harbor Symp Quant Biol. 1976;40:237–51.
19. Pestronk A, Drachman DB, Self S. Measurement of junctional acetylcholine receptors in myasthenia gravis: Clinical correlates. Muscle Nerve. 1985;8:245–51.
20. Engel AG, Tsujihata MT, Lindstrom JM, Lennon VA. The motor endplate in myasthenia gravis and in experimental autoimmmune myasthenia gravis. A quantitative ultrastructural study. Ann NY Acad Sci. 1976;274:60–79.
21. Molenaar PC, Polak RL, Miledi R, Alema S, Vincent A, Newsom-Davis J. The cholinergic synapse. Progr Brain Res. 1979;49:449–58.
22. Cull-Candy SG, Miledi R, Trautman A, Uchitel OD. On the release of transmitter at normal, myasthenia gravis and myasthenic syndrome affected human endplates. J Physiol Lond. 1980;299:621–38.
23. Cull-Candy SG, Miledi R, Trautman A. End-plate currents at normal and myasthenic human end-plates. J Physiol Lond. 1979;287:247–65.
24. Satyamurti S, Drachman DB, Slone F. Blockade of acetylcholine receptors at the neuromuscular junction. Ann NY Acad Sci. 1971;183:147–57.
25. Waud DR. A review of pharmacological approaches to the acetylcholine receptors at the neuromuscular junction. Ann NY Acad Sci. 1971;183:147–57.
26. Elmqvist D, Hofmann WW, Kugelberg J, Quastel DMJ. An electrophysiological and morphological study of the neuromuscular junctions in patients with myasthenia gravis. Exp Neurol. 1976;51:536–63.
27. Albuquerque EX, Rash JE, Mayer RF, Satterfield JR. An electrophysiological and morphological study of the neuromuscular junctions in patients with myasthenia gravis. Exp Neurol. 1976;51:536–63.
28. Stalberg E, Trontelj JV, Schwartz MS. Single muscle-fiber recording of the jitter phenomenon in patients with myasthenia gravis and in members of their families. Ann NY Acad Sci. 1976;274:189–202.
29. Barrett EF, Magleby KL. Physiology of cholinergic transmission. In: Goldberg AM, Hanin I, editors. Biology of Cholinergic Function. New York: Raven Press, 1976:29–100.
30. Kistler J, Stroud R, Klymkowsky M, Lalancette R, Fairclough R. Structure and function of an acetylcholine receptor. Biophys J. 1982;37:371–83.
31. Kubalek E, Ralston S, Lindstrom J, Unwin N. Location of subunits within the acetylcholine receptor by electron image analysis of tubular crystals from *Torpedo marmorata*. J Cell Biol. 1987;105:9–18.
32. Stevens CF. Channel families in the brain. Nature. 1987;328:198–9.
33. Ratnam M, Le Nguyen D, Rivier J, Sargent P, Lindstrom J. Transmembrane topography of the nicotinic acetylcholine receptor: immunochemical tests contradict theoretical predictions based on hydrophobicity profile. Biochemistry. 1986;25:2633–43.
34. Changeux JP. Functional architecture and dynamics of the nicotinic acetylcholine receptor: an allosteric ligand-gated ion channel. Fidia Research Foundation Neuroscience Award

Lectures. New York: Raven Press. 1990;4:21–168.
35. Thesleff S. Supersensitivity of skeletal muscle produced by botulinum toxin. J Physiol Lond. 1960;151:598–607.
36. Drachman DB, Stanley EF, Pestronk A, Price DL, Griffin JW. Neurotrophic regulation of two properties of skeletal muscle by impulse-dependent and spontaneous ACh transmission. J Neurosci. 1982;2:232–43.
37. Salpeter MM. Development and neural control of the neuromuscular junction and of the junctional acetylcholine receptor. In: Salpeter MM, editor. The Vertebrate Neuromuscular Junction. New York: Liss. 1987:55–15.
38. Schuetze SM, Role LW. Developmental regulation of nicotinic acetylcholine receptors. Annu Rev Neurosci. 1987;10:403–57.
39. Witzemann V, Brenner HR, Sakmann B. Neural factors regulate AChR subunit mRNAs at rat neuromuscular synapses. J Cell Biol. 1991;114:125–41.
40. Mishina M, Takai T, Imoto K, *et al.* Molecular distinction between fetal and adult forms of muscle acetylcholine receptor. Nature. 1986;321:406–11.
41. Witzemann V, Barg B, Nishikawa Y, Sakmann B, Numa S. Differential regulation of muscle acetylcholine receptor γ and ε-subunit mRNAs. FEBS Lett. 1987;242:419–24.
42. Steinbach JH. Structural and functional diversity in the vertebrate skeletal muscle nicotinic acetylcholine receptors. Annu Rev Physiol. 1989;51:353–65.
43. Ramsay DR, Drachman DB, Drachman RJ, Stanley EF. Stabilization of acetylcholine receptors at the neuromuscular synapse: The role of the nerve. Brain Res. 1992;581: 198–207.
44. Lipsky NG, Drachman DB, Pestronk A, Shih P-J. Neural regulation of mRNA for the α-subunit of acetylcholine receptors: Role of neuromuscular transmission. Exp Neurol. 1989;105:171–6.
45. Avila OA, Drachman DB, Pestronk A. Neurotransmission regulates stability of acetylcholine receptors at the neuromuscular junction. J Neurosci. 1989;9:2902–6.
46. Cohen JB, Changeux J-P. The cholinergic receptor protein in its membrane environment. Annu Rev Pharmacol. 1975;15:83–103.
47. Gotti C, Conti-Tronconi BM, Raftery MA. Mammalian muscle acetylcholine receptor purification and characterization. Biochemistry. 1982;21:3148–54.
48. Lindstrom J. An assay for antibodies to human acetylcholine receptor in serum from patients with myasthenia gravis. Clin Immunol Immunopathol. 1977;7:36–43.
49. Syapin P, Salvaterra P, Engelhardt J. Neuronal-like features of TE671 cells: presence of a functioning nicotinic cholinergic receptor. Brain Res. 1982;231:365–77.
50. Lindstrom J, Criado M, Ratnam M, *et al.* Using monoclonal antibodies to determine the structures of acetylcholine receptors from electric organs, muscles, and neurons. Ann NY Acad Sci. 1987;505:208–25.
51. Witzemann V, Stein E, Barg B, *et al.* Primary structure and functional expression of the α, β, γ, δ, and ε-subunits of the acetylcholine receptor from rat muscle. Eur J Biochem. 1990;194:437–48.
52. Drachman DB. How to recognize an antibody-mediated autoimmune disease: criteria. In: Waksman BH, editor. Immunologic Mechanisms in Neurologic and Psychiatric Disease. New York: Raven Press, 1990:183–6.
53. Lindstrom JM, Seybold ME, Lennon VA, Whittingham S, Duane DD. Antibody to acetylcholine receptor in myasthenia gravis: Prevalence, clinical correlates and diagnostic value. Neurology. 1976;26:1054–9.
54. Vincent A, Newsom-Davis J. Acetylcholine receptor antibody as a diagnostic test for myasthenia gravis: results in 153 validated cases and 2967 diagnostic assays. J Neurol Neurosurg Psychiatry. 1985;48:1246–52.
55. Howard FM Jr, Lennon VA, Finley J, Matsumoto J, Elveback LR. Clinical correlations of antibodies that bind, block, or modulate human acetylcholine receptors in myasthenia gravis. Ann NY Acad Sci. 1987;505:526–38.
56. Roses AD, Olanow CW, McAdams MW, Lane RJM. No direct correlation between serum antiacetylcholine receptor antibody levels and clinical state of individual patients with myasthenia gravis. Neurology. 1981;31:220–4.
57. Drachman DB, Adams RN, Josifek LF, Self SG. Functional activities of autoantibodies to acetylcholine receptors and the clinical severity of myasthenia gravis. N Engl J Med.

1982;307:769–75.
58. Engel AG, Sahashi K, Lambert EH, Howard FM. The ultrastructural localization of the acetylcholine receptor, immunoglobulin G and the third and ninth complement components at the motor endplate and their implications for the pathogenesis of myasthenia gravis. In: Aguayo AJ, Karpati G, editors. Current Topics in Nerve and Muscle Research. Amsterdam: Excerpta Medica. 1979:111–22.
59. Toyka KV, Drachman DB, Griffin DE, *et al.* Myasthenia gravis: Study of humoral immune mechanisms by passive transfer to mice. N Engl J Med. 1977;296:125–31.
60. Lambert EH, Lindstrom JM, Lennon VA. Endplate potentials in experimental autoimmune myasthenia gravis in rats. Ann NY Acad Sci. 1976;274:300–18.
61. Penn AS, Chang HW, Lovelace RE, Niemi W, Miranda A. Antibodies to acetylcholine receptors in rabbits: Immunological and electrophysiological studies. Ann NY Acad Sci. 1976;274:354–76.
62. Sanders DB, Schleifer LS, Eldefrawi ME, Norcross JL, Cobb ED. An immunologically induced defect of neuromuscular transmission in rats and rabbits. Ann NY Acad Sci. 1976;274:319–36.
63. Hertel G, Mertens HG, Reuther P, Ricker K. The treatment of myasthenia gravis with azathioprine. In: Dau PC, editor. Plasmapheresis and the Immunobiology of Myasthenia Gravis. Boston: Houghton Mifflin, 1979:315–28.
64. Dau PC, Lindstrom JM, Cassel CK, Clark EC. Plasmapheresis in myasthenia gravis and polymyositis. In Dau PC, editor. Plasmapheresis and the Immunobiology of Myasthenia Gravis. Boston: Houghton Mifflin, 1979:229–47.
65. Kao I, Drachman DB. Myasthenic immunoglobulin accelerates acetylcholine receptor degradation. Science. 1977;196:527–9.
66. Appel SH, Anwyl R, McAdams MW, Elias S. Accelerated degradation of acetylcholine receptor from cultured rat myotubes with myasthenia gravis sera and globulins. Proc Natl Acad Sci USA. 1977;74:2130–4.
67. Bevan S, Kullberg RW, Heinemann SF. Human myasthenic sera reduce acetylcholine sensitivity of human muscle cells in tissue culture. Nature. 1977;267:263–5.
68. Devreotes PN, Fambrough DM. Acetylcholine receptor turnover in membranes of developing muscle fibers. J Cell Biol. 1975;65:335–58.
69. Drachman DB, Angus CW, Adams RN, Michelson J, Hoffman GJ. Myasthenic antibodies cross-link acetylcholine receptors to accelerate degradation. N Engl J Med. 1978;298: 1116–22.
70. Lindstrom JM. The role of antibodies to the acetylcholine receptor protein and its component peptides in experimental autoimmune myasthenia gravis in rats. In: Dau PC, editor. Plasmapheresis and the Immunobiology of Myasthenia Gravis. Boston: Houghton Mifflin, 1979:3–19.
71. Pumplin DB, Drachman DB. Myasthenic patients' IgG causes redistribution of acetylcholine receptors: Freeze-fracture studies. J Neurosci. 1983;3:576–84.
72. Stanley EF, Drachman DB. Effect of myasthenic immunoglobulin on acetylcholine receptor of intact mammalian neuromuscular junctions. Science. 1978;200:1285–7.
73. Almon RR, Andrew CG, Appel SH. Serum globulin in myasthenia gravis: Inhibition of α-bungarotoxin binding to acetylcholine receptors. Science. 1974;186:55–7.
74. Bender AN, Engel WK, Ringel SP, Daniel MP, Vogel Z. Myasthenia gravis: A serum factor blocking acetylcholine receptors of the human neuromuscular junction. Lancet. 1975;1: 607–8.
75. Pachner AR. Anti-acetylcholine receptors antibodies block bungarotoxin binding to native human acetylcholine receptor on the surface of TE671 cells. Neurology. 1989;39:1057–61.
76. Engel AG, Arahata K. The membrane attack complex of complement at the endplate in myasthenia gravis. Ann NY Acad Sci. 1987;505:326–32.
77. Besinger UA, Toyka KV, Homberg M, Heininger K, Hohlfeld R, Fateh-Moghadam A. Myasthenia gravis: Long term correlation of binding and bungarotoxin blocking antibodies against acetylcholine receptors with changes in disease severity. Neurology. 1983;33: 1316–21.
78. Lefvert AK, Bergstrom K, Matell G, Osterman PO, Pirskanen R. Determination of acetylcholine receptor antibody in myasthenia gravis: Clinical usefulness and pathogenetic implications. J Neurol Neurosci Psychiatry. 1978;41:394–403.

79. Seybold M, Lindstrom J. Serial anti-acetylcholine receptor antibody titers in patients with myasthenia gravis. Effects of steroid therapy. In: Dau PC, editor. Plasmapheresis and the Immunobiology of Myasthenia Gravis. Boston; Houghton Mifflin, 1979:307–14.
80. Tzartos SJ, Sophianos D, Zimmermann K, Starzinski-Powitz A. Antigenic modulation of human muscle acetylcholine receptor by myasthenic sera. Serum titer determines receptor internalization. J Immunol. 1986;136:3231–7.
81. Eymard B, De la Porte S, Pannier C, *et al.* Effect of myasthenic patient sera on the number and distribution of acetylcholine receptors in muscle and nerve-muscle cultures from rat. Correlations with clinical state. J Neurol Sci. 1988;86:41–59.
82. Lindstrom J, Shelton D, Fujii Y. Myasthenia gravis. Adv Immunol. 1988;42:233–83.
83. Tzartos SJ, Seybold ME, Lindstrom JM. Specificities of antibodies to acetylcholine receptors in sera from myasthenia gravis patients measured by monoclonal antibodies. Proc Natl Acad Sci USA. 1982;79:188–92.
84. Vincent A, Whiting PJ, Schluep M, *et al.* Antibody heterogeneity and specificity in myasthenia gravis. Ann NY Acad Sci. 1987;505:106–20.
85. Tzartos SJ, Cung MT, Demange P, *et al.* The main immunogenic region (MIR) of the nicotinic acetylcholine receptor and the anti-MIR antibodies. Mol Neurobiol. 1991;5:1–29.
86. Ratnam M, Sargent P, Sarin V, *et al.* Location of antigenic determinants on primary sequences of the subunits of the nicotinic acetylcholine receptor by peptide mapping. Biochemistry. 1986;25:2621–32.
87. Lennon VA, Griesman GE. Evidence against acetylcholine receptor having a main immunogenic region as target for autoantibodies in myasthenia gravis. Neurology. 1989;39:1069–76.
88. Drachman DB, DeSilva S, Ramsay D, Pestronk A. Humoral pathogenesis of myasthenia gravis. Ann NY Acad Sci. 1987;505:90–104.
89. Lindstrom J, Campbell M, Nave B. Specificities of antibodies to acetylcholine receptors. Muscle Nerve. 1978;1:140–5.
90. Vincent A, Newsom-Davis J. Acetylcholine receptor antibody characteristics in myasthenia gravis. I. Patients with generalized myasthenia or disease restricted to ocular muscles. Clin Exp Immunol. 1982;49:257–65.
91. Nielsen EC, Rodgaard A, Djurup R, Somnier F, Gammeltoft M. A triple antibody assay for the quantitation of plasma IgG subclass antibodies to acetylcholine receptors in patients with myasthenia gravis. J Immunol. 1985;83:249–58.
92. Lefvert AK, Bergstrom K. Acetylcholine receptor antibody in myasthenia gravis: Purification and characterization. Scand J Immunol. 1978;8:525–33.
93. Lang B, Roberts AJ, Vincent A, Newsom-Davis J. Anti-acetylcholine receptor idiotypes in myasthenia gravis analyzed by rabbit anti-sera. Clin Exp Immunol. 1985;60:637–44.
94. Mossman S, Vincent A, Newsom-Davis J. Myasthenia gravis without acetylcholine-receptor antibody: A distinct entity. Lancet. 1986;1:116–19.
95. Drachman DB, DeSilva S, Ramsay D, Pestronk A. 'Sero-negative' myasthenia gravis: A humorally mediated variant of myasthenia. Neurology. 1987;37(Suppl.1):214.
96. Soliven BC, Lange DJ, Penn AS, *et al.* Seronegative myasthenia gravis. Neurology. 1988;38:514–17.
97. Evoli A, Bartoccioni E, Batocchi AP, Scuderi F, Tonali P. Anti-AChR-negative myasthenia gravis: clinical and immunological features. Clin Invest Med. 1989;12:104–9.
98. Brooks EB, Pachner AR, Drachman DB, Kantor FS. A sensitive rosetting assay for detection of acetylcholine receptor antibodies using BC3H1 cells: Positive results in 'antibody negative' myasthenia gravis. J Neuroimmunol. 1990;28:83–93.
99. Yamamoto T, Vincent A, Ciulla TA, Lang B, Johnston I, Newsom-Davis J. Seronegative myasthenia gravis: a plasma factor inhibiting agonist-induced acetylcholine receptor function copurifies with IgM. Ann Neurol. 1991;30:550–7.
100. Willcox N, Schluep M, Ritter MA, Newsom-Davis J. The thymus in seronegative myasthenia gravis patients. J Neurol. 1991;238:256–61.
101. Lennon VA, Lindstrom JM, Seybold ME. Experimental autoimmune myasthenia gravis: cellular and humoral aspects. Ann NY Acad Sci. 1976;274:283–99.
102. Hohlfeld R, Kalies I, Kohleisen B, Heininger K, Conti-Tronconi B, Toyka KV. Myasthenia gravis: Stimulation of antireceptor autoantibodies by autoreactive T cell lines. Neurology. 1986;36:618–21.

103. Abramsky O, Aharonov A, Webb C, Fuchs S. Cellular immune response to acetylcholine receptor rich fraction in patients with myasthenia gravis. Clin Exp Immunol. 1975;19: 11–16.
104. Richman DP, Antel JP, Patrick JW, Arnason BGW. Cellular immunity to acetylcholine receptor in myasthenia gravis: Relationship to histocompatibility type and antigenic site. Neurology. 1979;29:291–6.
105. Hohlfeld R, Toyka KV, Miner LL, Walgrave SL, Conti-Tronconi BM. Amphipathic segment of the nicotinic receptor alpha subunit contains epitopes recognized by T lymphocytes in myasthenia gravis. J Clin Invest. 1988;81:657–60.
106. Brocke S, Brautbar C, Steinman L, *et al.* *In vitro* proliferative responses and antibody titers specific to human acetylcholine receptor synthetic peptides in patients with myasthenia gravis and relation to HLA class II genes. J Clin Invest. 1988;82:1894–900.
107. Melms A, Chrestel S, Schalke BC, *et al.* Autoimmune T lymphocytes in myasthenia gravis. Determination of target epitopes using T lines and recombinant products of the mouse nicotinic acetylcholine receptor gene. J Clin Invest. 1989;83:785–90.
108. Protti MP, Manfredi AA, Straub C, Wu XD, Howard JF, Conti-Tronconi BM. Use of synthetic peptides to establish anti-human acetylcholine receptor CD4+ cell lines from myasthenia gravis patients. J Immunol. 1990;144:1711–20.
109. Newsom-Davis J, Harcourt G, Sommer N, Beeson D, Willcox N, Rothbard J-B. T cell reactivity in myasthenia gravis. J Autoimmunity. 1989;2(Suppl):101–8.
110. Berrih-Aknin S, Cohen-Kaminsky S, Lepage V, Neumann D, Bach J-F, Fuchs S. T-cell antigenic sites involved in myasthenia gravis: correlations with antibody titre and disease severity. J Autoimmunity. 1991;4:137–53.
111. Sommer N, Harcourt GC, Willcox N, Beeson D, Newsom-Davis J. Acetylcholine receptor-reactive T lymphocytes from healthy subjects and myasthenia gravis patients. Neurology. 1991;41:1270–6.
112. Sommer N, Willcox N, Harcourt GC, Newsom-Davis J. Myasthenic thymus and thymoma are selectively enriched in acetylcholine receptor reactive T cells. Ann Neurol. 1990;28: 312–19.
113. Schönbeck S, Chrestel S, Hohlfeld R. Myasthenia gravis: prototype of the antireceptor autoimmune diseases. Int Rev Neurobiol. 1990;32:175–200.
114. Schwartz RH. T-lymphocyte recognition of antigen in association with gene products of the major histocompatibility complex. Annu Rev Immunol. 1984;3:237–61.
115. Rudensky AY, Preston-Hurlburt P, Hong S-C, Barlow A, Janeway CA Jr. Sequence analysis of peptides bound to MHC class II molecules. Nature. 1991;353:622–7.
116. Melms A, Malcherek G, Gern U, *et al.* T cells from normal and myasthenic individuals recognize the human acetylcholine receptor: Heterogeneity of antigenic sites on the α-subunit. Ann Neurol. 1992;31:311–18.
117. Oshima M, Ashizawa T, Pollack MS, Atassi MZ. Autoimmune T cell recognition of human acetylcholine receptor: the sites of T cell recognition in myasthenia gravis on the extracellular part of the α-subunit. Eur J Imunol. 1990;20:2563–9.
118. Zhang Y, Schluep M, Frutiger S, *et al.* Immunological heterogeneity of autoreactive T lymphocytes against the nicotinic acetylcholine receptor in myasthenic patients. Eur J Immunol. 1990;20:2577–83.
119. Moiola L, Protti MP, Manfredi AA, Yuen MH, Howard JF, Conti-Tonconi BM. T helper epitopes on human nicotinic acetylcholine receptor in myasthenia gravis. Ann NY Acad Sci. 1993;681:198–218.
120. Berzofsky J, Brett SJ, Streicher HZ, Takahashi H. Antigen processing for presentation to T lymphocytes: function, mechanisms, and implications for the T cell repertoire. Immunol Rev. 1988;106:5–31.
121. Tesch H, Hohlfeld R, Toyka KV. Analysis of immunoglobulin and T cell receptor gene rearrangements in the thymus of myasthenia gravis patients. J Neuroimmunol. 1989;21: 169–76.
122. Grunewald J, Ahlberg R, Lefvert A-K, Dersimonian H, Wigzell H, Janson CH. Abnormal T cell expansion and V gene usage in myasthenia gravis patients. Scand J Immunol. 1991;34:161–8.
123. Castleman B. The pathology of the thymus gland in myasthenia gravis. Ann NY Acad Sci. 1966;135:496–503.

124. Buckingham JM, Howard FM, Bernatz PE, *et al.* The value of thymectomy in myasthenia gravis: computer assisted matched study. Ann Surg. 1976;184:453–8.
125. Drachman DB. Myasthenia gravis (2 parts). N Engl J Med. 1978;298:136–42 and 186–93.
126. Levine GD. Pathology of the thymus in myasthenia gravis: current concepts. In: Dau PC, editor. Plasmapheresis and the Immunobiology of Myasthenia Gravis. Boston: Houghton Mifflin, 1979:113–23.
127. Scadding GK, Vincent A, Newsom-Davis J, Henry K. Acetylcholine receptor antibody synthesis by thymic lymphocytes: correlation with thymic histology. Neurology. 1981;31:935–43.
128. Fujii Y, Monden K, Nakahara H, Hashimoto J, Kawashima Y. Antibody to acetylcholine receptor in myasthenia gravis: Production by lymphocytes from thymus and thymoma. Neurology. 1984;34:1182–6.
129. Van de Velde RL, Friedman NB. Thymic myoid cells and myasthenia gravis. Am J Pathol. 1970;59:247–68.
130. Wekerle H, Paterson B, Ketelsen UP, Feldman M. Striated muscle fibres differentiate in monolayer cultures of adult thymus reticulum. Nature. 1975;256:493–4.
131. Kao I, Drachman DB. Thymic muscle cells bear acetylcholine receptors: Possible relation to myasthenia gravis. Science. 1977;195:74–5.
132. Wheatley LM, Urso D, Tumas K, Matlzman J, Loh E, Levinson AI. Molecular evidence for the expression of nicotinic acetylcholine receptor α-chain in mouse thymus. J Immunol. 1992;148:3105–9.
133. Kirchner T, Hoppe F, Schalke B, Müller-Hermelink HK. Microenvironment of thymic myoid cells in myasthenia gravis. Virchows Arch B. 1988;52:237–57.
134. Marx A, O'Connor R, Geuder KI, *et al.* Characterization of a protein with an acetylcholine receptor epitope from myasthenia gravis-associated thymomas. Lab Invest. 1990;62: 279–86.
135. Willcox N. The third Euromyasthenia conference: meeting report and update on myasthenia research. Autoimmunity. 1992;11:209–12.
136. Datta SK, Schwartz RS. Infectious-myasthenia. N Engl J Med. 1974;291:1304–5.
137. Aoki T, Drachman DB, Asher DM, Gibbs CJ Jr, Bahmanyar S, Wolinsky JS. Attempts to implicate viruses in myasthenia gravis. Neurology. 1985;35:185–92.
138. Dieperink ME, Stefansson K. Molecular mimicry and microorganisms: a role in the pathogenesis of myasthenia gravis? Curr Topics Microbiol Immunol. 1989;145:57–65.
139. Schwimmbeck PL, Dyrberg T, Drachman DB, Oldstone MBA. Molecular mimicry and myasthenia gravis: An autoimmune site of the acetylcholine α-subunit that has biologic activity and reacts immunochemically with herpes simplex virus. J Clin Invest. 1989;84:1174–80.
140. Stefansson K, Dieperink ME, Richman DB, Gomez CM, Marton LS. Sharing of antigenic determinants between the nicotinic acetylcholine receptor and proteins in *Escherichia coli, Proteus vulgaris* and *Klebsiella pneumoniae.* N Engl J Med. 1985;312:221–5.
141. Simpson JA. Myasthenia gravis: A new hypothesis. Scott Med J. 1960;4:419–36.
142. Pirskanen R. Genetic aspects of myasthenia gravis, a family study of 264 Finnish patients. Acta Neurol Scand. 1977;56:365–88.
143. Oh SJ, Dwyer DS, Bradley RJ. Overlap myasthenic syndrome: combined myasthenia gravis and Eaton–Lambert syndrome. Neurology. 1987;37:1411–14.
144. Steinman L. Immunogenetic mechanisms in myasthenia gravis. In: Aquilonius S-M, Gillberg PG, editors. Progress in Brain Research. Amsterdam: Elsevier, 1990:117–24.
145. Carlsson B, Wallin J, Pirskanen R, Matell G, Smith CIE. Different HLA DR-DQ associations in subgroups of idiopathic myasthenia gravis. Immunogenetics. 1990;31: 285–90.
146. Bell J, Smoot S, Newby C, *et al.* HLA-DQ beta chain polymorphism linked to myasthenia gravis. Lancet. 1986;ii:1058–60.
147. Bucknall RC, Dixon A St J, Glick EN, Woodland J, Zutshi DW. Myasthenia gravis associated with penicillamine treatment for rheumatoid arthritis. Br Med J. 1975;1:600–2.
148. Kuncl RW, Pestronk A, Drachman DB, Rechthand E. The pathophysiology of penicillamine-induced myasthenia gravis. Ann Neurol. 1986;20:740–4.
149. Bever CT, Chang HW, Penn AS, Jaffe IA, Bock E. Penicillamine-induced myasthenia gravis: effects of penicillamine on acetylcholine receptor. Neurology. 1982;32:1077–82.

150. Smith CIE, Aarli JA, Biberfeld P, *et al.* Myasthenia after bone marrow transplantation: evidence for a donor origin. N Engl J Med. 1983;309:1565–8.
151. Kurtzke JF, Kurland LT. The epidemiology of neurologic disease. In: Joynt RT, editor. Clinical Neurology. Philadelphia: JB Lippincott, 1991:80–8.
152. Osserman KE. Myasthenia Gravis. New York: Grune and Stratton, 1958:80.
153. Ozdemir C, Young RR. The results to be expected from electrical testing in the diagnosis of myasthenia gravis. Ann NY Acad Sci. 1976;274:203–22.
154. Stalberg E, Trontelj J. Single Fibre Electromyography. Old Woking, Surrey: Mirvalle Press, 1979.
155. Sanders DE. The electrodiagnosis of myasthenia gravis. Ann NY Acad Sci. 1987;505: 539–56.
156. Vincent A, Newsom-Davis J. Anti-acetylcholine receptor antibody characteristics in myasthenia gravis. I. Patients with generalized disease and disease restricted to ocular muscles. Clin Exp Immunol. 1982;49:257–65.
157. Blalock A, Mason MF, Morgan HJ, Riven SS. Myasthenia gravis and tumors of the thymic region; report of a case in which the tumor was removed. Ann Surg. 1939;110: 544–59.
158. Lanska DJ. Indications for thymectomy in myasthenia gravis. Neurology. 1990;40:1828–9.
159. Keesey J. Indications for thymectomy in myasthenia gravis. In: Dau PC, editor. Plasmapheresis and the Immunology of Myasthenia Gravis. Boston: Houghton Mifflin, 1979:124–436.
160. Papatestas AE, Genkins G, Horowitz SH, Kornfeld P. Thymectomy in myasthenia gravis: Pathological, clinical and electrophysiological correlations. Ann NY Acad Sci. 1976;274:555–73.
161. Olanow CW, Wechsler AS, Sirotkin-Roses M, Stajich J, Roses AD. Thymectomy as primary therapy in myasthenia gravis. Ann NY Acad Sci. 1987;505:595–606.
162. Spath G, Brinkman A, Huth Ch, Witeholler H. Complications and efficacy of transternal thymectomy in myasthenia gravis. Thoracic Cardiovasc Surg. 1987;35:283–9.
163. Younger DS, Jaretzki A III, Penn AS, *et al.* Maximum thymectomy for myasthenia gravis. Ann NY Acad Sci. 1987;505:832–5.
164. Haynes RC Jr. Adrenocorticotropic hormone; adrenocortical steroids and their synthetic analogs; inhibitors of the synthesis and actions of adrenocortical hormones. In: Gilman AG, Rall TW, Nies AS, Taylor P, editors. Goodman and Gilman's The Pharmacological Basis of Therapeutics, eighth edn. New York: Pergamon Press, 1990:1431–62.
165. Handschumacher RE. Immunosuppressive agents. In: Gilman AG, Rall TW, Nies AS, Taylor P, editors. Goodman and Gilman's The Pharmacological Basis of Therapeutics, eighth edn. New York: Pergamon Press, 1990;1264–76.
166. Cupps TR, Fauci AS. Corticosteroid-mediated immunoregulation in man. Immunol Rev. 1982;65:133–54.
167. Dinarello CA, Mier JW. Lymphokines. N Engl J Med. 1987;317:940–5.
168. Balow JE, Rosenthal AS. Glucocorticoid suppression of macrophage migration inhibitory factor. J Exp Med. 1973;137:1031–9.
169. Parrillo JE, Faucei AS. Mechanisms of glucocorticoid action on immune processes. Annu Rev Pharmacol Toxicol. 1979;19:179–201.
170. Lew W, Oppenheim JJ, Matsushima K. Analysis of the suppression of IL-1α and IL-1β production in human peripheral blood mononuclear adherent cells by a glucocorticoid hormone. J Immunol. 1988;140:1895–902.
171. Gerard TL, Cupps TR, Jurgensen CH, Fauci AS. Hydrocortisone-mediated inhibition of monocyte antigen presentation: dissociation of inhibitory effect and expression of DR antigens. Cell Immunol. 1984;85:330–9.
172. Mokoena T, Gordon S. Human macrophage activation. Modulation of mannosyl, fucosyl receptor activity *in vitro* by lymphokines, gamma and alpha interferons, and dexamethasone. J Clin Invest. 1985;75:624–31.
173. Kaplan I, Blakely BT, Pavlath GK, Travis M, Blau HM. Steroids induce acetylcholine receptors on cultured human muscle: Implications for myasthenia gravis. Proc Natl Acad Sci. 1990;87:8100–4.
174. Braun S, Askansas V, Ibrahim E, Engel WK. Long-term treatment with hydrocortisone (HC) increases accumulation of acetylcholine receptors (AChRs) at human neuromuscular junctions (NMJs) in culture. Neurology. 1991;41(Suppl):154.

175. Van Wilgenburg H. The effect of prednisolone on neuromuscular transmission in the rat diaphragm. Eur J Pharmacol. 1979;55:355–61.
176. Arts WF, Oosterhuis HJ. Effect of prednisolone on neuromuscular blocking in mice *in vivo*. Neurology. 1975;25:1088–90.
177. Engel WK. Myasthenia gravis, corticosteroids, anticholinesterases. Ann NY Acad Sci. 1976;274:623–30.
178. Johns TR. Long-term corticosteroid treatment of myasthenia gravis. Ann NY Acad Sci. 1987;505:568–83.
179. Seybold ME, Drachman DB. Gradually increasing doses of prednisone in myasthenia gravis: reducing the hazards of treatment. N Engl J Med. 1974;290:81–4.
180. Warmoltz JR, Engel WK. Benefits from alternate-day prednisone in myasthenia gravis. N Engl J Med. 1972;286:17–20.
181. Pinelli P, Tonali P, Scopetta C. Long-term treatment of myasthenia gravis with alternate-day prednisone. Eur Neurol. 1974;12:129–41.
182. Scopetta C, Tonali P, Evoli A, David P, Crucitte F, Vaccario ML. Treatment of myasthenia gravis. J Neurol. 1979;222:11–21.
183. Sghirlanzoni A, Peluchette D, Fiacchino F, Mantagazza R, Cornelio F. Myasthenia gravis. Long term treatment with steroids. Neurology. 1984;34:170–4.
184. Okamoto S, Takegami T. Current concepts of steroid therapy in myasthenia gravis. In: Satoyoshi E, editor. Myasthenia Gravis. Tokyo: University of Tokyo Press, 1981;383.
185. Oosterhuis HJGH. Ergahrungen mit glykocorticoiden bei patienten mit myasthenia gravis. In: Hertel GUA, editor. Myasthenia Gravis. Stuttgart: Thième Verlag, 1977;246–51.
186. Arsura E, Brunner NC, Namba T, Grob D. High-dose intravenous methylprednisolone in myasthenia gravis. Arch Neurol. 1985;42:1149–53.
187. Sanders DB, Howard JF Jr, Johns TR, Campa JF. High dose daily prednisone in the treatment of myasthenia gravis. In: Dau PC, editor. Plasmapheresis and the Immunobiology of Myasthenia Gravis. Boston: Houghton Mifflin, 1979:289–306.
188. Witte AS, Cornblath DR, Parry GJ, Lisak RP, Schatz NJ. Azathioprine in the treatment of myasthenia gravis. Ann Neurol. 1984;15:602–5.
189. Mertens HG, Hertel G, Reuther P, Ricker K. Effect of immunosuppressive drugs (azathioprine). Ann NY Acad Sci. 1981;337:691–7.
190. Matell G. Immunosuppressive drugs: azathioprine in the treatment of myasthenia gravis. Ann NY Acad Sci. 1987;505:588–94.
191. Mantegazza R, Antozzi C, Peluchetti D, Sghirlanzoni A, Cornelio F. Azathioprine as a single drug or in combination with steroids in the treatment of myasthenia gravis. J Neurol. 1988;235:449–53.
192. Pirofsky B, Dawson PJ, Reid RH. Lack of oncogenicity with immunosuppressive therapy. Cancer. 1980;45:2096–101.
193. Whisnant JK, Pelkyelkey J. Rheumatoid arthritis: treatment with azathioprine (Imuran). Clinical side effects and laboratory abnormalities. Ann Rheum Dis. 1982;41:44–7.
194. Michels M, Hohlfeld R, Hartung H-P, Heininger K, Besinger UA, Toyka KV. Myasthenia gravis: discontinuation of long-term azathioprine. Ann Neurol. 1988;24:798.
195. Hohlfeld R, Toyka KV, Besinger VA, Gerhold B, Heininger K. Myasthenia gravis: reactivation of clinical disease and of autoimmune factors after discontinuation of long-term azathioprine. Ann Neurol. 1985;17:238–42.
196. Hohlfeld R, Michals M, Heininger K, Besinger U, Toyka KV. Azathioprine toxicity during long-term immunosuppression of generalized myasthenia gravis. Neurology. 1988;38: 258–61.
197. Kissel JT, Levy RJ, Mendel JR, Griggs RC. Azathioprine toxicity in neuromuscular disease. Neurology. 1986;36:35–9.
198. Borel JF, Feurer C, Gubler HU, Stahelin H. Biological effect of cyclosporin A: a new antilymphocyte agent. Agents Actions. 1976;6:468–75.
199. Kahn BD, Bach JF, editors. Proceedings of the Second International Congress on Cyclosporine. Transplant Proc. 1988;20(Suppl.3):1–1131.
200. Elliott JF, Lin Y, Mizel SB, Bleackley RC, Harnish DG, Paettkau V. Induction of interleukin 2 messenger RNA inhibited by cyclosporine A. Science. 1984;226:1439–41.
201. Kronke M, Leonard WJ, Depper JM, *et al.* Cyclosporine A inhibits T cell growth factor

gene expression at the level of mRNA transcription. Proc Natl Acad Sci USA. 1984;81: 5214–18.

202. Drachman DB, Adams RN, McIntosh K, Pestronk A. Treatment of experimental myasthenia gravis with cyclosporin A. Clin Immunol Immunopathol. 1985;34:174–88.
203. Goulon M, Elkharry D, Lokiec F, Gajdos PH. Results of a one-year open trial of cyclosporin in ten patients with severe myasthenia gravis. In: Kahan BD, editor. Cyclosporin: Applications in Autoimmune Diseases. Philadelphia: Grune and Stratton; 1988;211–17.
204. Nyberg-Hansen R, Gjerstad L. Myasthenia gravis. In Kahan BD, editor. Cyclosporin: Applications in Autoimmune Diseases. Philadelphia: Grune and Stratton, 1988;201–10.
205. Schalke B, Kappos L, Dommasch D, Rohrbach E, Mertens HG. Cyclosporin A treatment of myasthenia gravis: Initial results of a double blind trial of cyclosporin A versus azathioprine. Ann NY Acad Sci. 1988;505:872–5.
206. Tindall RSA, Rollins JA, Phillips JT, Greenlee RG, Wells L, Belendiuk G. Preliminary results of a double-blind, randomized, placebo-controlled trial of cyclosporine in myasthenia gravis. N Engl J Med. 1987;316:719–24.
207. Salamon JR, Griffin PJA. Immunosuppression with a combination of cyclosporin, azathioprine, and prednisolone may be unsafe. Lancet. 1985;2:1066–7.
208. Mihatsch MJ, Bach JF, Coovadia HM, *et al.* Cyclosporin-associated nephropathy in patients with autoimmune diseases. Klin Wschr. 1988;66:43–7.
209. The Multiple Sclerosis Study Group. Efficacy and toxicity of cyclosporine in chronic progressive multiple sclerosis: a randomized, double-blinded, placebo-controlled clinical trial. Ann Neurol. 1990;27:591–605.
210. Perez MC, Buot WL, Mercado-Danguilan C, Bagabaldo ZG, Renales LD. Stable remission in myasthenia gravis. Neurology. 1981;31:32–7.
211. Nouza K, Smat V. The favorable effect of cyclophosphamide in myasthenia gravis. Rev Fr Etudes Clin Biolog. 1968;13:161–3.
212. Niakan E, Harati Y, Rolak LA. Immunosuppressive drug therapy in myasthenia gravis. Arch Neurol. 1986;43:155–6.
213. Baker GL, Kahl LE, Zee BC, Stolzer BL, Agarwal AK, Medsger TA. Malignancy following treatment of rheumatoid arthritis with cyclophosphamide. Am J Med. 1987;83:1–9.
214. Pinching AJ, Peters DK, Newsom-Davis JN. Remission of myasthenia gravis following plasma exchange. Lancet. 1976;2:1373–6.
215. Dau PC, Lindstrom JM, Cassel CK, Denys EH, Shev EE, Spitler LE. Plasmapheresis and immunosuppressive drug therapy in myasthenia gravis. N Engl J Med. 1977;297: 1134–40.
216. Hawkey CJ, Newsom-Davis J, Vincent A. Plasma exchange and immunosuppressive drug treatment in myasthenia gravis: No evidence of synergy. J Neurol Neurosurg Psychiatry. 1981;44:469–75.
217. Keesey J, Buffkin D, Kebo D, Ho W, Herman C. Plasma exchange as therapy for myasthenia gravis. Ann NY Acad Sci. 1981;377:729–43.
218. Kornfeld P, Ambinder EP, Matta RJ, *et al.* Plasmapheresis in refractory generalized myasthenia gravis. Arch Neurol. 1981;38:478–81.
219. Newsom-Davis J, Ward CD, Wilson SG, Pinching AJ, Vincent A. Plasmapheresis: short- and long-term benefits? In: Dau PC, editor. Plasmapheresis and the Immunobiology of Myasthenia Gravis. Boston: Houghton Mifflin, 1979:199–208.
220. Miller RG, Milner-Brown HS, Dau PC. Antibody-negative acquired myasthenia gravis. Successful therapy with plasma exchange. Muscle Nerve. 1981;4:255.
221. Johns TR. Treatment of myasthenia gravis: long-term administration of corticosteroids with remarks on thymectomy. In: Griggs RC, Moxley RT III, editors. Treatment of Neuromuscular Diseases. New York: Raven Press, 1977:99.
222. Newsom-Davis J, Vincent A, Wilson SG, Ward CD. Long-term effects of repeated plasma exchange in myasthenia gravis. Lancet. 1979;1:464.
223. Newsom-Davis J, Pinching AJ, Wilson SG. Function of circulating antibody to acetylcholine receptor in myasthenia gravis: Investigated by plasma exchange. Neurology. 1978;28:266–72.
224. Complications of vascular access devices used for repeated haemodialysis. Br Med J. 1977;2:1373–4.

225. Arsura E. Experience with intravenous immunoglobulins in myasthenia gravis. Clin Immunol Immunopathol. 1989;53:S170.
226. Dwyer JM. Manipulating the immune-system with immune globulin. N Engl J Med. 1992;326:107–16.
227. Oats JA, Wood AJJ. The use of intravenous immune globulin in immunodeficiency diseases. N Engl J Med. 1991;325:110–17.
228. Killen JA, Lindstrom JM. Specific killing of lymphocytes that cause experimental autoimmune myasthenia gravis by ricin toxin-acetylcholine receptor conjugates. J Immunol. 1984;133:2549–53.
229. Sterz RK, Biro G, Rajki K, Filipp G, Peper K. Experimental autoimmune myasthenia gravis: Can pretreatment with ^{125}I-labeled receptor prevent functional damage at the neuromuscular junction? J Neuroimmunol. 1985;7:97–105.
230. Shizuru JA, Taylor-Edwards C, Banks B, Gregory AR, Fathman CG. Immunotherapy of the nonobese diabetic mouse: treatment with an antibody to T-helper lymphocytes. Science. 1988;240:659–62.
231. Brostoff SW, Mason DW. Experimental allergic encephalomyelitis: successful treatment *in vivo* with a monoclonal antibody that recognizes T helper cells. J Immunol. 1984;133:1938–42.
232. Bach J-F. Immunointervention in autoimmune diseases from cellular selectivity to autoantigen specificity. J Autoimmunity. 1992;5(Suppl A):3–10.
233. Cantrell DA, Smith KA. The interleukin 2 T cell system: A new cell growth model. Science. 1984;224:1312–16.
234. Waldmann TA. The structure, function, and expression of interleukin-2 receptors on normal and malignant lymphocytes. Science. 1986;232:727–32.
235. Williams DB, Parker K, Bacha P, *et al.* Diphtheria toxin receptor binding domain substitution with interleukin 2: genetic construction and properties of a diphtheria toxin-related interleukin-2 fusion protein. Protein Eng. 1987;1:493–8.
236. Balcer LJ, McIntosh KR, Nichols JC, Drachman DB. Suppression of immune responses to acetylcholine receptor by interleukin 2-fusion toxin: *In vivo* and *in vitro* studies. J Neuroimmunol. 1991;31:115–22.
237. Bacha P, Williams DB, Waters C, Williams JM, Murphy JR, Strom TB. Interleukin-2 receptor targeted cytotoxicity: interleukin-2 receptor-mediated action of a diphtheria toxin-related interleukin-2 fusion protein. J Exp Med. 1988;167:612–22.
238. Bacha P, Forte S, Kassam N, Thomas J, Akiyoshi D, Waters C, Nichols J, Rosenblum M. Pharmacokinetics of the recombinant fusion protein DAB 486-IL2 in animal models. Cancer Chemother Pharmacol. 1990;26:409–14.
239. Kiyokawa T, Williams DP, Snider CE, Strom TB, Murphy JR. Protein engineering of diphtheria-toxin-related interleukin-2 fusion toxins to increase cytotoxic potency for high-affinity IL-2-receptor-bearing target cells. Protein Eng. 1991;4:463–8.
240. Cohen IR, Ben-Nun A, Holoshitz J, Maron R, Zerubavel R. Vaccination against autoimmune disease with lines of autoimmune T lymphocytes. Immunol Today. 1983;4: 227–30.
241. Lider O, Reshef T, Beraud E, Ben-Nun A, Cohen IR. Anti-idiotypic network induced by T cell vaccination against experimental autoimmune encephalomyelitis. Science. 1988;239:181–3.
242. Ben-Nun A, Wekerle M, Cohen IR. Vaccination against autoimmune encephalomyelitis with T-lymphocyte line cells reactive against myelin basic protein. Nature. 1981;292: 60–1.
243. Maron R, Zerubavel R, Friedman A, Cohen IR. T lymphocyte line specific for thyroglobulin produces or vaccinates against autoimmune thyroiditis in mice. J Immunol. 1983;131: 2316–22.
244. Holoshitz J, Naparstek Y, Ben-Nun A, Cohen IR. Lines of T lymphocytes induce or vaccinate against autoimmune arthritis. Science. 1983;219:56–8.
245. Neilson EG, Phillips SM. Suppression of interstitial nephritis by auto-anti-idiotypic immunity. J Exp Med. 1982;155:179–89.
246. Kahn CR, McIntosh KR, Drachman DB. T-cell vaccination in experimental myasthenia gravis: a double-edged sword. J Autoimmunity. 1990;3:659–69.
247. Acha-Orbea H, Mitchell DJ, Timmerman L, *et al.* Limited heterogeneity of T cell

receptors from lymphocytes mediating autoimmune encephalomyelitis allows specific immunointervention. Cell. 1988;54:263–73.
248. Vandenbark AA, Chou YK, Bourdette DN, Whitman R, Hashim GA, Offner H. T cell receptor peptide therapy for autoimmune disease. J Autoimmunity. 1992:5(Suppl A): 83–92.
249. Howell MD, Winters ST, Olee T, Powell HC, Carlo DJ, Brostoff SW. Vaccination against experimental allergic encephalomyelitis with T cell receptor peptides. Science. 1989;246: 668–70.
250. Lehmann PV, Forsthuber T, Miller A, Sercarz EE. Spreading of T cell autoimmunity to cryptic determinants of an autoantigen. Nature. 1992;358:155–7.
251. Theofilopoulos AN, Balderas RS, Baccala R, Kono DH. T cell receptor genes in autoimmunity. Ann NY Acad Sci. 1993;681:33–46.
252. Fujii Y, Lindstrom J. Specificity of the T cell immune response to acetylcholine receptor in experimental autoimmune myasthenia gravis. J Immunol. 1988;140:1830–7.
253. Roitt I, Brostoff J, Male D. Immunology. St Louis: Mosby Co, 1986:8.5–8.7.
254. Reim J, McIntosh KR, Martin S, Drachman DB. Specific immunotherapeutic strategy for myasthenia gravis: targeted antigen-presenting cells. J Neuroimmunol. 1992;41:61–70.
255. Snider DP, Segal DM. Targeted antigen presentation using crosslinked antibody heteroaggregates. J Immunol. 1987;139:1609–16.
256. Jenkins MK, Schwartz RH. Antigen presentation by chemically modified splenocytes induces antigen-specific T cell unresponsiveness *in vitro* and *in vivo.* J Exp Med. 1987;165:302–19.
257. Palace J, Wiles CM, Newsom-Davis J. 3,4-Diaminopyridine in the treatment of congenital (hereditary) myasthenia. Neurol Neurosurg Psychiatry. 1991;54:1069–72.
258. Kuncl RW, Adams RN, Drachman DB. Inhibition of methyltransferase reduces the turnover of acetylcholine receptors. Proc Natl Acad Sci. 1988;85:4032–6.
259. Kuncl RW, Drachman DB, Wittstein I, *et al.* Novel therapy of experimental myasthenia gravis by reducing endocytosis of acetylcholine receptors. Neurology. 1991;41:154.
260. Heininger K, Hendricks M, Toyka KV. Myasthenia gravis: a new semi-selective procedure to remove acetylcholine receptor autoantibodies from plasma. Plasma Ther Transfus Technol. 1985;6:771–5.
261. DeSilva S, Blum JE, McIntosh KR, Order S, Drachman DB. Treatment of experimental myasthenia gravis with total lymphoid irradiation. Clin Immunol Immunopathol. 1988;48:31–41.
262. Pestronk A, Drachman DB. Dimethyl sulfoxide reduces titers of anti-receptor antibody in experimental myasthenia gravis. Nature. 1980;288:733–4.
263. Crain E, McIntosh KR, Gordon G, Pestronk A, Drachman DB. The effect of thalidomide on experimental autoimmune myasthenia gravis. J Autoimmunity. 1989;2:197–202.
264. Pestronk A, Drachman DB, Teoh R, Adams RN. Combined short-term immunotherapy cures experimental autoimmune myasthenia gravis. Ann Neurol. 1983;14:235–41.
265. Sterz RK, Biro G, Rajki K, Filipp G, Peper K. Experimental autoimmune myasthenia gravis: can pretreatment with ^{125}I-labeled receptor prevent functional damage at the neuromuscular junction? J Neuroimmunol. 1985;7:97–105.
266. Bogen S, Mozes E, Fuchs S. Induction of AChR-specific suppression: an *in vitro* model of antigen-specific immunosuppression in myasthenia gravis. J Exp Med. 1984;159:292–304.
267. Pachner AR, Kantor FS. Suppressor T-cell lines and hybridomas in murine myasthenia. Ann NY Acad Sci. 1987;505:619–27.
268. McIntosh KR, Drachman DB. Induction of suppressor cells specific for acetylcholine receptor in experimental autoimmune myasthenia gravis. Science. 1986;232:401–3.
269. McIntosh KR, Drachman DB, Kuncl RW. Antigen-specific suppressor macrophages induced by culture with cyclosporin A plus acetylcholine receptor. J Neuroimmunol. 1989;25:75–89.
270. Whitham RH, Vandenbark AA, Bourdette DN, Chou YK, Offner H. Suppressor cell regulation of encephalitogenic T cell lines: Generation of suppressor macrophages with cyclosporin A and myelin basic protein. Cell Immunol. 1990;126:290–303.
271. Waldor MS, Sriram S, McDevitt HO, Steinman L. *In vivo* therapy with monoclonal anti-Iα antibody suppresses immune responses to AChR. Proc Natl Acad Sci USA. 1983;80: 2713–17.

272. Aharoni RD, Teitelbaum D, Arnon R, Puri J. Immunomodulation of experimental allergic encephalomyelitis by antibodies to the antigen-Ia complex. Nature. 1991;351:147–50.
273. Adorini L. Inhibition of T cell activation by MHC blockade: A possible strategy for immunointervention in autoimmune diseases. J Autoimmunity. 1992;5(Suppl A):73–81.
274. Schonbeck S, Dwyer DS. Regulation of the immune response to acetylcholine-receptor after injection of anti-idiotypic antibodies. Immunobiology. 1984;168:184.
275. DeBaets MH, VanBreda Vriesman PJC. Immunomodulatory effects of anti-idiotypic antibodies in experimental autoimmune myasthenia gravis. Fed Proc. 1985;44:607.
276. Agius MA, Richman DP. Suppression of development of experimental autoimmune myasthenia gravis with isogeneic monoclonal antiidiotypic antibody. J Immunol. 1986;137:2195–8.
277. Souroujon MD, Fuchs S. Antiidiotypic antibodies in the regulation of experimental autoimmune myasthenia gravis. Ann NY Acad Sci. 1987;505:256–70.
278. Chiller JM, Habicht GS, Weigle WO. Cellular sites of immunologic unresponsiveness. Proc Natl Acad Sci USA. 1970;65:551–6.
279. Weiner HL, Zhang ZJ, Khoury SJ, *et al.* Antigen-driven peripheral immune tolerance. Suppression of organ-specific autoimmune diseases by oral administration of autoantigens. Ann NY Acad Sci. 1991;636:227–32.
280. DeSilva S, McIntosh KR, Blum JE, Order S, Mellits D, Drachman DB. Total lymphoid irradiation and antigen-specific tolerance: Treatment for experimental myasthenia gravis? J Neuroimmunol. 1990;29:93–103.
281. Waldman H, Qin S, Cobbold S. Monoclonal antibodies as agents to reinduce tolerance in autoimmunity. J Autoimmunity. 1992;5(Suppl A):93–102.
282. McIntosh KR, Drachman DB. Tolerance to acetylcholine receptor induced by AChR-coupled syngeneic cells. J Neuroimmunol. 1992;38:75–84.
283. Oki A, Sercarz E. T cell tolerance studied at the level of antigenic determinants. J Exp Med. 1985;161:897–911.

8
Immunological factors that influence disease severity in experimental autoimmune myasthenia gravis

K. A. KROLICK, P. A. THOMPSON, T. E. ZODA, S. MOHAN, R. J. BAROHN and T.-M. YEH

INTRODUCTION

In health, acetylcholine receptors (AChR) associated with muscle membrane at the endplate are designed to capture acetylcholine molecules released from vesicles at the motor nerve terminals. The AChR, complexed with transmitter, then acts as an ion channel to mediate cationic fluxes into innervated muscles, thereby initiating the chain of events leading to voluntary muscle contraction. Under certain circumstances, however, the AChR may be perturbed in a way that diminishes its ability to translocate ions effectively. Such is the case in myasthenia gravis (MG), an autoimmune disease mediated by antibodies with binding specificity for AChR; upon binding, anti-AChR antibodies may interfere with receptor function to varying degrees, impairing neuromuscular transmission and creating the commonly observed symptoms of weakness and easy fatigability. Much has been learned over the years with regard to the mechanisms underlying MG. However, much is still to be clarified. This is certainly due to the multifactorial nature of the disease: mechanisms for impaired neuromuscular function may be found at several levels. For example, as summarized in Figure 8.1, the induction and severity of disease symptoms might be influenced by the myophysiology of an individual, reflected by minor differences in AChR structure or numbers of receptors found on the post-junctional muscle membrane. Accessibility of AChR to antibody attack, determined by architectural features of the neuromuscular junction (which are even heterogeneous between different muscle fibre types within an individual), may also differ among individual patients. Together with these synaptic aspects, there are immunophysiological factors to be considered

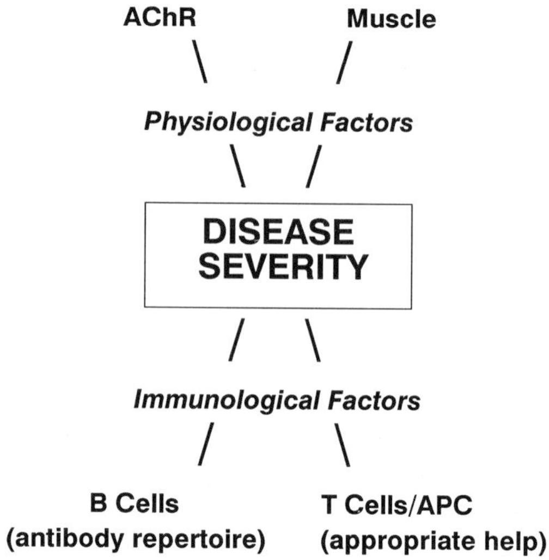

Figure 8.1 Factors affecting disease severity in myasthenia gravis.

when evaluating the induction and severity of symptoms in MG patients. For example, characteristics of the B lymphocyte/antibody response itself (directly responsible for interference with AChR function) need to be defined; these will lead to a better understanding of how the usual maintenance of immunological tolerance to self antigens has been circumvented and the exact immunopathological mechanisms that lead to perturbation of receptor function. Additional understanding of underlying mechanisms affecting disease induction and severity may be forthcoming as characteristics of the T lymphocyte response (indirectly responsible for interference of AChR function by serving as the regulator of the B cell response) continue to be defined. Due to the biochemical complexity of the self antigen involved (AChR), the biological complexity of the immune system, the complexity of the 'outbred' genetics of the human population, and the overall inability to perform the needed systematic evaluation of the immunopathological and neurophysiological aspects of the disease, animal models of MG (experimental autoimmune myasthenia gravis; EAMG) were developed in the early 1970s[1].

The detailed immunophysiological features of this useful model have been extensively reviewed elsewhere[2]; the purpose of this report is to summarize results of our own studies dealing with certain unresolved issues related to disease mechanisms. An initial problem, in the light of the proven ability of anti-AChR antibodies to damage or occlude the endplate receptor, is the lack of correlation between antibody titre and disease severity[3–6]. Some severely ill patients have barely detectable anti-AChR antibody titres, while certain other patients with very high antibody levels have very mild symptoms.

The working hypothesis and main premise on which our studies have been based is that some, but not all, anti-AChR antibodies produced in MG

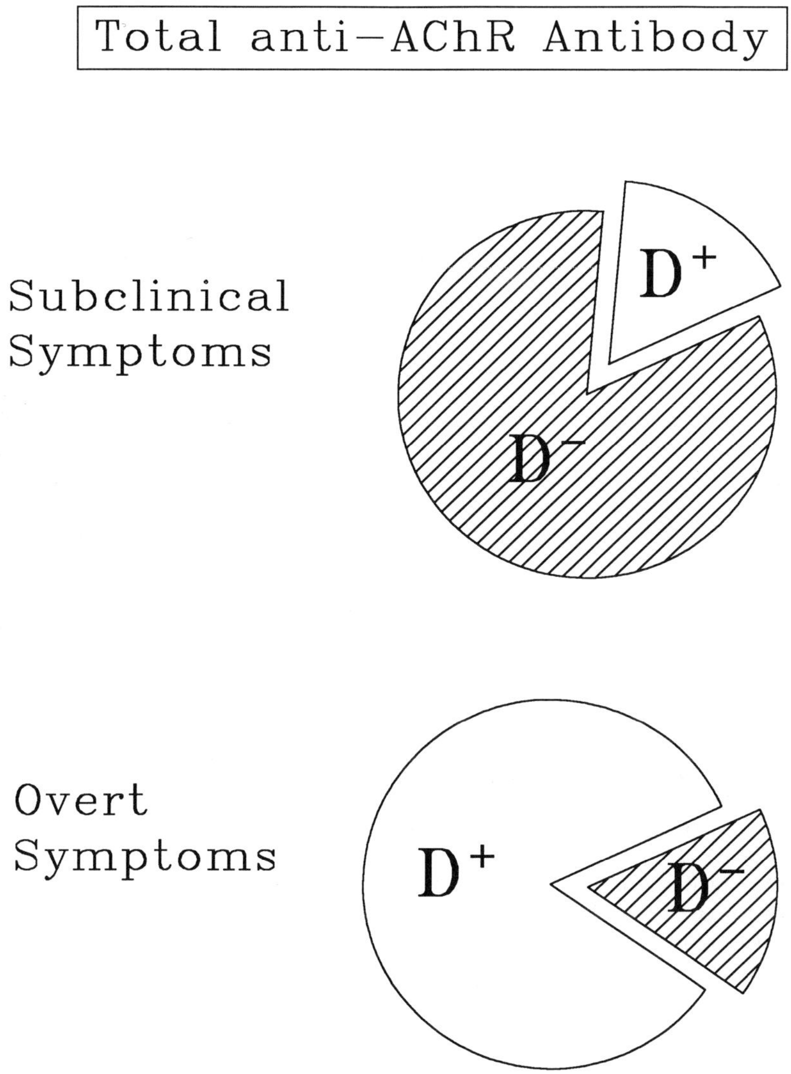

Figure 8.2 Hypothetical differences in the proportions of disease-causing (D^+) and benign (D^-) anti-AChR antibodies produced by two MG patients demonstrating differences in disease symptom severity. The explanation proposed here is that although both patients may have the same serum titre of anti-AChR antibodies, only that patient with a suprathreshold titre of the disease-causing antibody subset would demonstrate severe neuromuscular impairment

patients are directly responsible for neuromuscular disease; a certain proportion (differing from patient to patient) of the anti-AChR antibodies produced bear no direct relationship to disease (Figure 8.2). The ability to predict disease severity based on anti-AChR antibody titres would, therefore, be dependent on the determination of a minimal amount of the disease-causing antibody subset, or 'threshold' level of production, above which neuromuscular impairment could be detected, and the ability to identify and measure levels of the disease-causing antibody subset directly. Measurement of total anti-AChR antibody titres would likely be misleading unless the relevant subset accounted for the majority of the antibody.

NATURE OF THE PROBLEM: THE ANTI-AChR ANTIBODY RESPONSE

In general, the anti-AChR antibody response in MG patients and most experimental animal models is oligoclonal (see below); that is, a family of antibodies is produced, with reactivity directed at the AChR being the only characteristic required to be considered part of the family. The term anti-AChR does not specify whether the antibodies are of the IgM or IgG class, nor does it imply binding to any particular component of the receptor. Upon binding, these properties of an individual anti-AChR antibody molecule might, however, be very influential with regard to whether it has pathogenic potential and to the severity of the resulting disease state.

The biochemical and physical properties of immunoglobulins that deserve consideration include characteristics such as isotype (the class or subclass of the antibody), antigen-binding affinity, and antigen binding fine specificity (the exact site or epitope to which antigen binding occurs). Each characteristic will have varying importance in MG by establishing which antibody effector functions are activated during disease induction[3–14]. For example, the antibody isotype may confer on particular immunoglobulin classes or subclasses the ability to fix complement, resulting in focal membrane damage. Additionally, antibody isotype may determine the ability of antibodies to interact with Fc receptor-bearing effector cells following complement-dependent recruitment of inflammatory white cells into the junction. In combination with the appropriate antibody isotype, the exact location of binding determined by the fine specificity of the antibody may also influence the accessibility of the muscle membrane to complement attack. Furthermore, antibody binding affinity and fine specificity for particular AChR epitopes could determine the effectiveness of autoantibody binding and the cascade of other events that will follow; such qualities may have importance in determining the ability of anti-AChR antibodies to directly block acetylcholine-stimulated receptor function by binding at or near the acetylcholine binding site. Alternatively, autoantibodies directed against other sites on the AChR molecule may prevent proper function of the voltage-dependent ion channel, thus interfering with signal transmission. In addition to steric hindrance of AChR function, the autoantibodies can modulate the turnover and reinsertion of AChR at the surface of muscle fibres. The resulting loss of AChR density from the muscle membrane, dependent on the cross-linking of AChR molecules by bivalent antibody, would depend on the specificity of bound antibody with respect to the juxtaposition of epitopes on adjacent AChR molecules.

Thus, it would not be surprising to find that not all anti-AChR antibodies are equally capable of causing neuromuscular impairment. Characteristics of the anti-AChR antibodies such as isotype, affinity, and fine specificity would have potential importance by determining which of the pathogenic mechanisms described above play a determining role in induction of MG or EAMG. Furthermore, the repertoire of antibody specificity produced may show interpatient variability due to genetic differences between individuals with regard to available immunoglobulin variable region genes that dictate antibody specificity. If different MG patients produced different subsets of the total clonotypic spectrum of possible anti-AChR antibodies (some dominated by antibody species with disease-causing potential and some dominated by benign antibody species), one would expect interindividual differences in neuromuscular impairment to result. Identification of characteristics associated with the exact subset of antibodies directly responsible for impaired AChR function would likely lead to a more precise understanding of relationships between antibody titre and disease severity, as well as the opportunity to evaluate disease mechanisms more directly.

Finally, complex immunoregulatory phenomena, probably T cell-mediated, also influence the production and characteristics of anti-AChR antibodies. The complexities of immunopathology and immunoregulation obscure an understanding of the quantitative and qualitative relationships between the anti-AChR antibody response and the induction of AChR-dependent neuromuscular disease symptoms. Variability of disease severity may thus be explained by immunoregulatory activities that determine which anti-AChR antibodies are expressed or produced from within the potential anti-AChR antibody repertoire. These activities may involve major histocompatibility complex (MHC)-selected immunoregulatory T cell activities that direct the anti-AChR antibody response. In searching for an understanding of disease mechanisms that lead to an ability to predict disease state and progress, therefore, one must include not only parameters directly associated with the fine specificity repertoire of disease-causing antibodies, but also parameters associated indirectly with the regulation of the particular subset of the total anti-AChR response that causes perturbed AChR function. Over the past several years, this laboratory has employed various strategies to dissect the multifaceted immune response that leads to the neuromuscular impairment observed in experimental MG. This work has been greatly facilitated by the availability of rat strains whose differing sensitivity to immunization with AChR is partly based on known genetic factors.

EVALUATION OF ANTI-AChR ANTIBODIES IN RAT STRAINS THAT DIFFER IN THEIR SUSCEPTIBILITY TO EAMG

Isolectric focusing (IEF), in which antibody separations are based on their biochemical charge, has been the principal tool for assessing the clonotypic origins, heterogeneity, isotype, and relative antigen-binding avidity of serum anti-AChR antibodies[15–20]. IEF data obtained from this laboratory suggest that characteristics dictated by the clonal B cell origin of anti-AChR antibodies dramatically influence the myopathological effects seen in rats

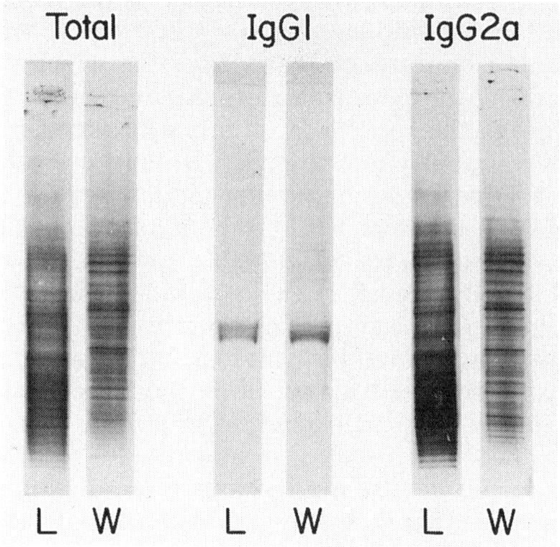

Figure 8.3 Isoelectric focusing analysis of antiserum from one representative Lewis (L) or Wistar Furth (W) rat immunized with AChR. AChR-specific antibody bands immunoblotted onto AChR-coated nitrocellulose paper were probed as indicated for total antibody, IgG1 antibody, or IgG2a antibody specific for AChR. Taken from reference 20

with EAMG. Immunopathological differences associated with different clonotypic species of anti-AChR antibodies identified in this way give a different perspective on disease mechanisms than studies of the bulk serum antibody response. For instance, clonally derived anti-AChR antibodies produced against different conformational states of the antigen[18], involving helper T cells of restricted fine specificity for AChR[17,19], and following treatments with idiotype-selective immunocytotoxic agents[21] can be examined. Characteristics of the anti-AChR antibodies produced in genetically different rat strains can also be compared[20,22]: AChR-immune Lewis rats demonstrate easily detectable neuromuscular dysfunction, while AChR-immune Wistar Furth (WF) rats demonstrate significant resistance to the induction of antibody-mediated muscle dysfunction (increased *in vitro* sensitivity to curare (seen as decreased RT_{50} values) reflects diminished AChR-dependent muscle contraction compared to normal muscles[23,24].

The complexity of IEF banding patterns reflects the number of AChR-reactive B cell clones making antibody: both Lewis and WF rats express similar clonotypic antibody heterogeneity and isotype preference (Figure 8.3). However, some antibody clonotypes from the two rat strains do not comigrate in pH gradients, indicating a lack of protein identity. Since the responses of both rat strains are dominated by the same IgG subclass (IgG2a) with no apparent allotypic differences[25], and there does not appear to be a clear distinction between Lewis and WF anti-AChR antibodies with regard to binding avidity, it is likely that many of the differences in net charge and isoelectric point (pI) between Lewis and WF antibodies are the result of variable region amino acid differences; this could indicate differences in

Table 8.1 Passive transfer of anti-AChR antibodies from Lewis rats can cause impaired muscle function in Wistar Furth rats

	RT_{50} (nM)[b]	
Amount of antibody transferred[a]	*Lewis*	*WF*
0	365 ± 30	437 ± 23
200	350 ± 6	400[c]
400	196 ± 37	140 ± 39
800[d]	< 100	< 100

[a]μg IgG fraction of AChR-immune Lewis rat serum transferred by intravenous injection

[b]Concentrations of tubocurarine required to inhibit AChR-dependent contractile tension of extensor digitorum longus muscles by 50%. Mean values (± SEM) represent determinations of muscles from rats of the indicated strain (3–6 rats/group). Evaluations of AChR-dependent contractile function of EDL muscles from many healthy and AChR-immunized rats (> 200 each) have indicated that healthy EDL muscles demonstrate RT_{50} values of 350–450 nM curare, while AChR-immune rats demonstrate RT_{50} values of 100–200 nM curare

[c]One rat tested at this dose of transferred antibody

[d]Both rat strains showed visible signs of muscle dysfunction following transfer of 800 μg Lewis antibody. RT_{50} values for these animals were not calculated because relative tensions were determined to be decreased by about 50–70% prior to the addition of any curare. Exposure to 100 nM curare resulted in no detectable contractile function (RT = 0)

antibody fine specificity and secondary differences in resulting AChR perturbations.

The main conclusion derived from this information is that, although the antibodies produced following a single AChR immunization of Lewis and WF rats are of similar clonotypic heterogeneity and avidity and dominated by the same IgG subclass, only Lewis rats develop impaired AChR-dependent neuromuscular function. Two possible explanations for this difference in disease induction are: first, the antibodies produced by the two rat strains may be of overlapping but non-identical fine specificities, and therefore express different degrees of disease-causing potential, or second, the antibodies produced by both rat strains include specificities that are associated with such a potential, but the biochemistry or presentation of junctional AChR in WF rats somehow differs from that in Lewis rats, resulting in resistance to antibody-mediated effects. This second possibility is less likely, since impaired muscle function has been demonstrated in WF rats after the passive transfer of preformed anti-AChR antibodies from Lewis donor rats (Table 8.1).

Following multiple injections of AChR, disease-resistant WF rats do finally demonstrate AChR-dependent neuromuscular dysfunction (Figure 8.4). There are at least two explanations for this: first, the early WF responses to AChR involve antibodies with no disease-causing activity, but hyperimmunization may result in mutations of antibody variable region genes that shift antibody binding fine specificity and/or avidity. Acquisition of these new antibody

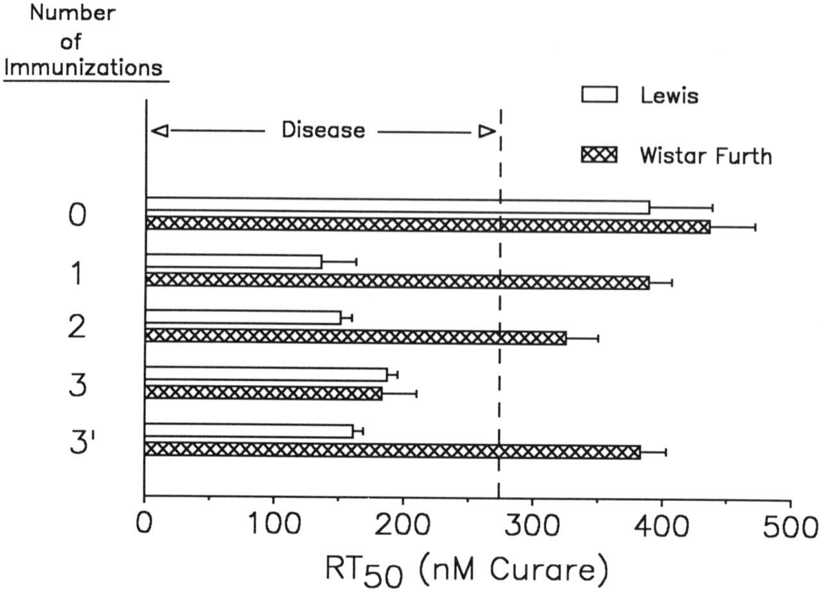

Figure 8.4 Disease induction in Lewis rats (□) and Wistar Furth rats (⊠) following multiple AChR immunizations. The dose of curare necessary to inhibit contractile force by 50% (RT_{50}), is thought to reflect the level of functional AChR expression and has been shown to be a sensitive reproducible indicator of antibody-mediated AChR perturbations[23,24]. The vertical dashed line has been arbitrarily placed to indicate the lowest RT_{50} value ever determined for EDL muscles from healthy control rats (i.e. 280 nM curare); in reality, after more than 200 assessments, control values are usually 350–500 nM, and diseased values 100–250 nM. Groups of four rats of each strain were injected (s.c.) with AChR emulsified in CFA, followed by one or two additional AChR booster injections given in saline. Three weeks following each injection a group of rats of each strain was sacrificed and tested for AChR-dependent muscle contractile function. Number of immunizations indicated is the sum of total injections given; 3′ indicates that rats were given 3 injections and allowed to wait 10 weeks, instead of the usual 3–5 weeks, before analysis of muscle function. Taken from reference 20

specificities could increase disease-causing potential. A second, but not mutually exclusive, explanation is that the disease-causing antibody fine specificities exist in the WF germline, but are initially expressed at very low frequency and/or are somehow immunosuppressed (possibly by T cell-mediated mechanism). Upon hyperimmunization, eventual activation and expansion of disease-causing B cell clones results in the production of enough anti-AChR antibody to exceed the threshold needed to result in impaired muscle function (Figure 8.2). Figure 8.5 demonstrates a simple disease *vs.* antibody titre relationship that suggests that this disease-causing threshold may exist; further, Lewis rat anti-AChR antibodies may simply contain a higher proportion of disease-causing antibody. It is also of note that the expression of disease symptoms in hyperimmunized WF rats is transient (< 10 weeks) (Figure 8.4), although the total anti-AChR antibody titre remains virtually constant during the same period of time. This may indicate that the production of the small subset of anti-AChR antibodies responsible

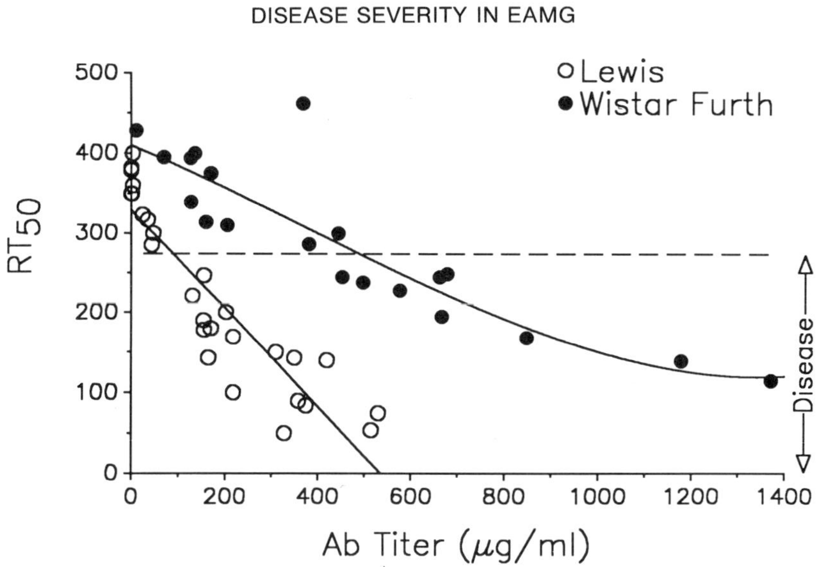

Figure 8.5 Relationship between serum anti-AChR antibody concentration and curare sensitivity (RT_{50}) demonstrated by EDL muscles from WF and Lewis rats. All rats were given an initial injection (s.c.) of 50 µg of AChR in CFA; some rats (groups of 4 rats each) were given one or two additional injections (s.c.) of 50 µg AChR in buffered saline at approximately 2 weeks and 4 weeks, respectively, following the first injection. Disregarding the exact immunization protocol, rats were then ranked according to resulting anti-AChR antibody titres and plotted as shown above against curare sensitivity (RT_{50}). Taken from reference 20

for disease symptoms in WF rats remains restricted by immunoregulatory factors. Changing IEF banding patterns that have been observed during a programme of multiple immunizations are consistent with this possibility and may provide a more sensitive way of monitoring relationships between anti-AChR antibody production and AChR-dependent myscle dysfunction[20].

DIFFERING DISEASE-CAUSING POTENTIALS ASSOCIATED WITH ANTI-AChR ANTIBODIES FROM EAMG-SUSCEPTIBLE RATS

Co-expression of benign and disease-causing anti-AChR antibodies in Lewis rats

Rat and mouse monoclonal antibody studies from several laboratories have been designed to examine disease-associated antibody characteristics and have, in fact, demonstrated the differential abilities of various AChR-specific monoclonal antibodies to passively transfer EAMG[26–30]. Although the use of monoclonal antibody techniques to study the immune response to particular antigenic determinants has proved extremely useful, there is still some confusion about relationships between antibody characteristics and their disease-causing potential. Such confusion may have arisen from the inherent biases produced by the inability to fuse, clone and expand B cells representing the entire expressed polyclonal anti-AChR antibody repertoire, or from biases introduced by screening strategies based on favoured antibody

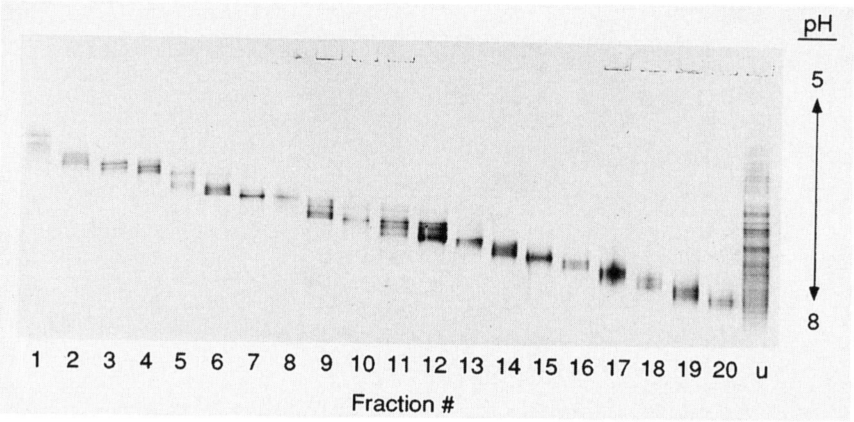

Figure 8.6 The polyclonal rat anti-AChR antibody response can be fractionated by preparative isoelectric focusing (pIEF) allowing the recovery of clonotypically restricted AChR-reactive antibodies. pIEF was performed as described in reference 16. Recovered protein from each fraction was then rerun on analytical IEF gels to assess purity and maintenance of binding activity against AChR. Numbers indicate the relative position in the pH gradient from which each fraction was recovered (increasing from the acidic to the alkaline range). Unfractionated antiserum is indicated by 'U'. Taken from reference 16

specificities. An alternative strategy, presented in a previous report[16], involves the identification of disease-causing clonal B cell products (AChR-reactive antibodies) present in immune rat serum using methods that are independent of the fine specificity, frequency, tissue distribution, and fusability of the responding B cells. Unfortunately, regardless of the method of antibody isolation, direct identification of important AChR determinants remains difficult because of the clear requirement of native AChR conformation for the binding of important disease-causing anti-AChR antibodies (see below). Conventional approaches to epitope mapping (such as synthetic peptide binding studies and Western blot analysis) may underestimate binding ability since these methods require antigen denaturation.

Our approach to assessing the heterogeneity and disease-causing potential of antibodies generated by immunization of rats with AChR is to purify antibodies directly from serum by preparative isoelectric focusing (pIEF) techniques[31] (Figure 8.6). Following electrofocusing, each purified pIEF fraction containing certain clonotypic antibody species, can be passively transferred into naïve recipient rats and tested for its ability to induce symptoms of impaired AChR-dependent neuromuscular function. Such studies aim to identify the disease-causing subset of anti-AChR antibodies from among the entire spectrum of AChR-reactive antibody clonotypes in Lewis rats with EAMG and to characterize individual antibody species capable of contributing to neuromuscular dysfunction.

Following transfer of antibodies obtained from the pIEF-fractionated sera of AChR-immunized Lewis rats to immunologically naïve, healthy recipient rats, two main subsets of AChR-specific antibody can be identified. One

Table 8.2 Relationships between disease-causing potential and reactivity with rat AChR[a]

	Disease-causing fractions	*Benign fractions*
Rat AChR$^+$	8, 9, 12, 13, 18	5, 10, 11, 14, 15, 16, 17, 19, 20
Rat AChR$^-$	None	1, 2, 3, 4, 6, 7

[a]Each pIEF antibody fraction described in Figure 8.6 was passively transferred into groups of naïve recipient rats and scored 24–48 h later for the ability to directly interfere with AChR-dependent contractile function of EDL muscles as described in Figure 8.4. Fractions that were determined to contain disease-causing AChR reactivity or benign AChR reactivity were then evaluated for their ability to bind AChR of rat muscle origin. Data are presented as pIEF fraction numbers assigned to each of these four groups

subset, representing about one-third of the expressed clonotypic antibody repertoire, is capable of directly perturbing AChR-dependent neuromuscular function (Table 8.2). A second subset has no detectable ability to induce disease symptoms. The anti-AChR antibodies used in these experiments are initially produced by immunization with electric ray (*Torpedo*) AChR: these are not 100% cross-reactive with rat AChR[16], but the inability of some antibody fractions to perturb AChR function cannot be explained by their inability to react with AChR of mammalian origin. Furthermore, the ability of certain pIEF fractions to transfer disease symptoms does not correspond with a particular antibody isotype (although the response is dominated by IgG2a) and does not depend solely on high relative binding avidity (benign reactivities with high relative binding avidity are also observed). Nonetheless, an anti-AChR antibody subset that is likely to contain reactivities that are most directly responsible for neuromuscular disease symptoms demonstrated by rats with EAMG can be directly identified and purified from immune serum.

Conformation dependence of important AChR epitopes

Studies of disease-sensitive Lewis rats and disease-resistant Wistar Furth rats suggest that a particular set of anti-AChR antibodies prominently produced by Lewis rats but absent in WF rats, appears to be required for induction of neuromuscular disease. Lewis anti-AChR antibodies are not all equally capable of impairing AChR-dependent neuromuscular function. What are the characteristics of anti-AChR antibodies that allow disease-causing potential to be expressed? Early studies by other investigators[32–35] demonstrated the importance of the three-dimensional conformation of AChR in determining anti-AChR antibody fine specificity for AChR epitopes. In the EAMG model, for example, serum antibody responses to denatured AChR differ from those to native AChR in terms of the ability to cause neuromuscular interference. Studies from this laboratory later also demonstrated clonotypic distinctions between disease-causing and non-disease-causing anti-AChR antibodies in Lewis rats immunized with either conformationally intact AChR, or reduced and SDS-denatured AChR[18]. Antibodies directed against linear (as opposed to conformational) epitopes are often incapable of eliciting symptoms; however, although reactivity of serum antibodies with AChR epitopes demonstrating native conformation appears to be one prerequisite for inducing disease, it is not necessarily sufficient. Antibodies produced as a result of immunization with denatured AChR (dAChR) but cross-reactive with native AChR (nAChr), are similar to, but not identical with, those produced directly against nAChR; dAChR-stimulated antibodies are skewed to the acidic end of the IEF pH gradient (in contrast to the more alkaline nature of antibodies stimulated with native AChR) and are clearly incapable of causing detectable impairment of AChR-dependent muscle contractile function[18]. These observations suggest that certain antibody subsets owe their disease-causing potential to the properties of the immunogen, though similar levels of anti-AChR, isotype distribution, and clonotypic antibody heterogeneity can be evoked with either native or denatured AChR. It should also be noted that although the antibody response to dAChR is considerably skewed in favour of determinants associated with the cytoplasmic region of the receptor[36–38], other antibodies are clearly capable of recognizing extracellular regions (K. Krolick, unpublished observations).

In conclusion, the repertoire of rat anti-AChR antibodies expressed in Lewis rats is composed of at least two main subsets of antibody, one capable of directly perturbing AChR function and the other incapable of such an effect. Compared to IEF banding patterns of identified disease-causing antibodies, IEF banding patterns of anti-AChR antibodies that have no detectable disease-causing potential (e.g., those produced by immunization of rats with denatured AChR[18] or a rat strain that demonstrates resistance to disease induction[20]) show an apparent absence of disease-causing clonotypes, but maintenance of many of the benign antibody clonotypes. This offers possible explanations for the lack of detectable disease in the face of easily detectable anti-AChR antibodies following immunization under these circumstances.

SELECTIVE EXPRESSION OF THE DISEASE-CAUSING ANTI-AChR ANTIBODY SUBSET

In light of the clear differences in disease-causing potential possessed by particular subsets of anti-AChR antibodies, it is of great interest to be able to predict when the activity of the highly immunopathological antibodies is likely to be expressed. We discuss below two possible influences that may be involved: first, immunoregulatory helper T lymphocytes may be capable of steering the antibody specificity repertoire towards or away from disease-causing specificities, and second, additional antibody reactivities may be produced in some individuals that are capable of counteracting the effects of disease-causing reactivities.

Role of helper T lymphocytes

Major histocompatibility complex (MHC) class II molecules are thought to influence the specificity repertoire of T cells, which may then indirectly affect subsequent B cell activities[39,40]. Protein antigens are taken up by specialized antigen-presenting cells (APC) and processed in an intracellular compartment into an immunogenic form. The processing step appears to involve denaturation and limited proteolysis[41]. An immunogenic fragment of the antigen becomes associated with the MHC molecule[42] by binding to a specific site[43], binding being mediated by allele-specific amino acid residues. Different MHC allele-encoded molecules in outbred individuals or in different rodent strains may differ in the fragments of a given antigen that are presented to T cells. This process has been termed 'determinant selection'[44]. The complex formed by the antigen fragment and MHC molecule is then displayed on the APC cell surface and, if recognized by a T cell receptor[45], leads to activation of that T cell. In health, T cell unresponsiveness (tolerance) to particular antigen fragments of host (self) origin probably results either from a failure of processed self antigen to bind to MHC[46], or from the deletion or inactivation of these antigen-specific T cells[47].

The anti-AChR antibody response in EAMG is polyclonal at the B cell level, as described above, and is T cell-dependent. Even in inbred animals, direct demonstration of the importance of helper T cell specificity in EAMG is difficult, complicated by restricted antigen recognition governed by the genes of the MHC. Different strains of mice and rats demonstrate different patterns of MHC-dependent reactivity for AChR and panels of AChR peptides[48–60]; these MHC-determined differences in the expressed and activated T cell specificity repertoire may be the basis, in part, for differences in the severity of disease observed. Studies from this laboratory point to T cell reactivity directed at a restricted region of the α-subunit as being most effective in stimulating anti-AChR antibody production[17,19,61] and eventual neuromuscular dysfunction.

The influence of T cell specificity on the clonotypic heterogeneity and disease-causing potential of antibodies against the AChR has been evaluated[18]. The fact that anti-AChR antibody response is oligoclonal/polyclonal, and that only a subset of these antibodies is able to directly interfere with AChR-dependent function, raises the question of whether restricting the activated AChR-specific helper T cell repertoire would subsequently result in a similar restriction in the antibody repertoire, and whether such a T cell-restricted anti-AChR antibody response would continue to elicit neuromuscular symptoms.

Adoptive transfer studies using T cells from rats immunized with the purified AChR subunits (α, β, γ, and δ) and with B cells from donor rats immunized with the intact AChR suggest that T cell specificity for antigen may influence the exact subset of antibody clonotypes produced; however resulting antibody titres, affected by which T cells are used, also appear to influence the degree of disease observed. The results of such studies are therefore ambiguous in that, regardless of the AChR subunit specificity of the T cells, all recipient animals demonstrate AChR-dependent muscle dysfunction if adequate anti-AChR antibody titres are reached. One conclusion is that if the importance of T cell specificity is to be fully appreciated, the activated anti-AChR T cell repertoire must be further restricted.

The rat anti-AChR immune response has been shown to be dominated by T cell reactivity directed toward a small number of biochemical regions[53]. The region including the α-subunit amino acid residues at positions 100–116 appears to be important in determining T cell reactivity to AChR. Furthermore, significant cross-reactivity is known to exist between this α-subunit sequence and determinants associated with the other AChR subunits. For these reasons it appears likely that α100–116 T cell determinant(s) plays an important role in the anti-AChR antibody response, and probably in generating disease symptoms. We have studied the immunogenicity of the α100–116 peptide with regard to the regulation of the production of the disease-causing subset of AChR-reactive antibody[20]. Although regulation of the anti-AChR antibody response by peptide-reactive helper T cells results in lower antibody titres than those produced in responses regulated by T cells reactive with the whole AChR, the clonotypic heterogeneity of the antibodies examined by IEF is similar to those regulated by unrestricted AChR-reactive T cells. This suggests that the spectrum of antibody specificities produced is probably similar and of similar disease-causing potential. The disease-causing potential of the anti-AChR antibodies produced with the help of peptide-reactive T cells can be verified by adoptive transfers followed by tests of AChR-dependent muscle function. Thus, T cells reactive with the small (17 amino acids) synthetic peptide are capable of helping virtually all possible anti-AChR antibody clonotypes, including those involved in inducing neuromuscular disease.

The virtually complete expression of the entire repertoire of antibodies reactive with AChR, in spite of the highly restricted T cell reactivity, was not predicted. It had been assumed that restriction of the T cell specificity repertoire to a very small subset of total possible reactivities, would similarly limit the antibody specificity repertoire. Clearly, this is not the case. The observation that a single small immunogenic peptide can stimulate T cells that effectively help all AChR-reactive B cells to produce a heterogeneous antibody response is difficult to reconcile with the various proposed mechanisms that require antigen bridging to obtain T cell to B cell signalling[62]. However, the region associated with α100–116, as well as other homologous regions, is represented more than once in each AChR monomer. There are at least two α-subunits per AChR monomer each containing the α100–116 sequence. Moreover, there appears to be significant T cell cross-reactivity between α-derived peptide and the other three AChR subunits[53,61]. This may also help to explain previous observations using AChR-reactive T hybridomas, in which over 50% of a panel of 32 clones produced IL-2 on *in vitro* challenge with any of the four purified AChR subunits[63].

Differences in disease severity caused by manipulations of the T cell specificities involved may therefore have only a quantitative basis. That is, in studies performed thus far, influences of T cell specificity on disease severity in rats appear to be directly related to the levels of circulating anti-AChR antibody attained, not to influences on the selection of particular B cell specificities. The effectiveness by which T cells transmit helper signals certainly determines the frequency, but not necessarily the specificity, of B cells activated. It is noteworthy that, as in other systems[64], T cell helper activity may not correlate directly with other T cell activities such as proliferation. Thus, a single amino acid substitution in the α100–116 peptide (proline for threonine at position 106) results in a virtually unaffected ability to stimulate proliferation, while nearly all ability to stimulate the help of AChR-reactive B cells with subsequent disease induction is lost. This may imply that at least two T cells with differing fine specificities can react with the α100–116 peptide and cross-react with native AChR. One T cell can proliferate when challenged with the original peptide and the cross-reactive proline-substituted peptide, but is not capable of activating the appropriate B cells. The second T cell stimulates B cells, and may or may not be easily stimulated to proliferate by the peptides.

Taking all of these observations together, the specificity of T cell reactivities is unlikely to be a clear predictor of subsequent disease severity or the key to future immunotherapies. Assessment of T cell reactivity (in terms of proliferation) without careful evaluation of its potential helper activity may be misleading with regard to antibody responses that follow. Even T cells confirmed to have relevant helper activity may demonstrate promiscuous selectivity with regard to the B cell clones activated. Furthermore, the prominence of particular antigenic determinants in T cell activation is likely to vary between patients[65–67], dependent on mechanisms related to antigen processing events and the role of the MHC in the recognition of antigen by T cells. Thus, the factor more likely to account for variations in disease severity is in the efferent arm of the immune response and related to the fine specificity of anti-AChR antibodies.

Role of blocking antibodies

As described above, although many of the antibodies against denatured AChR epitopes can cross-react with native AChR[18], immunization of rats with dAChR does not cause neuromuscular dysfunction. In light of this observation, it was of interest to ask whether the anti-dAChR response was simply and passively missing key fine specificities required for disease induction, or perhaps was associated with an antibody activity that was capable of actively interfering with a second antibody activity with disease-causing potential. Experimental strategies for approaching this question involved the evaluation of disease induced by mixtures of the serum activities produced by rats following immunization with nAChR and following immunization with dAChR. Three examples of such experiments are shown in Table 8.3. In experiment 1, rats were hyperimmunized with a primary injection (s.c.) of dAChR in complete Freund's adjuvant (CFA) followed 1 month later by two additional injections of dAChR in saline. They were then challenged with nAChR in CFA for an additional month. Rats immunized with dAChR in this way demonstrated substantial anti-AChR antibody titres and, as shown, were refractory to disease induction by challenge with

Table 8.3 Inhibition of anti-nAChR antibody induction of neuromuscular dysfunction by anti-dAChR antibodies

Experiment 1. Standard immunization with nAChR does not induce disease in rats previously hyperimmunized with dAChR

Immunization status[a]	*Pre-challenge antibody injected*[b]	*nAChR challenge*[c]	RT_{50}[d]
Naïve (6)	None	nAChR/CFA (s.c.)	115 ± 21
DAChR-immune (4)	None	nAChR/CFA (s.c.)	450 ± 39

Experiment 2. Passive transfer of preformed anti-nAChR antibodies does not induce disease in rats previously hyperimmunized with dAChR

Immunization status	*Pre-challenge antibody injected*	*nAChR challenge*	RT_{50}
Naïve (4)	None	Anti-nAChR antibody	98 ± 21
dAChR-immune (4)	None	Anti-nAChR antibody	391 ± 39

Experiment 3. Passive transfer of serum Ig fractions containing anti-nAChR antibodies does not induce disease in rats pretreated with serum Ig fractions from dAChR-immunized rats

Immunization status	*Pre-challenge antibody injected*	*nAChR challenge*	RT_{50}
Naïve (4)	None	Anti-nAChR antibody	98 ± 21
Naïve (3)	Anti-dAChR antibody	Anti-nAChR antibody	363 ± 15

[a]Immunization status of rats prior to any challenge with anti-nAChR antibodies; dAChR-immune rats had been injected (s.c.) with 50 μg dAChR in CFA followed by two additional booster doses of dAChR prior to nAChR antibody challenge. Numbers in parentheses indicate the number of rats evaluated.

[b]400–500 μg of AChR-specific antibody injected (i.v.) 24–48 h prior to anti-nAChR antibody challenge.

[c]nAChR antibody challenge was performed, as indicated, either by active immunization with 50 μg nAChR in CFA (s.c.) 1 month prior to examination of muscle function or by passive injection (i.v.) of 400 μg preformed anti-nAChR antibodies 48 h prior to examination of muscle function.

[d]EDL muscles from the indicated rats were evaluated for AChR-dependent muscle contraction by determining their curare sensitivity (indicated as RT_{50} values (± SEM)) as described in the text. Decreasing RT_{50} values (i.e. increasing sensitivity to curare) indicates the onset of impaired AChR function. EDL muscles from immunologically naïve, healthy rats demonstrate RT_{50} values of 350–450 nM.

nAChR. In experiment 2, rats demonstrating ongoing anti-AChR antibody responses against dAChR (as in experiment 1) were injected (i.v.) with 0.5 mg of anti-nAChR antibody. These rats were apparently resistant to the neuromuscular effects of injected anti-nAChR antibody, unlike immunologically naïve rats that showed the usual induction of impaired AChR-dependent muscle function. The results of experiment 3 were consistent with the 'protective' effects of antibodies present during an active immunization. A disease-resistant state was observed following the passive injection of the Ig fraction of anti-dAChR antiserum 24 h prior to injection of anti-nAChR antibody. When the Ig fractions of sera from rats immunized against nAChR and dAChR were injected into naïve rats in varying proportions, a relatively more potent effect of the protective activity was observed over the effects of the disease-causing activity. Thus, a 3–5 × molar excess of anti-nAChR antibodies was required to induce impaired AChR function (not shown).

In order for the anti-nAChR antibody effect to be neutralized, either the binding of antibodies to the conformation-dependent determinant(s) must be blocked or, once bound, the subsequent change to receptor function must not occur. One might speculate, therefore, that a subset of anti-dAChR antibody(s) may bind to the AChR in such a way as to sterically or allosterically interfere with anti-nAChR antibody binding, or may bind in such a way as to prevent the anti-nAChR antibody-induced structural alterations of the AChR that leads to impaired receptor function. Alternatively, anti-dAChR antibody-induced AChR perturbations may stimulate AChR biosynthesis and increase AChR membrane density; evidence for this possibility has been suggested by studies demonstrating refractoriness to disease induction in animals following administration of suboptimal doses of disease-causing antibodies[68]. However, no increased resistance to the antagonistic effects of curare was observed, as might have been expected if a significant increase in AChR density had occurred. Finally, since the source of transferred antibody was the Ig fraction of anti-dAChR antiserum, other AChR-nonreactive antibody specificities may also play a role. Therefore, the explanation may not directly involve anti-dAChR antibody activity at all: it may be that the dAChR hyperimmunization required to achieve high titres of antibody against this antigen of relatively low immunogenicity (compared to the highly immunogenic nAChR) might have resulted in the production of idiotype-reactive antibodies capable of binding back onto disease-causing anti-AChR antibodies present in the response.

The present studies may point to another explanation for the confusing inconsistencies observed in attempts to relate anti-AChR antibody titres to disease severity and progression in human patients with myasthenia gravis. Evaluation of total anti-AChR antibody concentrations may be very misleading if disease outcome is actually dependent on the presence of particular subsets of those antibodies. Not only may disease severity depend on the titre of a small subset of disease-causing antibody(s) reactive with a particular conformation-dependent AChR region, but it may also depend on the relative contribution of an additional subset of antibody(s) with potential protective activity.

SOME OBSERVATIONS CONCERNING ANTIBODY SPECIFICITIES DEMONSTRATED BY HUMAN MG PATIENTS

Recently, co-existing antibody responses against both AChR and myosin have been described in patients with MG[69–72]. Although the association of MG with anti-AChR antibodies has long been known, the characteristics of MG-related antibodies with additional reactivity against myosin have not been clearly delineated. In light of the potential significance of anti-myosin reactivity with regard to mechanisms of disease induction in MG, we initiated a study[73] to assess the level of clonotypic heterogeneity associated with the anti-myosin antibodies, similar to the evaluations of anti-AChR antibodies described above for EAMG in rats. During the course of these studies, clonotypic antibody species with the unexpected ability to bind both AChR and myosin were observed.

Isoelectric focusing analyses performed on sera obtained from 45 MG patients revealed clonotypic antibody heterogeneity comparable to that seen in the rat. This is true of IEF banding patterns of antibodies from MG patient sera that specifically bind to either AChR-coated or to myosin-coated nitrocellulose paper; however, IEF patterns produced by binding to either AChR or myosin were for the most part, and unexpectedly, the same. Identity in the isoelectric points of many of the antibodies examined is consistent with their amino acid compositions being equivalent. In other words, a single set of antibodies present in patient serum recognizes both AChR and myosin, in contrast to the expected finding of two independent sets of antibodies, each with individual reactivities against each of the antigens in question.

Amino acid sequences of AChR and myosin have been compared in an effort to explain the observed cross-reactivity. Quite unexpectedly, the greatest sequence identity is found between amino acid residues 67–76 of the AChR α-subunit, a region associated with great immunogenicity[74] and in close proximity to the acetylcholine and toxin binding sites[75,76], and a region in the myosin domain (MHC-S1) that lies adjacent to a portion of both the actin binding site (approximately 30 amino acids away[77,78]) and the ATP binding site (approximately 50 amino acids away[79]). The physiological significance of these cross-reactive determinants being in the vicinity of biologically important regions of their respective molecules remains unknown. The validity of the binding studies is supported, however, by the finding that patient antibodies with reactivity to both myosin and the synthetic AChR α-subunit peptide (α61–76) also co-purify on antigen columns, co-migrate in IEF gels (Figure 8.7), and clearly demonstrate inhibited antigen binding when either myosin or the AChR peptide is used as the inhibitor (Figure 8.8).

The observations described above lead to several important questions. First, what stimulates the production of these cross-reactive antibodies? Second, what role do they play in the course and progress of MG? Third, and most perplexing, what is the explanation for the existence of this antigenic/structural relationship between two complex proteins with strikingly dissimilar functions?

In identifying the initial stimulus for antibody production with reactivity for both AChR and myosin, one might question whether anti-AChR antibodies are cross-reacting with myosin or vice versa. An exogenous antigen may play a role[80]: for example, administration of certain drugs or infection by certain microbial agents may stimulate antibody reactivities that are directly cross-reactive with the AChR or that may perturb the idiotypic network in such a way as to generate AChR reactivities indirectly[81–88]. Unpredicted cross-reactivities have also been found between myosin and certain microbial antigens[89–91], raising the possibility that myosin-reactive autoantibodies produced during infection might also cross-react with antigenically related self antigens, including the AChR. Is it possible that the 'immunodominance' of the main immunogenic region associated with the AChR region α67–76 is only apparent, reflecting a cross-reactivity with a set of autoantibodies stimulated by a myosin-like antigen associated with certain microorganisms?

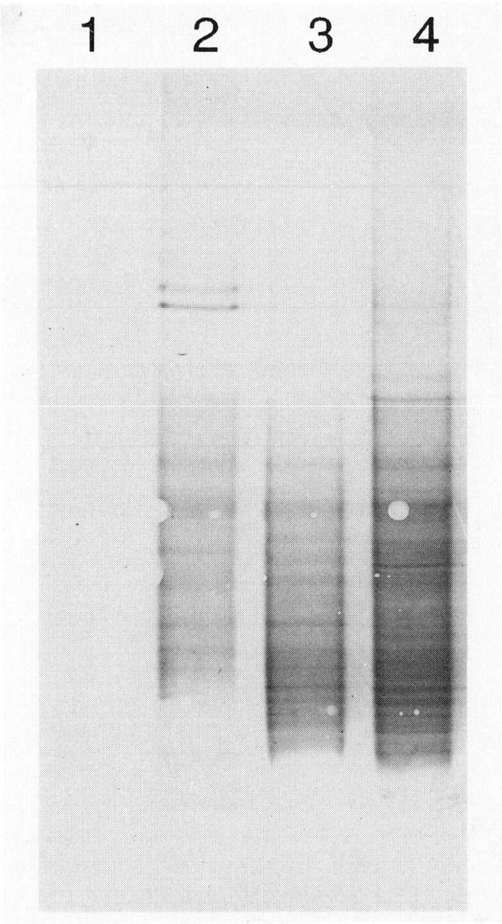

Figure 8.7 Electrofocused MG patient antibodies bound to myosin-coated paper demonstrate similar banding patterns whether originally obtained by affinity purification on columns coupled with myosin or the MIR-containing peptide (α61–76). Following electrofocusing in a pH 5–8 gradient, antibodies were blotted onto nitrocellulose paper coated with purified myosin. The blot was then probed with HRP-conjugated rabbit anti-human Ig and developed with diaminobenzidine. Lane 1: normal non-immune human Ig; Lane 2: affinity-purified patient anti-myosin; Lane 3: affinity-purified patient anti-MIR peptide; Lane 4: unfractionated patient Ig. Taken from reference 73

Studies of the potential importance, if any, of AChR/myosin cross-reactivity in MG must take into account the fact that whole AChR is clearly extracellular, myosin is intracellular. It is difficult to envisage the pathological role played by antibodies against an intracellular protein. Some initial perturbation of the junctional muscle membrane by antibodies newly synthesized to AChR may lead to the exposure of internal cytoskeletal elements, after which damage to the junction would be compounded by the binding of the same antibodies to the now accessible myosin. Alternatively,

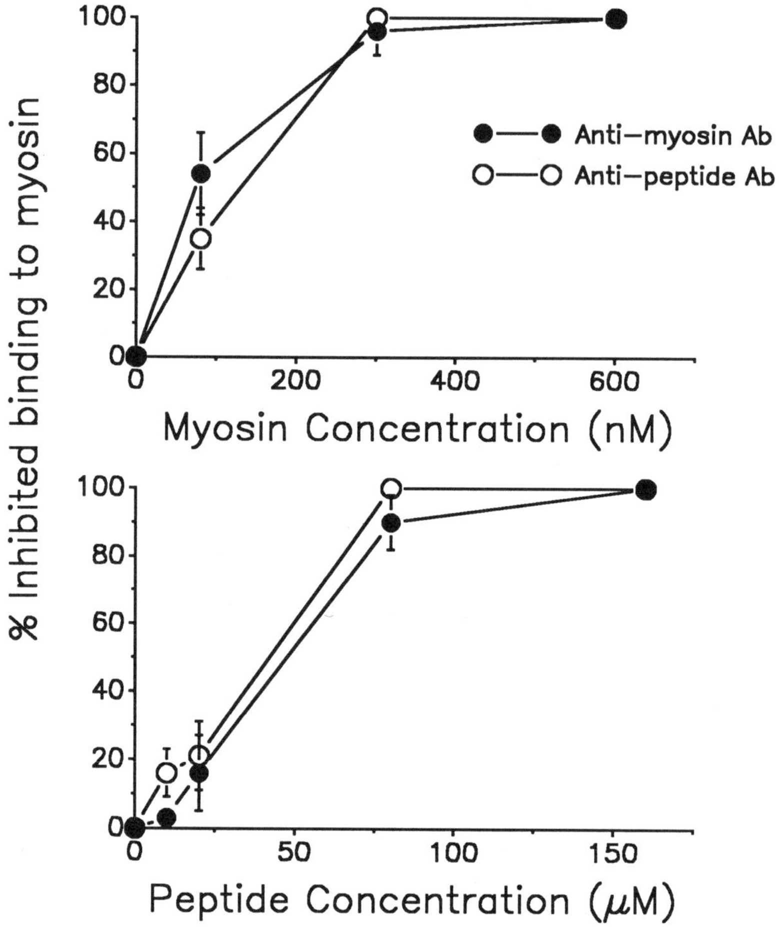

Figure 8.8 AChR α61–76 peptide can inhibit myosin-reactive antibodies from binding to myosin. Patient antibodies affinity-purified on either myosin columns (●) or AChR α61–76 peptide columns (○) were preincubated for 45 min at room temperature with the indicated inhibitor concentrations of either myosin (upper panel) or the AChR peptide (lower panel) before exposure to 5 μg of solid-phase myosin. In each case, binding by patient antibodies was probed using ^{125}I-labelled rabbit anti-human Ig; percentage inhibited binding is given as mean values of triplicate samples (± SEM) for which 100% (uninhibited) binding resulted in CPM bound that ranged from about 4500 to 6500 c.p.m. bound. Inhibition of antibody binding to myosin by equivalent concentrations of an unrelated control peptide (N-terminal region of the SV40 T antigen) never exceeded 5%. Taken from reference 73

cross-reactive antibodies newly synthesized against damaged myosin or AChR–myosin complexes[92–96], may then bind to AChR displayed on the intact junctional membrane. Once this point is reached, one can imagine a circular perpetuation of this antibody response in which either AChR or myosin can serve as the primary stimulus.

FINAL CONCLUSIONS

The strategies of the experimentation described above were designed to address the confusion resulting from observations concerning the lack of correlation between antibody titres and disease severity in MG patients. Lessons learned from these studies indicate that if the proportion of the total expressed/produced anti-AChR antibody repertoire with disease-causing potential differs between patients, then assessment of the total antibody titre becomes meaningless unless a particular patient produces disease-causing reactivities that make up a major portion of the total titre. In contrast, a patient could produce a very high anti-AChR antibody titre but remain in relatively good health because the vast majority of the autoantibody is biologically benign. The key to exploiting the existence of antibody subsets with differing disease-causing potential will be to create probes that allow the easy monitoring of the relevant reactivities. These probes may be anti-idiotypic antibodies that specifically recognize idiotopes associated with disease-causing anti-AChR antibodies that are under-represented on antibodies unable to cause disease.

Alternatively, molecular (DNA) probes that identify activated lymphocytes expressing particular antibody-associated complementarity determining regions (CDR) might assess very precisely the contribution made by a disease-causing antibody subset in MG patients. Identification of all characteristics associated with antibodies responsible for impaired muscle function would probably lead to a more precise understanding of relationships between antibody titre and disease severity, as well as the opportunity to more directly evaluate disease mechanisms and to develop more effective immunotherapeutic strategies.

ACKNOWLEDGEMENTS

This research is currently supported by NIH grants NS28172 and NS24954, and a grant from the Muscular Dystrophy Association.

References

1. Patrick J, Lindstrom JM. Autoimmune response to acetylcholine receptor. Science. 1973;180:871–2.
2. Lindstrom J, Shelton D, Fujii Y. Myasthenia gravis. Adv Immunol. 1988;42:233–84.
3. Lindstrom J, Seybold ME, Lennon VA, Whittingham S, Duane DD. Antibody to acetylcholine receptor in myasthenia gravis: Prevalence, clinical correlates, and diagnostic value. Neurology. 1976;26:1054–9.
4. Tindall RSA. Humoral immunity in myasthenia gravis: clinical correlations of anti-receptor antibody avidity and titer. Ann NY Acad Sci. 1981;377:316–29.
5. Drachman DB, Adams RN, Josifek LF, Self SG. Functional activities of autoantibodies to acetylcholine receptors and the clinical severity of myasthenia gravis. N Engl J Med. 1982;307:769–75.
6. Hohlfeld R, Sterz R, Kalies I, Wekerle H, Peper K. Experimental myasthenia: Lack of correlation between the autoantibody titer and the reduction of acetylcholine-controlled ionic channels measured at functioning endplates. Muscle Nerve. 1983;6:160–3.

7. Lefvert AK, Cuenoud S, Fulpius BW. Binding properties and subclass distribution of anti-acetylcholine receptor antibodies in myasthenia gravis. J Neuroimmunol. 1981;1:125–35.
8. Lennon VA, Seybold ME, Lindstrom J, Cochrane C. Role of complement in the pathogenesis of experimental autoimmune myasthenia gravis. J Exp Med. 1978;147:973–83.
9. Bray JJ, Drachman DB. Binding affinities of anti-acetylcholine receptor autoantibodies in myasthenia gravis. J Immunol. 1982;128:105–10.
10. Eldefrawi ME, Aronstam RS, Bakry NM, Eldefrawi AT, Albuquerque EX. Activation, inactivation, and desensitization of acetylcholine receptor channel complex detected by binding of histrionicotoxin. Proc Natl Acad Sci USA. 1980;77:2309–13.
11. Marzo AL, Garlepp MJ, Schon-Hegrad M, Dawkins RL. Susceptibility to murine experimental autoallergic myasthenia gravis: The role of antibody specificity. Clin Exp Immunol. 1986;64:101–6.
12. Heinemann S, Bevan S, Kullberg R, Lindstrom J, Rice J. Modulation of acetylcholine receptor by antibody against the receptor. Proc Natl Acad Sci USA. 1977;74:3090–4.
13. Drachman DB, Angus CW, Adams RN, Kao I. Myasthenic antibodies crosslink acetylcholine receptors to accelerate degradation. N Engl J Med. 1978;298:1116–22.
14. Tzartos SJ, Sophianos D, Efthimiadis A. Role of the main immunogenic region of acetylcholine receptor in myasthenia gravis. An Fab monoclonal antibody protects against modulation by human sera. J Immunol. 1985;134:2343–9.
15. Brown RM, Krolick KA. Clonotypic analysis of the antibody response to the acetylcholine receptor in experimental autoimmune myasthenia gravis. J Neuroimmunol. 1988;19:205–22.
16. Thompson PA, Krolick KA. Acetylcholine receptor-reactive antibodies in experimental autoimmune myasthenia gravis differing in disease-causing potential: subsetting by preparative isoelectric focusing. Clin Immunol Immunopathol. 1992;62:199–209.
17. Yeh T, Krolick KA. Influence of T cell specificity on the heterogeneity and disease-causing capability of antibody against the acetylcholine receptor. J Neuroimmunol. 1987;17:17–34.
18. Yeh T, Krolick KA. Clonotypic analysis of anti-acetylcholine receptor antibodies produced against native and denatured antigen. J Neuroimmunol. 1989;24:133–43.
19. Yeh TM, Krolick KA. T cells reactive with a small synthetic peptide of the acetylcholine receptor can provide help for a clonotypically heterogeneous antibody response and subsequently impaired muscle function. J Immunol. 1990;144:1654–60.
20. Zoda T, Yeh TM, Krolick KA. Clonotypic analysis of anti-acetylcholine receptor antibodies from EAMG-sensitive Lewis rats and EAMG-resistant Wistar Furth rats. J Immunol. 1991;146:663–70.
21. Brown RM, Krolick KA. Selective idiotype suppression of an adoptive secondary anti-acetylcholine receptor antibody response by immunotoxin treatment prior to transfer. J Immunol. 1988;140:893–8.
22. Biesecker G, Koffler D. Resistance to experimental autoimmune myasthenia gravis in genetically inbred rats: association with decreased amounts of in situ acetylcholine receptor–antibody complexes. J Immunol. 1988;140:3406–10.
23. Olsberg CA, Maxwell LC, Mikiten TM, Krolick KA. Analysis of contractile properties of muscles from rats immunized with purified acetylcholine receptor. J Neuroimmunol. 1987;14:253–66.
24. Thompson PA, Barohn RJ, Krolick KA. Repetitive nerve stimulation vs. twitch tension in rats with EAMG. Muscle Nerve. 1991;15:94–100.
25. Gutman GA. Rat immunoglobulin allotypes. In: Weir DM, editor. Genetics and Molecular Immunology. Oxford: Blackwell Scientific Publications, 1986: Chap 98.
26. Lennon V, Lambert E. Myasthenia gravis induced by monoclonal antibodies to acetylcholine receptor. Nature. 1980;285:238–40.
27. Lennon VA, Lambert EH. Monoclonal antibodies to acetylcholine receptors: Evidence for a dominant idiotype and requirement of complement for pathogenicity. Ann NY Acad Sci. 1981;377:77–96.
28. Gomez C, Richman D. Anti-acetylcholine receptor antibodies directed against the α-bungarotoxin binding site induce a unique form of experimental myasthenia. Proc Natl Acad Sci USA. 1983;80:4089–93.
29. Gomez C, Richman D. Monoclonal anti-acetylcholine receptor antibodies with differing capacities to induce experimental autoimmune myasthenia gravis. J Immunol. 1985;135: 234–41.

30. Tzartos S, Hochschwender S, Vasquez P, Lindstrom J. Passive transfer of experimental autoimmune myasthenia gravis by monoclonal antibodies to the main immunogenic region of the acetylcholine receptor. J Neuroimmunol. 1987;15:185–94.
31. Thompson PA, Krolick KA. Subsetting of acetylcholine receptor-reactive antibodies by preparative isoelectric focusing. Prep Biochem. 1991;21:229–35.
32. Bartfeld D, Fuchs S. Immunological characterization of an irreversibly denatured acetylcholine receptor. FEBS Lett. 1977;77:214–18.
33. Bartfeld D, Fuchs S. Specific immunosuppression of experimental autoimmune myasthenia gravis by denatured acetylcholine receptor. Proc Natl Acad Sci USA. 1978;75:4006–10.
34. Bartfeld D, Fuchs S. Fractionation of antibodies to acetylcholine receptor according to antigenic specificity. FEBS Lett. 1979;105:303–6.
35. Lindstrom JM, Lennon VA, Seybold ME, Whittingham S. Experimental autoimmune myasthenia gravis: biochemical and immunochemical aspects. Ann NY Acad Sci. 1976;274:254–74.
36. Froehner SC. Identification of exposed and buried determinants of the membrane-bound acetylcholine receptor from *Torpedo californica*. Biochemistry. 1981;20:4905–15.
37. Ratnam M, Sargent PB, Sarin V, *et al.* Location of antigenic determinants on primary sequences of subunits of nicotinic acetylcholine receptor by peptide mapping. Biochemistry. 1986;25:2621–32.
38. Ralston S, Sarin V, Thanh HL, Rivier J, Fox JL, Lindstrom J. Synthetic peptides used to locate the bungarotoxin binding site and immunogenic regions on a subunit of the nicotinic acetylcholine receptor. Biochemistry. 1987;26:3261–6.
39. Guillet J-G, Lai MZ, Briner TJ, *et al.* Immunological self, nonself discrimination. Science. 1987;235:865–70.
40. Buus S, Sette A, Miles C, Grey HM. The relation between major histocompatibility complex restriction and the capacity of Ia to bind immunogenic peptides. Science. 1987;235:1353–8.
41. Berzofsky JA, Brett SJ, Streicher HZ, Takahashi H. Antigen processing for presentation to T lymphocytes: Function, mechanisms, and implications for the T cell repertoire. Immunol Rev. 1988;106:5–31.
42. Babbitt BP, Allen PM, Matsueda G, Haber E, Unanue ER. The binding of immunogenic peptides to Ia histocompatibility molecules. Nature. 1985;317:359–61.
43. Brown JH, Jardetzky T, Saper MA, Samaraoui B, Bjorkman PJ, Wiley DC. A hypothetical model of the foreign antigen binding site of class II histocompatibility molecules. Nature. 1988;332:845–50.
44. Rosenthal A. Determinant selection and macrophage function in genetic control of the immune response. Immunol Rev. 1978;40:136–52.
45. Davis M, Bjorkman P. T cell antigen receptor genes and T cell recognition. Nature. 1988;334:395–402.
46. Lorenz RG, Tyler AN, Allen PM. T cell recognition of ribonuclease: Self/nonself discrimination at the level of binding to the I-A^k molecule. J Immunol. 1988;141:4124–8.
47. Lorenz RG, Allen PM. Direct evidence for functional self protein/Ia-molecule complexes *in vivo*. Proc Natl Acad Sci USA. 1988;85:5220–4.
48. Fuchs S, Nevo D, Tarrah-Hazdai R, Yaar I. Strain differences in the autoimmune response of mice to acetylcholine receptors. Nature. 1976;263:329–30.
49. Christadoss P, Lennon VA, David C. Genetic control of experimental autoimmune myasthenia gravis in mice. I. Lymphocyte proliferative response to acetylcholine receptor is under H-2-linked Ir gene control. J Immunol. 1979;123:2540–3.
50. Christadoss P, Lindstrom J, Melvold R, Talal N. Mutation at I-A beta chain prevents experimental autoimmune myasthenia gravis. Immunogenetics. 1985;21:33–8.
51. Berman PW, Patrick J. Linkage between the frequency of muscular weakness and loci that regulate immune responsiveness in murine experimental myasthenia gravis. J Exp Med. 1980;152:507–20.
52. Biesecker G, Koffler D. Resistance to experimental autoimmune myasthenia gravis in genetically inbred rats: Association with decreased amounts of in situ acetylcholine receptor-antibody complexes. J Immunol. 1988;140:3406–10.
53. Fujii Y, Lindstrom J. Specificity of the T cell immune response to acetylcholine receptor in experimental myasthenia gravis. Response to subunits and synthetic peptides. J Immunol. 1988;140:1830–7.

54. Zhang Y, Barkas T, Juillerat M, Schwendimann B, Wekerle H. T cell epitopes in experimental myasthenia gravis of the rat: Strain-specific epitopes and cross-reaction between two distinct segments of the α chain of the acetylcholine receptor (*Torpedo californica*). Eur J Immunol. 1988;18:551–7.
55. Yokoi T, Mulac-Jericevic H, Atassi MZ. T lymphocyte recognition of acetylcholine receptor. Localization of the full T cell recognition profile on the extracellular part of the α chain of *Torpedo californica* acetylcholine receptor. Eur J Immunol. 1987;17:1697–702.
56. Atassi MZ, Biserka M, Yokoi T, Manshouri Y. Localization of the functional sites on the α chain of acetylcholine receptor. Fed Proc. 1988;46:2538–47.
57. Lennon VA, McCormick DJ, Lambert EH, Griesmann GE, Atassi MZ. Region of peptide 125-147 of acetylcholine receptor alpha subunit is exposed at neuromuscular junction and induces experimental autoimmune myasthenia gravis, T cell immunity, and modulating autoantibodies. Proc Natl Acad Sci USA. 1985;82:8805–9.
58. Hohlfeld R, Kalies I, Heinz F, Kalden JR, Werkele H. Autoimmune rat T lymphocytes monospecific for acetylcholine receptor: Purification and fine specificity. J Immunol. 1981;126:1355–9.
59. Infante AJ, Thompson PA, Krolick KA, Wall KA. Determinant selection in murine experimental autoimmune myasthenia gravis: effect of the bm12 mutation on T cell recognition of acetylcholine receptor epitopes. J Immunol. 1991;146:2977–82.
60. Infante AJ, Levcovitz H, Wall KA, Thompson PA, Krolick KA. Preferential use of a T cell receptor Vβ gene by acetylcholine receptor-reactive T cells from myasthenia gravis susceptible mice. J Immunol. 1992;148:3385–90.
61. Krolick KA, Urso OE. Influence of T cell specificity on the antibody response to the acetylcholine receptor. J Neuroimmunol. 1986;13:75–81.
62. Celada F, Sercarz EE. Preferential pairing of T–B specificities in the same antigen: the concept of directional help. Vaccine. 1988;6:94–8.
63. Tami JA, Urso OE, Krolick KA. T cell hybridomas reactive with the acetylcholine receptor and its subunits. J Immunol. 1987;138:732–8.
64. Arthur R, Mason D. T cells that help B cell responses to soluble antigen are distinguishable from those producing interleukin 2 on mitogenic or allogeneic stimulation. J Exp Med. 1986;163:774–86.
65. Hohlfeld R, Toyka KV, Heininger K, Gross-Wilde H, Kalies I. Autoimmune human T lymphocytes specific for acetylcholine receptor. Nature. 1984;310:244–6.
66. Hohlfeld R, Toyka KV, Miner LL, Walgrave SL, Conti-Tronconi BM. Amphipathic segment of the nicotinic receptor alpha subunit contains epitopes recognized by T lymphocytes in myasthenia gravis. J Clin Invest. 1988;81:657–60.
67. Melms A, Chrestel S, Schalke BC, *et al.* Autoimmune T lymphocytes in myasthenia gravis. Determination of target epitopes using T lines and recombinant products of the mouse nicotinic acetylcholine receptor gene. J Clin Invest. 1989;83:785–90.
68. Corey AL, Richman DP, Agius MA, Wollmann RL. Refractoriness to a second episode of experimental myasthenia gravis: correlation with AChR concentration and morphologic appearance of the postsynaptic membrane. J Immunol. 1987;138:3269–75.
69. Williams CL, Lennon VA. Thymic B lymphocyte clones from patients with myasthenia gravis secrete monoclonal striational autoantibodies reacting with myosin, a actinin, or actin. J Exp Med. 1986;164:1043–59.
70. Penn AS, Schotland DL, Lamme S. Anti-muscle and anti-acetylcholine receptor antibodies in myasthenia gravis. Muscle Nerve. 1986;9:407–15.
71. Zimmermann CW, Weiss G. Antibodies not directed against the acetylcholine receptor in myasthenia gravis: an immunoblot study. J Neuroimmunol. 1987;16:225–36.
72. Connor RI, Lefvert AK, Benes SC, Lang RW. Incidence and reactivity patterns of skeletal and heart (SH) reactive autoantibodies in the sera of patients with myasthenia gravis. J Neuroimunol. 1990;26:147–57.
73. Mohan S, Barohn RJ, Krolick KA. Unexpected crossreactivity between myosin and a main immunogenic region (MIR) of the acetylcholine receptor: isoelectric focusing analysis of antisera obtained from myasthenia gravis patients. Clin Immunol Immunopathol. 1992;64:218–26.
74. Tzartos S, Kokla A, Walgrave SL, Conti-Tronconi BM. Localization of the main

immunogenic region of human muscle acetylcholine receptor to residues 67-76 of the α subunit. Proc Natl Acad Sci USA. 1988;85:2899–903.
75. Claudio T, Raftery MA. Inhibition of bungarotoxin binding to acetylcholine receptors by antisera from animals with experimental autoimmune myasthenia gravis. J Supramol Structure. 1980;14:267–79.
76. Pachner AR. Anti-acetylcholine receptor antibodies block bungarotoxin binding to native human acetylcholine receptor on the surface of TE671 cells. Neurology. 1989;39:1057–61.
77. Dan-Goor M, Muhlrad A. Antibody directed against the 142–148 sequence of the myosin heavy chain interferes with myosin–actin interaction. Biochemistry. 1991;30:400–5.
78. Tong SW, Elzinga M. The sequence of the NH_2-terminal 204-residue fragment of the heavy chain sequence of rabbit skeletal muscle myosin. J Biol Chem. 1983;258:13100–10
79. Warrick HM, Spudich JA. Myosin structure and function in cell motility. Annu Rev Cell Biol. 1987;3:379–421.
80. Oldstone MBA. Molecular mimicry and autoimmune disease. Cell. 1987;50:819–20.
81. Albers J, Hodach R, Kimmel D, Treacy W. Penicillamine associated myasthenia gravis. Neurology. 1980;30:1246–50.
82. Aoki T, Drachman DB, Asher DM, Gibbs CJ, Bahmanyar S, Wolinsky JS. Attempts to implicate viruses in myasthenia gravis. Neurology. 1985;35:185–92.
83. Lentz TL, Benson RJJ, Klimowicz D, Wilson PT, Hawrot E. Binding of rabies virus to purified *Torpedo* acetylcholine receptor. Mol Brain Res. 1986;1:211–19.
84. Lefvert A, James RW, Alliod C, Fulpius BW. A monoclonal anti-idiotypic antibody against anti-receptor atibodies from myasthenic sera. Eur J Immunol. 1982;12:790–6.
85. Dwyer DS, Bradley RJ, Urquhart CK, Kearney JF. Naturally occurring anti-idiotypic antibodies in myasthenia gravis patients. Nature. 1983;301:611–14.
86. Strickland FM, Hamilton SL, Blalock E, Cerny J. Shared idiotype between phosphoryl-choline-specific antibody and acetylcholinesterase detectable by a monoclonal antibody. J Immunol. 1985;134:1053–8.
87. Lang B, Roberts AJ, Vincent A, Newsome-Davis J. Anti-acetylcholine receptor idiotypes in myasthenia gravis analyzed by rabbit antisera. Clin Exp Immunol. 1985;60:637–44.
88. Lefvert A, Holm G, Pirskanen R. Autoantiidiotypic antibodies in myasthenia gravis. Ann NY Acad Sci. 1986;505:133–54.
89. Cunningham MW, McCormack JM, Fenderson PG, Ho M, Beachey EH, Dale JB. Human and murine antibodies cross-reactive with streptococcal M protein and myosin recognize the sequence GLN-LYS-SER-LYS-GLN in M protein. J Immunol. 1989;143:2677–83.
90. Cunningham MW, Antone SM, Fulizia JM, McManus BM, Fischetti VA, Gauntt CJ. Molecular mimicry between streptococcal M protein, coxsackie viruses, and human cardiac myosin: A link to cytotoxic autoimmunity. Proc Natl Acad Sci USA. 1992;89:1320–4.
91. Beisel KW, Srinivasappa J, Prabhakar BS. Identification of a putative shared epitope between coxsackie virus B4 and alpha cardiac myosin heavy chain. Clin Exp Immunol. 1991;86:49–55.
92. Prives J, Fulton A, Penman S, Daniels MP, Christian CN. Interaction of the cytoskeletal framework with acetylcholine receptor on the surface of embryonic muscle cells in culture. J Cell Biol. 1982;92:231–6.
93. Gotti C, Conti-Tronconi BM, Raftery MA. Mammalian muscle acetylcholine receptor purification and characterization. Biochemistry. 1982;21:3148–54.
94. Froehner SC. The submembrane machinery for nicotinic acetylcholine receptor clustering. J Cell Biol. 1991;114:1–7.

9
Autoimmune diseases of muscle

R. HOHLFELD and A. G. ENGEL

INTRODUCTION

This chapter focuses primarily on the immunopathogenesis, clinical features and treatment of polymyositis (PM), inclusion body myositis (IBM) and dermatomyositis (DM), the commonly encountered inflammatory myopathies. Parasitic, bacterial, spirochaetal and viral infectious myopathies are not discussed. For recent general reviews, the reader may wish to refer to references 1–5.

PATHOGENESIS

Hypothetically, the immune effector mechanism(s) in the inflammatory myopathies could be humoral, cell-mediated, or both (Table 9.1). The possible targets in muscle consist of the muscle fibre, the vascular components, and the connective tissue elements. Current evidence suggests that in DM the effector response is mediated predominantly by humoral factors and that the muscle microvasculature is an early, and probably primary, target. By contrast, in PM and IBM there is evidence for T cell-mediated cytotoxicity directed against the muscle fibre.

Table 9.1 Possible immune effector mechanisms in autoimmune myopathies

Antibody-dependent cytotoxicity
Complement-mediated
Cell-mediated (macrophages, NK cells)
Cell-dependent cytotoxicity
Antigen-specific, MHC-restricted (Tc cells)
Broad specificity and MHC unrestricted (NK cells)
Immune complex-mediated cytotoxicity

Humoral effector mechanisms in DM

Several observations suggest that circulating antibodies or immune complexes induce vascular injury in DM. Severe injury to the intramuscular blood vessels has been demonstrated by light and electron microscopy[6–9]. Further, immune complexes (immunoglobulins and complement C3) were observed in the mural elements of perimysial venules, and C5b-9 complement membrane attack complex (MAC) neoantigens were shown to be localized to the walls of intramuscular arterioles and capillaries[10,11]. These observations suggest that the microvascular injury in DM is mediated by complement, and that the lytic complement pathway is triggered either by a pathogenic antibody that binds to a vascular element, or by the deposition of immune complexes on or around the vessel walls. The muscle fibre injury may arise secondary to ischaemia; alternatively, immune complexes could injure muscle fibres and blood vessels concurrently. An inflammatory exudate is commonly present in DM, and at least some of the tissue damage could be mediated by inflammatory cells.

Immunophenotype analysis of mononuclear cells in DM has helped to clarify the role of the inflammatory cells[12]. The inflammatory exudate is predominantly perivascular and perimysial, and to a lesser extent endomysial. B cells are most abundant at perivascular and least abundant at endomysial sites. At all three sites B cells are more abundant in DM than in PM or IBM. By contrast, the proportion of T cells is lowest at perivascular and highest at endomysial sites. The CD4/CD8 ratio is the highest at perivascular and lowest at endomysial sites. Although many inflammatory cells display HLA class II (HLA-DR) antigen, less than 20% of the perivascular and endomysial T cells are HLA-DR$^+$, that is, activated. Macrophages account for 25–30% of all mononuclear cells at the different sites. Natural killer (NK) cells are sparse and present only at perivascular sites. Invasion of non-necrotic muscle fibres by mononuclear cells is not a feature of DM: it was observed in only a few fibres in less than half of the patients. The distribution of mononuclear cell subsets is similar in childhood and adult DM.

The high percentage of B cells, the high CD4/CD8 ratios and the close proximity of CD4$^+$ cells to B cells at all sites of cell accumulation suggest T helper cell-dependent stimulation of B cells to secrete immunoglobulin. The close proximity of macrophages to CD4$^+$ cells at all sites of accumulation further suggests that T helper cells may be triggered to respond to an antigen by antigen-presenting cells. These features, the fact that invasion of non-necrotic muscle fibres by mononuclear cells is essentially absent, and the paucity of mature NK cells imply that DM is humorally mediated, and that a local humoral response is probably occurring in muscle itself. However, the presence of a diffuse endomysial infiltrate containing CD8$^+$ cells and macrophages could still indicate a cell-mediated effector response against a vascular or connective tissue component.

Further support for a primary microvascular insult in DM derives from studies of the earliest pathological alterations in DM[13,14]. In six DM muscle specimens that appeared normal on routine analysis of cryostat sections, electron microscopy revealed microtubular inclusions and microvacuoles in

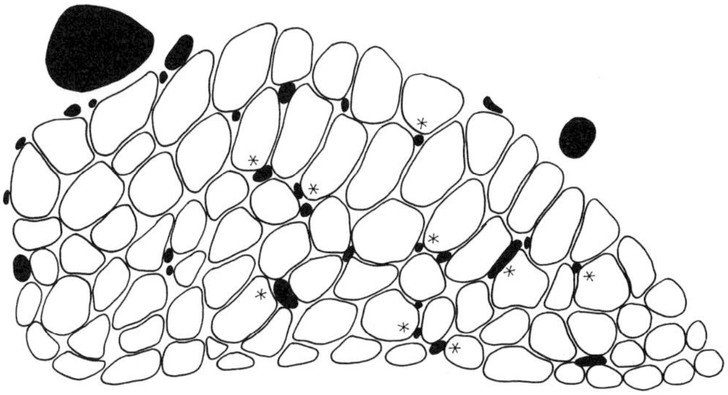

Figure 9.1 Characteristic changes in DM. Muscle fibres are shown white, blood vessels black. Note atrophic fibres at the bottom edge of the fascicle (perifascicular atrophy). Clusters of capillaries and venules react for complement membrane attack complex (MAC). MAC^+ vessels are marked with an asterisk. The capillary density (number of capillaries/mm^2 of fibre area) and the capillary index (number of capillaries/1000 μm^2 area of each fibre) are significantly reduced. Modified from reference 14

a proportion of endomysial capillaries, and pale swollen endothelial cells were seen in three of the six specimens[13]. In another study, 10 DM muscle specimens in which routine examination of cryostat sections revealed no diagnostic abnormality, were analysed quantitatively for the density and distribution of capillaries. Capillaries were localized using the lectin *Ulex europaeus* agglutinin I, and the proportion of MAC-positive capillaries was determined with a polyclonal antiserum against neoantigenic determinants of the C5b-9 complement membrane attack complex (MAC)[14]. The study revealed a marked capillary depletion. The mean capillary density (number/mm^2 muscle fibre area) was 275 in the 10 patients and 393 in eight normal controls ($p < 0.001$), and the capillary frequency distribution in $100 \times 100\,\mu m$ squares was significantly shifted to the left, compared with the control distribution ($p < 0.001$)[14]. Further, in all 10 cases, a proportion of the capillaries were positive for MAC (Figure 9.1). The findings indicate that in DM capillary lysis precedes other pathological changes in muscle, and that the capillary endothelium is an early, and possibly primary, target of the autoimmune response[14]. Consistent with this notion is the recent demonstration of circulating antibodies recognizing human umbilical vein endothelial cells in eight of 18 DM patients[15].

Cellular effector mechanisms in PM and IBM

Immunohistochemical studies have provided strong evidence for a role of cellular effector mechanisms in the pathogenesis of PM and IBM[12,16–21]. In both diseases, the inflammatory exudate is predominantly endomysial, and in the endomysium it is selectively enriched in $CD8^+$ cells. The exudate is also prominent at perivascular and perimysial sites in PM, but less marked at these sites in IBM.

$CD8^+$ cytotoxic T lymphocytes (CTL) account for an increasing proportion

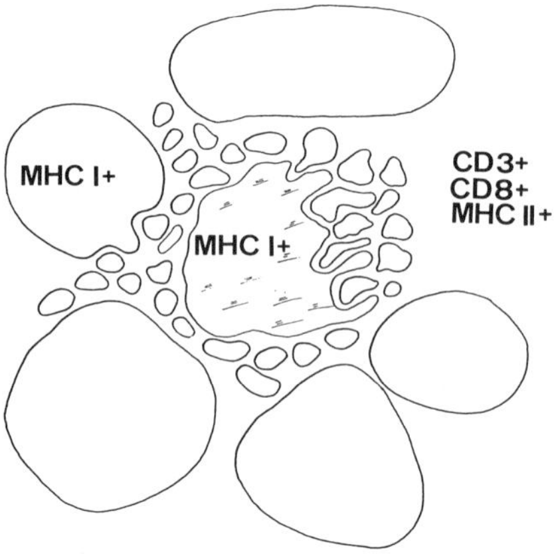

Figure 9.2 Characteristic endomysial lesion in polymyositis. T cells surround and focally invade a non-necrotic muscle fibre. The majority of the autoinvasive T cells have the phenotype $CD3^+$, $CD8^+$, HLA class II^+. All invaded and some non-invaded muscle fibres show surface reactivity for HLA class I antigens. Some invaded fibres also show cytoplasmatic reactivity for HLA class I antigens. From reference 5, with permission

of T cells and of all mononuclear cells as one proceeds from perivascular to perimysial to endomysial sites, and the proportion of activated T cells is nearly twice as high at endomysial as at perivascular sites. By contrast, B cells are more abundant at perivascular and absent or nearly absent from endomysial sites. Macrophages account for nearly the same proportion of cells at all three sites of accumulation. $CD16^+$ NK cells are virtually absent in IBM and PM, indicating that NK-type myocytotoxicity does not play an important role in these diseases[19]. However, a subtype of $CD3^+CD8^+$ T cells expressing CD57 accounted for 29% and 23% of all $CD3^+$ cells in IBM and PM, respectively[19]. *In vitro*, T cells with this phenotype show lectin-dependent cytotoxicity, but little or no spontaneous (NK-like) cytotoxicity[22,23].

A characteristic finding of both PM and IBM is non-necrotic muscle fibres that are focally invaded and destroyed by $CD8^+$ CTL (Figure 9.2). The CTL are accompanied by a lesser number of macrophages. Quantitative analysis revealed that in IBM, these non-necrotic invaded fibres, which can be regarded as indicators of cell-mediated cytotoxicity, are 5.5 times more frequent than necrotic fibres[19]. In PM, the two mechanisms of fibre destruction are detected at comparable frequencies[19].

The invading cells consist essentially of $CD8^+$ cells and macrophages in a ratio of 2–3 to 1[16]. Only a few $CD4^+$ cells occur among the invading cells, but approximately one-quarter of the cells that surround the invaded fibres are $CD4^+$. Close to 34% of the invading $CD8^+$ cells and 17–25% of the surrounding $CD8^+$ cells are activated, as suggested by their expression of HLA-DR antigens. The distribution of the identified phenotypes is similar in PM and IBM except for the slightly but significantly higher percentage of $CD8^+$ cells among either the invading or surrounding cells in IBM than in PM.

An interesting question is whether the endomysial T cells observed in PM and IBM are monoclonal, oligoclonal, or polyclonal. Using the polymerase chain reaction, it has recently become possible to isolate mRNA coding for T cell receptor (TCR) directly from autoimmune lesions[24,25]. The TCR $V\alpha$ and $V\beta$ repertoire has been examined in muscle biopsy specimens from 15 patients with PM and 16 controls, including six patients with Duchenne muscular dystrophy[25]. In PM, the most commonly rearranged TCR variable genes were $V\alpha1$, $V\alpha5$, $V\beta1$, and $V\beta15$. By contrast, the spectrum of TCR α or β rearrangements noted in patients with Duchenne muscular dystrophy was much broader. No TCR rearrangements were found in muscles from the other controls. Sequence analysis revealed the presence of the $J\beta2.1$ region in 90% of the $V\beta15$-positive clones studied, absence of random additions in the TCR diversity region, and a common motif in the CDR3 region of the TCR. Although these results are consistent with the notion that the effector cells in PM represent a relatively small number of distinct (oligoclonal) autoreactive T cell clones, the results of PCR analyses of TCR have been highly controversial in other diseases[24]. Therefore, in future studies, it will be essential to combine PCR analyses with morphological (immunocytochemical) analyses to identify the type of TCR expressed by the autoaggressive T cells observed *in situ*.

The different stages of CTL-mediated myocytotoxicity have been analysed by immunoelectron microscopy[17]. Initially, $CD8^+$ cells and macrophages abut onto and send spike-like processes into non-necrotic muscle fibres. Subsequently, an increasing number of $CD8^+$ cells and macrophages traverse the basal lamina, focally replace, displace or compress the fibre, and spikes from these cells honeycomb the adjacent fibre regions. The macrophages contain only few heterophagic vacuoles and therefore act in a cytotoxic rather than phagocytic capacity. Either the integrity of the muscle fibre surface membrane facing the invading cells is maintained, or the membrane is damaged and rapidly repaired, or the damage cannot be detected by electron microscopy. Nearby fibre regions often show either degenerative changes (increased rough endoplasmic reticulum, polyribosomes, proliferating T-tubules) or degenerative changes (mitochondrial loss and degenerating myofibrils).

Antigen-specific T cell-mediated cytotoxicity in PM and IBM would require expression of major histocompatibility complex class I antigens (HLA class I) on the surface of the target cell[26]. Increased HLA class I antigens are expressed on muscle fibres in both inflammatory and non-inflammatory myopathies[27,28]. It is now fully established that HLA class I antigen expression is consistently increased on the non-necrotic muscle fibres invaded by T cells in PM and IBM (Figure 9.2). However, HLA class I antigen expression in itself is not sufficient to attract CTL because many HLA class I antigen-positive fibres are not invaded by CTL in PM and IBM, and because HLA class I antigen-positive muscle fibres can be observed in DM, and in other myopathies in which evidence of T cell-mediated muscle fibre injury is absent[27,28].

Taken together, the results of the immunohistochemical studies provide strong evidence for HLA-restricted, antigen-specific, T cell-mediated myocytotoxicity in PM and IBM. This implies that the α/β antigen receptor of the cytotoxic CD8$^+$ T cells recognizes antigen(s) presented by HLA-class I molecules on the sarcolemma. According to the rules of antigen presentation via the endogenous pathway[29], these antigens are usually peptides of 8–11 amino acids that are derived from proteins synthesized in the antigen-presenting (target) cell. These proteins may be viral components or genuine self proteins. It is now well established that the vast majority of HLA class I molecules expressed on the surface of any cell are loaded with endogenous self peptides, including peptides derived from heat shock proteins[30]. Furthermore, most attempts to demonstrate viral antigens or genome in muscle fibres in the 'idiopathic' inflammatory myopathies have failed[31]. Therefore we favour the hypothesis that a T cell-mediated autoimmune reaction against endogenous self-antigen(s) rather than viral antigens plays a role in the pathogenesis of PM and IBM.

Cellular effector mechanisms in PM mediated by γ/δ T cells and expression of heat shock proteins by muscle fibres

In most cases of PM, DM and IBM, only very few T cells express the γ/δ receptor. A notable exception is a patient with PM in whom myocytotoxicity was mediated by autoaggressive CD4$^-$CD8$^-$ γ/δ T cells[32]. The vast majority of muscle-infiltrating T cells were reactive with a pan-γ/δ T cell receptor-specific monoclonal antibody, but unlike more than 90% of peripheral blood γ/δ T cells, these lymphocytes did not react with monoclonal antibodies specific for the Vδ1 or Vγ9 variable chain of the γ/δ T cell receptor. In addition, the autoaggressive T cells showed a very unusual differential reactivity with two different monoclonal antibodies against Vδ2. These immunocytochemical observations indicated that the infiltrating T cells expressed a Vδ2-containing T cell receptor with unusual structural features. Using conventional and anchored polymerase chain reaction (PCR) for the analysis of T cell receptor transcripts, we found a striking predominance of one unusual Vδ2/Jδ3 recombination and one Vγ3/Jγ1 recombination in the muscle biopsy specimen from this patient[33]. Both the unusual phenotype and the dominance of distinct T cell receptor transcripts are compatible with the assumption that one T cell clone, which expresses a Vγ3/Jγ1/Cγ1/Vδ2/Jδ3/Cδ disulphide-linked TCR, dominates among the infiltrating T cells in this patient[33].

The fact that some γ/δ T cells recognize heat shock proteins (hsp) prompted us to study the muscular expression of 65 kDa hsp in PM mediated by γ/δ T cells, in other inflammatory myopathies, and in normal muscle[34]. In PM mediated by γ/δ T cells, essentially all muscle fibres showed intense surface reactivity and frequently intermyofibrillar and subsarcolemmal reactivity for 65 kDa hsp. Some of the inflammatory cells, capillary endothelial cells, and the mural elements of larger blood vessels also reacted with the anti-65 kDa hsp monoclonal antibody. Similarly, in other inflammatory myopathies, the

65 kDa hsp was detected on inflammatory cells, degenerating and regenerating fibres, and on many but not all non-necrotic muscle fibres invaded by T cells. In normal muscle, 65 kDa hsp was detected on capillary endothelial cells, the mural elements of larger vessels, and some intracellular organelles, probably mitochondria[34].

In vitro models of T cell-mediated muscle fibre injury

Human myoblasts can be isolated from muscle biopsy specimens by mechanical dissociation and trypsinization[35–37], and can be expanded in culture. Purity of the myoblast preparations can be assessed by reactivity with a monoclonal antibody against CD56 (Leu 19/NKH-1), which reacts with an isoform of the neural cell adhesion molecule N-CAM not expressed on fibroblasts[36,38,39]. The same monoclonal antibody can be used to purify myoblasts by fluorescence-activated or magnetic cell sorting. Myoblasts can be induced to fuse into multinucleated myotubes by culturing the cells in a fusion supporting medium[35–37].

Expression of HLA and adhesion molecules on myoblasts and myotubes

Several different groups of investigators have examined which immunologically relevant surface molecules are either constitutively expressed on myoblasts and myotubes, or can be induced by inflammatory cytokines known to be locally secreted during inflammatory responses[36,40–47]. Table 9.2 summarizes the present knowledge of the phenotypic properties of human myoblasts and myotubes. Myoblasts constitutively express HLA class I antigens[36] and a low level of lymphocyte function-associated (LFA) molecule 3 (LFA-3, CD58)[40]. Both molecules are members of the immunoglobulin superfamily and have a broad tissue distribution[48]. LFA-1 (CD11a/CD18) and LFA-2 (CD2) are not expressed[40]. Tumour necrosis factor (TNF)-α, a cytokine secreted by macrophages, T cells and NK cells[49], induces myoblasts to express the intercellular adhesion molecule-1 (ICAM-1, CD54)[40]. ICAM-1, also a member of the immunoglobulin family, is absent from most cells in normal, non-lymphoid tissue but is expressed on diverse cell types in response to inflammatory mediators[48]. Interferon-γ (IFN-γ), a cytokine secreted by T cells and natural killer cells[50], induces myoblasts to express HLA-DR and ICAM-1[36,40–43], reaching a plateau after 48 h. HLA-DP and HLA-DQ can also be induced by IFN-γ but the kinetics of cytokine induction and the levels of expression vary between the different HLA class II molecules[40,42]. Like myoblasts, myotubes constitutively express HLA class I but not HLA class II antigens[5,36]. Unlike myoblasts, only a subpopulation of myotubes can be induced by IFN-γ to express HLA-DR[51]. Further, unlike myoblasts, myotubes do not express detectable levels of HLA-DP or HLA-DQ (Table 9.2).

Table 9.2 Constitutive and cytokine-induced expression of HLA and cell adhesion molecules by human myoblasts and myotubes (from reference 51)

Surface antigen	*Constitutive expression*	*Cytokine-induced expression*	
		TNF-α	*IFN-γ*
Myoblasts			
HLA-class I	(+)	N.D.	+
HLA-class II			
DR	−	−	+
DP	−	−	+
DQ	−	−	(+)
ICAM-1	−	+	+
LFA 1	−	−	−
LFA 2	−	N.D.	−
LFA 3	(+)	(+)	(+)
Myotubes			
HLA-class I	(+)	+	+
HLA-class II			
DR	−	−	+*
DP	−	−	−
DQ	−	−	−
ICAM-1	−	+	+
LFA-1	−	−	−
LFA-2	−	−	−
LFA-3	−	−	−

*Positive staining varied between 40 and 95% in different experiments; − negative, (+) weak, + positive staining

CTL-mediated lysis of myoblasts and myotubes

Cultured myotubes and myoblasts express HLA class I molecules. This qualifies them as potential targets of $CD8^+$ CTL[26]. CTL-mediated lysis of myotubes has been shown in two different experimental situations. First, myotubes were lysed by allogeneic $CD8^+$ CTL lines raised against the allogeneic histocompatibility antigens expressed by the donor of the myotubes[52]. Second, myotubes were lysed by autologous $CD8^+$ CTL isolated from muscle of a small number of patients with inflammatory myopathy[37].

The lysis of myotubes by alloreactive $CD3^+CD8^+$ CTL involved the recognition of allogeneic class I HLA antigens because it was completely blocked with a monoclonal antibody against a monomorphic determinant of HLA class I antigens[52]. Autologous control myotubes were not lysed. Further, the alloreactive CTL had no detectable nonspecific (NK-like) killing properties. The results obtained in this model system clearly establish that cultured myotubes are fully susceptible to HLA class I-restricted lysis by $CD8^+$ CTL. This has obvious implications for myoblast transfer therapies and for gene therapy based on myoblast transfer[53–55].

Perhaps more interestingly, myotubes can be also killed by autologous $CD8^+$ CTL. This observation was made in the course of a systematic study of polyclonal T cell lines which were directly isolated from the muscle of patients with different inflammatory myopathies[37]. Sixteen cell lines that consisted predominantly of $CD8^+$ cells were obtained from six patients with PM, four with IBM, four with DM, and one with other muscle disease. None of the lines displayed NK-like cytotoxicity, but all were capable of lectin-dependent cytotoxicity. Three of six PM, one of four IBM, and one of five DM lines showed low but statistically significant lysis against autologous myotubes (6–27% specific lysis at an effector to target ratio of 20:1).

The autoreactive myocytotoxicity observed in this *in vitro* system is consistent with the hypothesis that some of the CTL isolated from muscle recognize the same antigen on myotubes *in vitro* that they recognize on muscle fibres *in vivo*. This could be a genuine autoantigen, or a foreign (viral?) antigen. At present, we cannot distinguish between the two possibilities. However, together with the other evidence discussed above, the first possibility appears more likely.

Antigen presentation to $CD4^+$ T cells

Antigen presentation to $CD8^+$ T cells requires the expression of HLA class I antigen, whereas antigen presentation to $CD4^+$ T cells depends on the constitutive or induced expression of HLA class II antigen on the surface of the antigen-presenting cell[56–62]. The observation that myoblasts can be induced to express HLA class II by IFN-γ[36,41–43] raised the interesting possibility that cytokine-induced myoblasts can present antigen to $CD4^+$ helper/inducer T cells. We tested human myoblasts, cultured from muscle biopsy specimens and more than 95% pure, for their capacity to present various protein antigens to $CD4^+$ T cells. In co-culture experiments we compared the antigen-presenting properties of cytokine-induced and non-induced myoblasts using autologous T cell lines specific for tuberculin, tetanus toxoid or myelin basic protein[40]. Non-induced myoblasts or myoblasts treated with TNF-α alone could not present any of these antigens to T cells. However, IFN-γ-treated myoblasts induced antigen-specific T cell proliferation. Further, in the presence of the relevant antigen, IFN-γ induced myoblasts were killed by the T cells[40]. In the absence of antigen, specific lysis did not occur. The lytic potential of the T cells was demonstrated with lectin-induced lysis, which was observed with all types of target myoblasts. Control experiments with K562 cells as target cells did not show significant lysis, excluding NK-like activity of the $CD4^+$ T-cell lines used. Antigen specific lysis was reduced to background level by adding anti-HLA-DR mAb L-243, whereas lectin (PHA)-induced ^{51}Cr release was not inhibited.

These results suggest that HLA class II antigen-positive human myoblasts may act as facultative local antigen-presenting cells in muscle by providing both the signals necessary to trigger antigen-specific lysis and T cell proliferation. It should be noted, however, that HLA-DR has not been demonstrated on the surface of human muscle fibres in inflammatory lesions in PM, DM, or IBM[12,19,27]; however the level of HLA class II antigens expression *in vivo* may be so low that it escapes detection by immunofluorescence microscopy. Using a sensitive peroxidase technique, HLA class II expression was noted on some muscle fibres in one patient with human T-cell lymphotropic virus (HTLV) I-negative PM, three patients with HTLV-I-positive PM, and five patients with PM and HTLV-I-associated myelopathy[63]. These findings await confirmation.

If muscle fibres do express HLA-DR *in vivo*, it is conceivable that they could present not only viral or bacterial antigens to $CD4^+$ T cells, but also muscular autoantigens or alloantigens. Furthermore, the expression and presentation of allogeneic histocompatibility antigens by myoblasts and myotubes could be a major obstacle for 'myoblast transplantation', an experimental therapy for degenerative muscle diseases currently being studied in clinical trials[53–55].

NK cell-mediated muscle fibre injury *in vitro*

Cultured myotubes are susceptible to lysis by freshly isolated allogeneic and autologous peripheral blood mononuclear cells[52]. The lysis is not due to cytotoxic macrophages because macrophage-depleted cell preparations retain the cytotoxic potential. In addition the lysis of myotubes by peripheral blood mononuclear cells is not mediated by HLA class I-restricted CTL because it is not inhibited in the presence of monoclonal antibody directed against the HLA class I antigens[52]. The cytotoxicity is, however, mediated by $CD16^+$ NK cells, since it is abrogated by depletion of $CD16^+$ cells.

It is not known whether NK cells can attack normal myotubes *in vivo*. If regenerating myotubes *in vivo* were as susceptible to NK cell-mediated lysis as are cultured myotubes, normal muscle regeneration could not occur. One possibility is that myotubes are intrinsically more resistant to autologous NK cells *in vivo*. Regenerating muscle fibres are known to express high levels of CD56 *in vivo*[38,39], so that N-CAM expression on myotubes is probably not a regulating factor. However, there may be other mechanisms preventing the lysis of myoblasts and myotubes by NK cells *in vivo*. These factors might act at the level of effector cells, target cells, or both.

CLINICAL FEATURES AND DIFFERENTIAL DIAGNOSIS

PM and DM

PM and DM are characterized by proximal, often symmetrical, muscle weakness which typically develops over weeks to months and may be associated with transient muscle pain. Extraocular and facial muscles are typically spared. The clinical feature that differentiates DM from PM is a typical skin rash consisting of a blue-purple discoloration of the upper eyelids and erythematous lesions on the face, upper trunk, knuckles and other joints. Later in the course of the disease, these lesions may suffer scaling, depigmentation and/or hyperpigmentation, leaving tell-tale scars. Extramuscular manifestations are more frequent in children than in adults; these may include subcutaneous calcifications and joint contractures.

The single most useful laboratory test is the serum level of the muscle enzyme creatine kinase (CK). The enzyme is released from necrotic muscle fibres, and the serum level usually parallels disease activity.

Needle electromyography shows a myopathic pattern with low voltage motor unit potentials and abnormal spontaneous activity, usually in the form of increased insertional activity, fibrillation potentials, and positive sharp waves[64]. This pattern can be seen in a variety of myopathies and is not diagnostic for those associated with autoimmune, or any other, inflammatory processes.

The most obvious changes on light microscopy include the presence of inflammatory cells, necrosis and regeneration of muscle fibres, and increased connective tissue. A finding that is highly characteristic of DM, but not of PM, is perifascicular atrophy (atrophy of the muscle fibres at the periphery of fascicles). Small zones of muscle infarction may be observed in childhood DM, but not in the adult forms of either PM or DM. In DM, in contrast to PM, the intramuscular blood vessels show endothelial hyperplasia and sometimes obliteration of capillaries. Other characteristic changes that have provided important clues to the pathogenesis of PM and DM are reviewed on pages 236–240.

PM may be associated with retrovirus (HIV, HTLV-1) infections. In these cases, there is good evidence that the virus does not directly infect the muscle but triggers a T cell-mediated cytotoxic process similar to that seen in other forms of the disease[65]. It is important to note that zidovudine, an agent used to treat HIV-infected patients, can itself cause a toxic myopathy which may be difficult to distinguish from the primary, virus-associated PM[2,3,66].

As many as 40% of patients with PM or DM (but not IBM) have cardiac involvement, which may lead to conduction defects and dilated cardiomyopathy. Pulmonary disease occurs in up to 50% of patients as the result of respiratory muscle weakness, pneumonitis as a result of methotrexate treatment, or interstitial lung disease. The latter condition is associated with anti-Jo-1 antibodies and develops in up to 10% of patients with PM[67]. The features of DM may overlap those of certain connective tissue diseases, such as systemic lupus erythematosus, Sjögren's syndrome, rheumatoid arthritis, systemic sclerosis, or mixed connective tissue disease ('overlap syndrome').

The possible association of myositis with malignant tumours has been the subject of a longstanding debate. A recent epidemiological study[68] concluded that the incidence of cancer was increased both in patients with DM and in those with PM. The mortality rate from the malignancy was, however, only increased in the patients with DM. A thorough search for an occult neoplasm is advisable in patients with any inflammatory myopathy, especially DM[69].

IBM

The typical clinical features of IBM are insidious onset after 50 with painless, proximal lower extremity weakness, a 3:1 male:female ratio, slow but relentless progression with selectively severe involvement of quadriceps, iliopsoas, tibialis anterior, biceps and triceps muscles, relatively early depression of the knee reflex, and a normal or mildly elevated serum creatine kinase level[70]. Distal weakness occurs in about 50% of patients, but in only

35% is it as great or greater than proximal weakness. External ocular muscles are usually spared. Significant associated illnesses include other autoimmune disorders (15%), diabetes mellitus (20%) and diffuse peripheral neuropathy (18%).

The typical light microscopic features of IBM include rimmed vacuoles, eosinophilic intranuclear and cytoplasmic inclusions, small groups of atrophic fibres without fibre type grouping, and an inflammatory exudate involving endomysial and, to a lesser extent, perivascular tissue sites. Immunocytochemical characterization of the inflammatory cells has provided important clues to the pathogenesis of IBM (see pages 238–239). Electron microscopic demonstration of the characteristic filamentous inclusions resembling myxovirus nucleocapsids confirms the diagnosis but is rarely needed, as the predictive value of the light microscopic criteria is more than 90%[70].

Immunoelectron microscopy shows cytoplasmic tubulo-filaments that are reactive for ubiquitin[71,72], and β-amyloid protein is localized in proximity to cytoplasmic tubulofilaments[73]. The accumulations of β-amyloid protein in IBM muscle share many features with the amyloid accumulations in brain of patients with Alzheimer's disease, but the total amount of amyloid accumulating in muscle is minute and it is yet uncertain that these deposits affect the course of the disease.

Differential diagnosis

The differential diagnosis of PM, DM and IBM can be clarified by appropriate clinical, EMG and histopathological studies. For example, in acid maltase deficiency the muscle biopsy demonstrates a vacuolar myopathy with high glycogen content and acid phosphatase reactivity in the vacuoles. Limb-girdle dystrophies develop more slowly and lack inflammatory changes in the muscle biopsy. In glucocorticosteroid-induced myopathy the serum creatine kinase level is normal and the muscle biopsy shows selective type II muscle fibre atrophy. In zidovudine-induced myopathy the muscle biopsy shows ragged-red fibres. A more detailed review of differential diagnosis is presented in Table 9.3 and references 2–4.

MANAGEMENT

Prednisone is the first-line drug for the treatment of PM and DM[1–4]. Initial therapy with 1 mg/kg prednisone in a single daily dose is maintained for 4 weeks or longer until the CK level and the clinical status improve. After this the dose is tapered slowly over approximately 10 weeks to 1 mg/kg every other day. If improvement continues, the dose is further reduced by 5–10 mg every 4 weeks until the maintenance dose (the lowest possible dose that controls the disease) is reached. In a favourable case, the dose will eventually range from 10 to 20 mg every other day.

A problem of treatment is that the long-term use of corticosteroids may itself induce a myopathy that can be difficult to distinguish from an

Table 9.3 Differential diagnosis of idiopathic inflammatory myopathies

Sporadic muscular dystrophy
Necrotizing myopathy with carcinoma
Late-onset congenital myopathy
Proximal spinal muscular atrophy
Polymyalgia rheumatica
Chronic fatigue syndrome
Metabolic myopathies
Mitochondrial myopathy
Acid maltase deficiency (children, adults)
Debranching enzyme deficiency
Primary carnitine deficiency
Short-chain acyl-CoA dehydrogenase deficiency
Endocrine myopathies
Thyrotoxic and myxoedema myopathies
Corticosteroid-induced myopathy
Drug-induced and toxic myopathies
Myopathies induced by emetine, chloroquine, colchicine, lovastatin/gemfibrozil, zidovudine, cocaine, alcohol, etc.

exacerbation of the inflammatory component. If weakness increases following tapering of steroids and is accompanied by an increase of the CK, the clinical deterioration is probably due to exacerbation of myositis. If such clear evidence is lacking, it may nevertheless be advisable first to increase the dose of steroids temporarily. If the patient then fails to improve, steroid myopathy is more likely than exacerbation of the inflammatory process[2].

An objective increase in muscle strength usually occurs by the third month of therapy[2]. If prednisone fails to produce a clear benefit after this period, or if the patient requires > 25 mg/day, or develops side-effects, a second-line drug is required. It is reasonable first to try the least toxic immunosuppressive drug, azathioprine (2.5–3 mg/kg daily for 4–6 months) and then, if treatment is still ineffective, to use methotrexate (15–25 mg/week orally). Cyclosporin may be a useful alternative or adjunctive third-line drug (reviewed in reference 3). High-dose immunoglobulins may be useful as an adjunctive immunomodulatory agent for acute exacerbations or for selected cases of severe chronic disease refractory to conventional therapy (reviewed in references 2, 3).

Polymyositis in HIV-positive patients presents a special therapeutic challenge. Although this form of PM is probably triggered by the virus, there is no evidence that muscle cells are directly infected[65]: it appears that the virus initiates a T cell-mediated cytotoxic response against muscle fibres. The therapeutic dilemma derives mainly from two considerations[66]: first, treatment with prednisone is itself potentially dangerous in immunocompromised patients; second, the anti-virus agent, zidovudine, can cause a mitochondrial myopathy[66] which may worsen the patient's weakness. The following strategy for the management of HIV-associated polymyositis has been recommended[66]. Before using prednisone, a nonsteroidal anti-inflammatory agent should be tried. If this fails, zidovudine should be discontinued for 3–4 weeks and the clinical response (muscle strength, CK) observed. If strength increases, another retroviral agent should be substituted for zidovudine. If strength decreases or does not change, prednisone should be started at a dose of 40–60 mg/day.

Patients with fulminant PM or DM may require intensive care, particularly if there is significant respiratory and/or pharyngeal involvement or if respiratory failure ensues. The latter may be precipitated suddenly, even in patients with long-standing, slowly progressive disease, by pulmonary infections or aspiration. In the presence of any severe, systemic complication, especially cardiac involvement or interstitial lung disease, it is best to treat the patient in the intensive care unit.

In patients with an acute course in whom oral corticosteroids have failed, high-dose corticosteroids (e.g. 500 mg methylprednisolone/day) may be given intravenously for 5–10 days in combination with methotrexate (25 mg/week orally). In addition, high-dose intravenous immunoglobulin (0.4 g/kg/day) should be administered for 4–5 days[74]. There is no convincing evidence that plasmapheresis or leukapheresis are effective in either PM or DM[75], although this has been debated[76]. The response to therapy with cyclophosphamide and cyclosporin is also disappointing[2].

Patients with chronic disease in whom respiratory failure has been precipitated by an infection should be treated with appropriate antibiotics plus high-dose intravenous immunoglobulin. Further, the original treatment plan should be revised, depending on the presumed cause of the deterioration. If the pulmonary infection appears to be a complication of immunosuppression, cytotoxic drugs may have to be stopped entirely or sharply reduced. In some cases it will be necessary to change to another immunosuppressive agent. If the infection is due to aspiration in a very weak 'undertreated' patient, more aggressive immunosuppressive treatment is needed, and it may be necessary to provide temporary mechanical respiratory assistance.

In patients with cardiac and pulmonary complications other than interstitial lung disease the myositis is treated according to the same principles as in patients without these complications. In patients with interstitial lung disease, cyclophosphamide may be beneficial[67,77].

Corticosteroid therapy is ineffective in IBM. Nevertheless, one cannot confidently assume that IBM is always refractory to immunotherapy: a transient response to therapy has been observed in some patients, and the total number of patients with IBM who have received immunotherapy is still relatively small, and only a few of these have had a systematic and sustained trial of one or more immunotherapeutic agents at the maximum tolerated dose. In addition, as the disease progresses slowly, a therapeutic effect that consists of an arrest of disease progression rather than reversal of deficits could be easily overlooked. Withholding treatment because the majority of patients fail to respond will deny the chance of improvement to a small minority who might respond.

A pilot study in four IBM patients indicated that treatment with high-dose intravenous immunoglobulin may have a beneficial effect in some patients[78]. Improvement of muscle strength was reported to last from 2 to 4 months after 2 monthly infusions (total of 2 g/kg per month). Controlled, blind trials of a larger number of patients are needed to assess the usefulness of IV immunoglobulin therapy in IBM.

SUMMARY

Cell-mediated immune mechanisms play a prominent role in inclusion body myositis (IBM) and polymyositis (PM). In both IBM and PM, $CD8^+$ cytotoxic T cells expressing the α/β receptor surround and focally invade non-necrotic muscle fibres. This lesion can be considered the hallmark of cell-mediated myocytotoxicity. Essentially the same type of lesion is observed in a variant form of PM, in which $CD4^-CD8^-$ T cells bearing the γ/δ receptor surround and invade non-necrotic muscle fibres.

In both IBM and PM, all of the invaded and some of the non-invaded muscle fibres strongly express HLA class I. This is consistent with the hypothesis that the $CD8^+$ autoinvasive cytotoxic T cells recognize antigenic peptide(s) bound to HLA-class I molecules on the muscle fibre surface. According to the rules of antigen-processing, these peptides derive from proteins synthesized in the muscle fibre. Theoretically, the proteins could be viral components or genuine self proteins. The first possibility appears less likely, since most attempts to demonstrate viral antigens or genome in muscle fibres have failed. On the other hand, it is well established that the majority of HLA class I molecules expressed on the surface of any cell are loaded with endogenous self peptides. Therefore it seems plausible that the auto-aggressive T cells recognize muscle-specific autoantigen(s) in the inflammatory myopathies.

In contrast to PM and IBM, humoral immunity is an early and probably initiating event in DM. The concept that humorally mediated damage to blood vessels initiates the angiopathy of DM is supported by distinctive capillary changes, endomysial capillary necrosis, significantly reduced capillary numbers relative to muscle fibre area, and immunolocalization of complement, including C5b-9 membrane attack complex (MAC), to capillaries in DM muscle.

Recently, it has become possible to study the interactions between muscle cells and cytotoxic effector cells *in vitro*. Myoblasts and myotubes can be induced to express a variety of immunologically important histocompatibility and cell adhesion molecules. Myotubes are highly susceptible to lysis by allogenic $CD8^+$ cytotoxic T cells sensitized against HLA-class I alloantigens. Interestingly, cultured myotubes are also susceptible to lysis by antigen-non-specific natural killer cells. Further, myoblasts induced by IFN-γ to express HLA class II antigens acquire the full potential to process and present complex protein antigens to $CD4^+$ T cells. This may indicate that myoblasts can actively participate in local immune reactions by presenting (auto)antigens to helper/inducer T cells.

$CD8^+$ T cells have been expanded directly from muscle of patients with various inflammatory myopathies and their interactions with autologous myotubes have been investigated *in vitro*. In several cases, a low but significant autoreactive cytotoxic effect was observed. This is consistent with the hypothesis that some cytotoxic effector T cells recognize an autoantigen on myotubes. One of the major goals for future studies is to define the autoantigens that are relevant in the pathogenesis of the inflammatory myopathies.

Because PM and DM are considered to be autoimmune diseases of muscle, the therapeutic aim is to suppress the autoimmune process. Corticosteroids are first-line agents, and azathioprine is the most widely used second-line agent. Lifelong immunosuppressive treatment may be required in some patients. Preliminary clinical evidence indicates that treatment with high dose intravenous immunoglobulin may be helpful in some patients with PM and DM. Plasmapheresis is probably not efficient. Most cases of IBM are refractory to treatment with corticosteroids or immunosuppressive agents. A preliminary study suggests that high dose intravenous immunoglobulin may have a beneficial effect in some patients with IBM.

ACKNOWLEDGEMENTS

This work was supported by NIH grant NS-6277, a grant from the Muscular Dystrophy Association, and by grants from the Deutsche Forschungsgemeinschaft (SFB 217/C13), the Wilhelm Sander Stiftung and the Max-Planck Society.

References

1. Engel AG, Hohlfeld R, Banker BQ. The polymyositis and dermatomyositis syndromes. In: Engel AG, Franzini-Armstrong C, editors. Myology, 2nd Edn. New York: McGraw-Hill; 1994:1335–83.
2. Dalakas MC. Polymyositis, dermatomyositis, and inclusion body myositis. N Engl J Med. 1991;325:1487–98.
3. Dalakas MC. Inflammatory and toxic myopathies. Curr Opin Neurol Neurosurg. 1992;5:645–54.
4. Engel AG. Inflammatory myopathies. In: Wyngaarden JB, Smith LH, Bennett JC, editors. Cecil Textbook of Medicine. Philadelphia: Saunders, 1992:2256–8.
5. Hohlfeld R, Engel AG. Immune responses in muscle. Semin Neurosci. 1992;4:249–55.
6. Banker BQ, Victor M. Dermatomyositis (systemic angiopathy) of childhood. Medicine. 1966;45:261–89.
7. Banker BQ. Dermatomyositis of childhood. Ultrastructural alterations of muscle and intramuscular blood vessels. J Neuropathol. Exp Neurol. 1975;34:46–75.
8. Carpenter S, Karpati G, Rothman S, Watters G. The childhood type of dermatomyositis. Neurology. 1976;26:952–62.
9. Jerusalem F, Rakusa M, Engel AG, MacDonald RD. Morphometric analysis of skeletal muscle capillary ultrastructure in inflammatory myopathies. J Neurol Sci. 1974;23:391–401.
10. Whitaker JN, Engel WK. Vascular deposits of immunoglobulin and complement in idiopathic inflammatory myopathy. N Engl J Med. 1972;286:333–8.
11. Kissel JT, Mendell JR, Rammohan KW. Microvascular deposition of complement membrane attack complex in dermatomyositis. N Engl J Med. 1986;314:331–4.
12. Arahata K, Engel AG. Monoclonal antibody analysis of mononuclear cells in myopathies. I. Quantitation of subsets according to diagnosis and sites of accumulation and demonstration and counts of muscle fibres invaded by T cells. Ann Neurol. 1984;16:193–208.
13. De Visser M, Emslie-Smith AM, Engel AG. Early ultrastructural changes in adult dermatomyositis. Capillary abnormalities precede other structural changes in muscle. J Neurol Sci. 1989;94:181–92.
14. Emslie-Smith A, Engel AG. Microvascular changes in early and advanced dermatomyositis. A quantitative study. Ann Neurol. 1990;27:343–56.
15. Cervera R, Ramirez G, Fernandez-Sola J, *et al.* Antibodies to endothelial cells in dermatomyositis: association with interstitial lung disease. Br Med J. 1991;302:880–1.
16. Engel AG, Arahata K. Monoclonal antibody analysis of mononuclear cells in myopathies.

II. Phenotypes of autoinvasive cells in polymyositis and inclusion body myositis. Ann Neurol. 1984;16:209–16.
17. Arahata K, Engel AG. Monoclonal antibody analysis of mononuclear cells in myopathies. III. Immunoelectron microscopy aspects of cell-mediated muscle fiber injury. Ann Neurol. 1986;19:112–25.
18. Engel AG, Arahata K. Mononuclear cells in myopathies. Quantitation of functionally distinct subsets, recognition of antigen-specific cell-mediated cytotoxicity in some diseases, and implications for the pathogenesis of the different inflammatory myopathies. Hum Pathol. 1986;17:704–21.
19. Arahata K, Engel AG. Monoclonal antibody analysis of mononuclear cells in myopathies. IV. Cell-mediated cytotoxicity and muscle fibre necrosis. Ann Neurol. 1988;23:168–73.
20. Arahata K, Engel AG. Monoclonal antibody analysis of mononuclear cells in myopathies. V. Identification and quantification of T8+ cytotoxic and T8+ suppressor cells. Ann Neurol. 1988;23:493–9.
21. Engel AG, Arahata K, Emslie-Smith AM. Immune effector mechanisms in inflammatory myopathies. Res Pub Assoc Res Nerv Ment Dis. 1990;68:141–57.
22. Phillips JH, Lanier LL. Lectin-dependent and anti-CD3 induced cytotoxicity are preferentially mediated by peripheral blood cytotoxic T lymphocytes expressing Leu7 antigen. J Immunol. 1986;136:1579–85.
23. Rüthlein JH, James SP, Strober W. Role of CD2 in activation and cytotoxic function of CD8/Leu7-positive T cells. J Immunol. 1988;141:3791–7.
24. Marguerie C, Lunardi C, So A. PCR-based analysis of the TCR repertoire in human autoimmune diseases. Immunol Today. 1992;13:336–8.
25. Mantegazza R, Andreetta F, Bernasconi P, Baggi F, Oksenberg JR, Simoncini O, Mora M, Cornelio F, Steinman L. Analysis of T cell receptor repertoire of muscle-infiltrating T lymphocytes in polymyositis: Restricted $V\alpha/\beta$ rearrangements may indicate antigen-driven selection. J Clin Invest. 1993;91:2880–6.
26. Hohlfeld R. Neurological autoimmune disease and the trimolecular complex of T-lymphocytes. Ann Neurol. 1989;25:531–8.
27. Karpati G, Pouliot Y, Carpenter S. Expression of immunoreactive major histocompatibility complex products in human skeletal muscles. Ann Neurol. 1988;23:64–72.
28. Emslie-Smith AM, Arahata K, Engel AG. Major histocompatibility complex class I antigen expression, immunolocalization of interferon subtypes, and T cell-mediated cytotoxicity in myopathies. Hum Pathol. 1989;20:224–31.
29. Braciale TJ. Antigen processing for presentation by MHC class I molecules. Curr Opin Immunol. 1992;4:59–62.
30. Jardetzky TS, Lane WS, Robinson RA, Madden DR, Wiley DC. Identification of self peptides bound to purified HLA-B27. Nature. 1991;353:326–9.
31. Leff RL, Love SJ, Miller FW, *et al.* Viruses in idiopathic inflammatory myopathies: Absence of candidate viral genomes in muscle. Lancet. 1992;339:1192–5.
32. Hohlfeld R, Engel AG, Kunio I, Harper MC. Polymyositis mediated by T lymphocytes that express the γ/δ receptor. N Engl J Med. 1991;13:877–81.
33. Pluschke G, Rüegg D, Hohlfeld R, Engel AG. Autoaggressive myocytotoxic T-lymphocytes expressing an unusual γ/δ T-cell receptor. J Exp Med. 1992;176:1785–9.
34. Hohlfeld R, Engel AG. Expression of 65-kd heat shock proteins in the inflammatory myopathies. Ann Neurol. 1992;32:821–3.
35. Blau HM, Webster C. Isolation and characterization of human muscle cells. Proc Natl Acad Sci USA. 1981;78:6523–7.
36. Hohlfeld R, Engel AG. Induction of HLA-DR expression on human myoblasts with interferon-γ. Am J Pathol. 1990;136:503–8.
37. Hohlfeld R, Engel AG. Coculture with autologous myotubes of cytotoxic T cells isolated from muscle in inflammatory myopathies. Ann Neurol. 1991;29:498–507.
38. Schubert W, Zimmermann K, Cramer M, Starzinsky-Powitz A. Lymphocyte antigen Leu-19 as a marker of regeneration in human skeletal muscle. Proc Natl Acad Sci USA. 1989;86:307–11.
39. Illa I, Leon-Monzon M, Dalakas MC. Regenerating and denervated human muscle fibers and satellite cells express neural cell adhesion molecules recognized by monoclonal antibodies to natural killer cells. Ann Neurol. 1992;31:46–52.

40. Goebels N, Michaelis D, Wekerle H, Hohlfeld R. Human myoblasts as antigen presenting cells. J Immunol. 1992;149:661–7.
41. Bao S, King NJC, Dosremedios CG. Elevated MHC class-I and class-II antigens in cultured human embryonic myoblasts following stimulation with γ-interferon. Immunol Cell Biol. 1990;68:235–42.
42. Mantegazza R, Hughes SM, Mitchell D, Travis M, Blau HM, Steinman L. Modulation of MHC class II antigen expression in human myoblasts after treatment with IFN-γ. Neurology. 1991;41:1128–32.
43. Roy R, Dansereau G, Tremblay JP, *et al.* Expression of major histocompatibility complex antigens on human myoblasts. Transplant Proc. 1991;23:799–801.
44. Beauchamp JR, Abraham DJ, Bou-Gharios G, Partridge TA, Olsen I. Expression and function of heterotypic adhesion molecules during differentiation of human skeletal muscle in culture. Am J Pathol. 1992;140:387–401.
45. Cifuentes-Diaz C, Delaporte C, Datreaux B, Charron D, Fardeau M. Class II MHC antigens in normal skeletal muscle. Muscle Nerve. 1992;15:295–302.
46. Kalovidouris AE. The role of cytokines in polymyositis: Interferon-γ induces class II and enhances class I major histocompatibility complex antigen expression on cultured human muscle cells. J Lab Clin Med. 1992;120:244–51.
47. Hardiman O, Faustman D, Li X, Sklar RM, Brown RH. Expression of major histocompatibility complex antigens in cultures of clonally derived human myoblasts. Neurology. 1993;43:604–8.
48. Springer TA. Adhesion receptors of the immune system. Nature. 1990;346:425–34.
49. Jäättelä M. Biologic activities and mechanisms of action of tumor necrosis factor-α/cachectin. Lab Invest. 1991;64:724–42.
50. Nathan C, Yoshida R. Cytokines: interferon-γ. In: Gallin JI, Goldstein IM, Snyderman R, editors. Inflammation: Basic Principles and Clinical Correlates. New York: Raven Press, 1988:229–51.
51. Michaelis D, Goebels N, Hohlfeld R. Constitutive and cytokine-induced expression of HLA and cell adhesion molecules by human myotubes. Am J Pathol. 1993;143:1142–9.
52. Hohlfeld R, Engel AG. Lysis of myotubes by alloreactive cytotoxic T cells and natural killer cells. Relevance to myoblast transplantation. J Clin Invest. 1990;86:370–4.
53. Karpati G. The principles and practice of myoblast transfer. In Griggs R, Kaspar G, editors. Myoblast Transfer Therapy. New York: Plenum Press, 1990.
54. Karpati G, Ajdukovic D, Arnold D, *et al.* Myoblast transfer in Duchenne muscular dystrophy. Ann Neurol. 1993;34:8–17.
55. Engel AG. Gene therapy for Duchenne dystrophy. Ann Neurol. 1993;34:3–4.
56. Wekerle H, Linington C, Lassmann H, Meyermann R. Cellular immune reactivity within the CNS. Trends Neurosci. 1986;9:271–7.
57. Unanue ER, Allen PM. The basis for the immunoregulatory role of macrophages and other accessory cells. Science. 1987;236:551–8.
58. Pober JS. Cytokine-mediated activation of vascular endothelium. Am J Pathol. 1988;133:426–33.
59. Berzofsky JA, Brett SJ, Streicher HZ, Takahashi H. Antigen processing for presentation to T lymphocytes: function, mechanisms and implications for the T cell response. Immunol Rev. 1989;106:5–31.
60. Weaver CT, Unanue ER. The costimulatory function of antigen-presenting cells. Immunol Today. 1990;11:49–55.
61. Braciale TJ, Braciale VL. Antigen presentation: structural themes and functional variations. Immunol Today. 1991;12:124–9.
62. Brodsky FM, Guagliardi L. The cell biology of antigen processing and presentation. Ann Rev Immunol. 1991;9:707–44.
63. Higuchi I, Montmayor E, Izumo S, Inose M, Osame M. Immunohistochemical characteristics of polymyositis in patients with HTLVI-associated myelopathy and HTLVI carriers. Muscle Nerve. 1993;16:472–6.
64. Robinson LR. AAEM case report #22: polymyositis. Muscle Nerve. 1991;14:310–15.
65. Illa I, Nath A, Dalakas MC. Immunocytochemical and virological characteristics of HIV-associated inflammatory myopathies: similarities with seronegative polymyositis. Ann Neurol. 1991;29:474–81.

66. Dalakas MC, Illa I, Pezeshkpour GH, Laukaitis JP, Cohen B, Griffin JL. Mitochondrial myopathy caused by long-term zidovudine therapy. N Engl J Med. 1990;322:1098–105.
67. Tazelaar HD, Viggiano RW, Pickersgill J, Colby TV. Interstitial lung disease in polymyositis and dermatomyositis: clinical features and prognosis as correlated with histologic findings. Am Rev Resp Dis. 1990;141:727–33.
68. Sigurgeirsson B, Lindelöf B, Edhag O, Allander E. Risk of cancer in patients with dermatomyositis or polymyositis – a population-based study. N Engl J Med. 1992;326: 363–7.
69. Bernard P, Bonnetblanc JM. Dermatomyositis and malignancy. J Invest Dermatol. 1993;100:128S–132S.
70. Lotz BP, Engel AG, Nishino H, Stevens JC, Litchy WJ. Inclusion body myositis. Brain. 1969;112:727–42.
71. Massa R, Weller B, Karpati G, Shoubridge E, Carpenter S. Familial inclusion body myositis among Kurdish-Iranian Jews. Arch Neurol. 1991;48:519–22.
72. Askanas V, Serdaroglu P, Engel WK, Alvarez RB. Immunolocalization of ubiquitin in muscle biopsies of patients with inclusion body myositis and oculopharyngeal muscular dystrophy. Neurosci Lett. 1991;130:73–6.
73. Askanas V, Engel WK, Alvarez RB. Light and electron microscopic localization of β-amyloid protein in muscle biopsies of patients with inclusion body myositis. Am J Pathol. 1992;141:31–6.
74. Jann S, Beretta S, Moggio M, Adobbati L, Pellegrini G. High-dose intravenous human immunoglobulin in polymyositis resistant to treatment. J Neurol Neurosurg Psychiatry. 1992;55:60–2.
75. Miller FW, Leitman SF, Cronin ME, *et al.* Controlled trial of plasma exchange and leukapheresis in polymyositis and dermatomyositis. N Engl J Med. 1992;326:1380–4.
76. Dau PC. Plasma exchange in polymyositis and dermatomyositis. N Engl J Med. 1992;327:1030.
77. Al-Janadi M, Smith CD, Karsh J. Cyclophosphamide treatment of interstitial pulmonary fibrosis in polymyositis/dermatomyositis. J Rheumatol. 1989;16:1592–6.
78. Soueidan SA, Dalakas MC. Treatment of inclusion-body myositis with high-dose intravenous immunoglobulin. Neurology. 1993;43:876–9.

10
Retrovirus-related neuromuscular diseases

M. C. DALAKAS, I. ILLA and M. MONZON

INTRODUCTION

Muscle or peripheral nerve is frequently involved in patients with HIV infection. Neuropathy or myopathy may accompany seroconversion, may represent the first clinical manifestation of an established or undiagnosed HIV infection or may complicate full-blown AIDS[1–13]. The HIV-related neuromuscular disorders, although rarely life-threatening, are often disabling; hence the need for early diagnosis and initiation of therapy. While pathological studies show that neuromuscular pathology is almost universal in patients dying of AIDS[14–17], clinical studies estimate the frequency of symptomatic myopathy at up to 30%[18] and that of neuropathy at 35%[19]. Such clinical under-recognition is probably related to the dysfunction of other organs, commonly affected in this multisystem disease, which overshadows co-existent neuromuscular complications. Because a myopathy or neuropathy may coincide with seroconversion for HIV[12,13] or may be the only indication of a chronic, undiagnosed HIV infection, every patient who comes to a neurology clinic with acquired myopathy or neuropathy is now requested to consent to HIV screening.

Apart from the morbidity caused by these neuromuscular diseases, their occurrence in the setting of a viral infection provides a unique opportunity to examine how a known retrovirus triggers the development of an acquired inflammatory myopathy or demyelinating neuropathy. Advances in the molecular virology of retroviruses and in molecular immunological techniques offer additional opportunities to study the mechanism of viral persistence in muscles and nerves.

This chapter presents the present knowledge on the clinical spectrum, pathogenesis, and treatment of the myopathies and neuropathies associated

Table 10.1 Clinicopathological spectrum of HIV-related muscle diseases

HIV-myopathy with histological features of:
Inflammation (HIV polymyositis)*
Necrosis with minimal primary inflammation*
Nemaline (rod) bodies*
Subclinical neuromuscular involvement with histological features of:
inflammation
denervation
type II muscle fibre atrophy
HIV-wasting (cachectic) syndrome with histological features of:
type II muscle fibre atrophy
Myoglobinuria
Myasthenia gravis
Pyomyositis

*These features may co-exist in various degrees

with retroviruses, and describes the myotoxicity or neurotoxicity of the anti-retroviral drugs currently in use.

HIV MYOPATHY

HIV-positive patients may develop a frank myopathy with subacute onset and slow progression, characterized histologically by endomysial inflammation (HIV-polymyositis), muscle fibre necrosis with minimal primary inflammation and, rarely, nemaline (rod) bodies[2–7]. As these histological features often co-exist in various degrees, we prefer the term HIV myopathy as an all-inclusive designation for the morphological spectrum of clinically homogeneous myopathy seen in patients with HIV infection (Table 10.1). HIV myopathy may be present early in the course of HIV infection but more often complicates full-blown AIDS[1–12]. It may co-exist with other neurological manifestations, such as peripheral neuropathy and, rarely, with dementia or myelopathy. HIV myopathy is seen almost exclusively in adults: well documented cases of primary HIV myopathy in children with AIDS have not been reported[6,7]. Although HIV myopathy was generally rare prior to the introduction of azathioprine (AZT), reports have increased since AZT became the drug of choice in the treatment of AIDS due to its myocytotoxicity[20–23] and to the patients' longer survival. Because endomysial inflammation is often seen in patients with AZT-induced myopathy, a primary inflammatory muscle disease related to HIV infection may be easily attributed to, or overshadowed by, the myocytotoxic effect of the drug[20–23].

HIV myopathy begins with the subacute onset of proximal, often symmetrical muscle weakness, with or without wasting of the arms and, more often, the legs. The serum creatine kinase level is elevated by as much as 10–15 times. Myalgia may be present. The clinical presentation is similar to that seen in adult-onset acquired polymyositis[24–26]. In two cases, a facial rash aroused suspicion of a dermatomyositis-like disorder[27,28] but the classical skin lesions and the histological signs of dermatomyositis were not present. The electromyogram shows spontaneous activity with fibrillation and positive

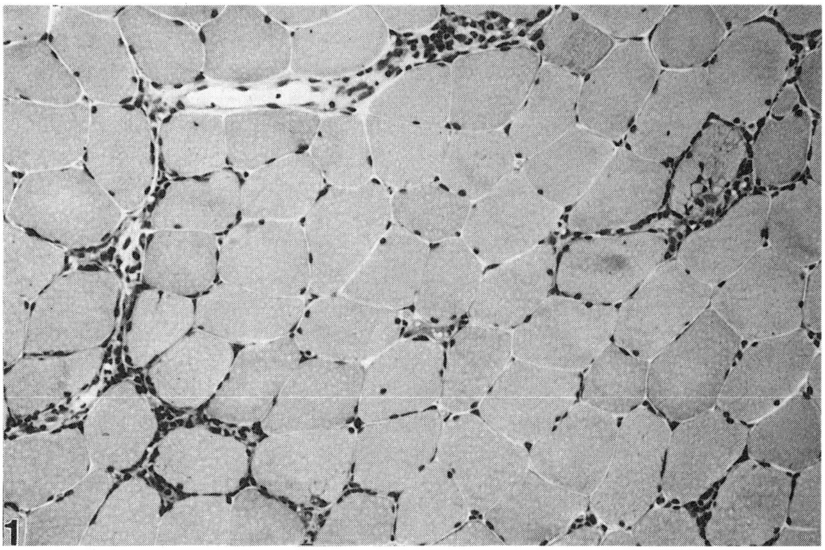

Figure 10.1 Transverse frozen section of a muscle biopsy specimen from a patient with HIV myopathy. Note perivascular and endomysial inflammation with cells surrounding healthy muscle fibres and phagocytosis (trichrome, × 120)

sharp waves and brief, low-amplitude, polyphasic (myopathic) units. Nerve conduction studies are normal or may show a mild, axonal sensory neuropathy.

The muscle biopsy shows perivascular, perimysial, or endomysial inflammatory cells, mostly lymphocytes and macrophages surrounding healthy, non-necrotic, muscle fibres, as well as phagocytosis and degeneration or necrosis of muscle fibres (Figure 10.1). In more severe cases, there is an increase in connective tissue. While true vasculitis is not present, perivascular inflammation is not uncommon[1–3]. Rarely, a few cytoplasmic bodies and rods can be seen. Occasionally, muscle fibre degeneration predominates and endomysial inflammation appears sparse[9,11]; in such cases, overlooked endomysial infiltrates can be visualized using immunocytochemistry. Scattered angulated fibres are not uncommon and, if present, they raise suspicion of a co-existing axonal neuropathy. Electron microscopy shows disorganization of the myofibrillar structures and inflammatory cells consisting of macrophages, plasma cells, and lymphocytes[29]. Some specimens may show evidence of osmiophilic destruction of the muscle fibres with numerous tubuloreticular profiles in the endothelial cells, and brisk inflammation that may include lymphoplasmatoid cells[2,29]. Mitochondria and other membrane-bound elements of the cell, as well as thick and thin filaments, are normal. Viral particles have not been seen.

Although nemaline (rod) bodies can be found in the muscle fibres of some patients with HIV myopathy[2,4,8,11], they can occasionally be the predominant histological finding[30]. In the first patient with HIV myopathy and rods that we reported[30], the rods were abundant in the centre of type I muscle fibres and appeared similar to those seen in congenital nemaline myopathy. Rods are occasionally seen in patients with polymyositis. However, the muscle biopsy in our original patient did not show inflammation. Subsequently, other cases of rods in HIV-positive patients with or without endomysial inflammation, have been reported[8,11,31]. In contrast, rods are very frequently seen in patients with AZT myopathy[5–7,20–23]. Rods originate in the Z discs[32] and consist of actin and α-actinin, the major proteins through which actin filaments are attached to the Z discs[33]. Their presence without other associated myopathic features could suggest that the virus or released cytokines and lymphokines are toxic to the structural and contractile muscle proteins. It is of interest that elevated serum levels of immunoglobulins (IgG, IgA, and IgM), as seen in AIDS, and high levels of circulating immune complexes and anti-nuclear antibodies may be present in HIV-negative patients with adult-onset nemaline myopathy[34]. Whether viruses or immunotoxins acting *in utero* or later in life play a role in the development of congenital or acquired nemaline myopathy is only speculative.

OTHER HIV-RELATED MYOPATHIC CONDITIONS

Subclinical neuromuscular involvement

The muscles, and more often the peripheral nerves, are affected in almost all patients who die of AIDS[14,17]. In one prospective and another retrospective clinicopathological study[16,35], 60–96% of untreated HIV-positive patients without neuromuscular symptoms and with normal neurological examination had abnormal histological signs consisting of denervation in 76% of the patients, type II muscle fibre atrophy (the histological correlate of the HIV wasting syndrome) in 58% of the patients, endomysial inflammation in 36% and necrosis with phagocytosis in 30%. These changes, presumably multifactorial in origin, may provide a histological correlate for the non-specific symptoms that many HIV-positive patients with normal strength experience, such as myalgia, fatigue, diminished endurance, or transient elevation of creatine kinase levels.

Myoglobinuria

Myoglobinuria, elevation of serum creatine kinase levels up to 400 000 units and myalgia with or without mild muscle weakness, may develop in some HIV-positive patients[2,10,36]. Myoglobinuria may coincide with seroconversion for HIV[12] and can be recurrent. In one case, it was associated with disseminated cytomegalovirus infection and presented with a necrotizing myopathy and rhabdomyolysis[2].

Myasthenia gravis

Myasthenia gravis has been reported in three HIV-positive patients: a 15-year-old boy[37], a 36-year-old man[38] and an 18-year-old man[39], all of whom had relatively mild disease that responded to pyridostigmine. One patient[38] improved spontaneously as the levels of antibody to the acetylcholine receptor (AChR) fell concomitantly with the decrease of $CD4^+$ cells and the reduction in cell-mediated immune responses. This confirms that in myasthenia gravis the antibody response to AChR is regulated by T cells, and implies that the HIV-induced global immunodeficiency state can also result in specific immunosuppression, associated with clinical improvement.

Pyomyositis

Pyomyositis, a disease common in the tropics but extremely rare in the Western hemisphere, is being seen with increasing frequency in patients with AIDS[40,41], and is the most common myopathy in HIV-positive children[7]. Pyomyositis is suspected when patients have low-grade fever, even without leukocytosis, localized pain and swelling in a large muscle group and possible elevation of creatine kinase levels. Ultrasound, magnetic resonance imaging, or computed tomography with contrast reveals an enhancing lesion, often with fluid density[42]. The implicated organism is usually *Staphylococcus aureus* and rarely gram-negative organisms. Risk factors for the disease include underlying muscle abnormalities, exercise-induced trauma or haematogenous spread of a bacterial infection, even in the presence of negative blood cultures. The pathogenesis of pyomyositis is unknown, but defects of neutrophil function[40] and the common colonization of HIV-positive patients by *S. aureus* may result in infection of the muscle. It is of relevance that neutrophils from HIV-positive patients show reduced chemotaxis and bactericidal activity against *S. aureus*[43]. Furthermore, the HIV envelope glycoprotein, gp160, can inhibit neutrophil chemotaxis[40].

PATHOGENESIS OF HIV MYOPATHY

In a persistent viral infection such as that caused by HIV, an inflammatory myopathy must be caused either by direct, acute or chronic, infection of the muscle by the virus or by an autoimmune response against muscle antigens triggered by the virus. Demonstrating that the virus is present within the affected muscle fibres will lend credence to the long-standing theory that viruses are causally related to inflammatory myopathies. Alternatively, demonstrating that HIV triggers an autoimmune mechanism similar to that described for the polymyositis in HIV-negative patients[26,44–46] will support the view that viruses are capable of inducing an autoimmune attack by exposing muscle antigens against which there is no self-tolerance. Therefore, we searched for both the virus and the induction of autoimmunity in the muscles of patients with HIV myopathy.

Virological studies in muscle biopsy specimens

We examined muscle biopsy specimens from 21 patients with HIV myopathy by electron microscopy, immunocytochemistry, *in situ* hybridization, muscle

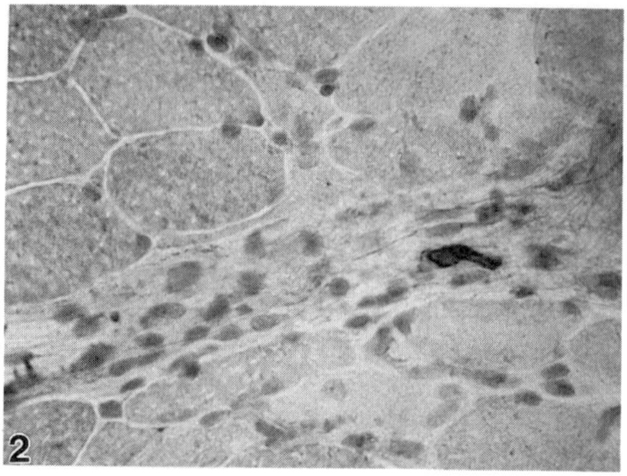

Figure 10.2 Transverse frozen section of a muscle biopsy specimen from a patient with HIV myopathy. Staining with antibodies to HIV antigen gp41 shows the antigen in a mononuclear cell within the endomysial septae in the proximity of a muscle fibre. No HIV antigens were found within the muscle fibres (avidin–biotin immunoperoxidase technique counterstained with 1% haematoxylin, ×475)

cultures and the polymerase chain reaction (PCR). We, and others, found no electron microscopic evidence of viral particles within the muscle or infiltrating lymphoid cells[2,4,8,29]. Using specific antibodies against various HIV proteins, including gp120 and gp41, we could not immunolocalize viral antigens within the muscle fibres but only within occasional endomysial lymphoid cells surrounding muscle fibres or within the endomysial septae[47] (Figure 10.2a,b). Similarly, using a ^{35}S-labelled HIV RNA transcript of the virus, we identified signals of viral nucleic acids within occasional endomysial lymphoid cells surrounding the muscle fibres (but not within the muscle fibres) in up to two consecutive sections from six of the 10 muscle biopsy specimens examined[48,49] (Figure 10.3A,B). Others have reported similar findings[50,51]. Using primers amplifying a 115 bp sequence from the *gag* gene and a 262 bp DNA fragment from the *pol* gene of the HIV genome, we found HIV-specific amplification products within the nucleic acids extracted from 4 μm thick serial sections in only two of the 10 muscle biopsy specimens and in only two of eight consecutive sections examined with PCR[49,52] (Figure 10.4). As would be expected from the size of the endomysial lymphoid cells and the low probability of the same cell occurring in more than two consecutive 4 μm serial sections, the HIV sequences detected within these consecutive sections probably belonged to the HIV-positive sparse lymphoid cells rather than to muscle fibres.

To determine whether integrated HIV sequences are replicated within the myonuclei and the satellite cells in the absence of lymphoid cells, we used the PCR technique to search for the presence of viral sequences in cultures established from six muscle biopsy specimens of patients with HIV myopathy. We were unable to find HIV-specific amplification bands within the genomic DNA extracted from these cultures[49].

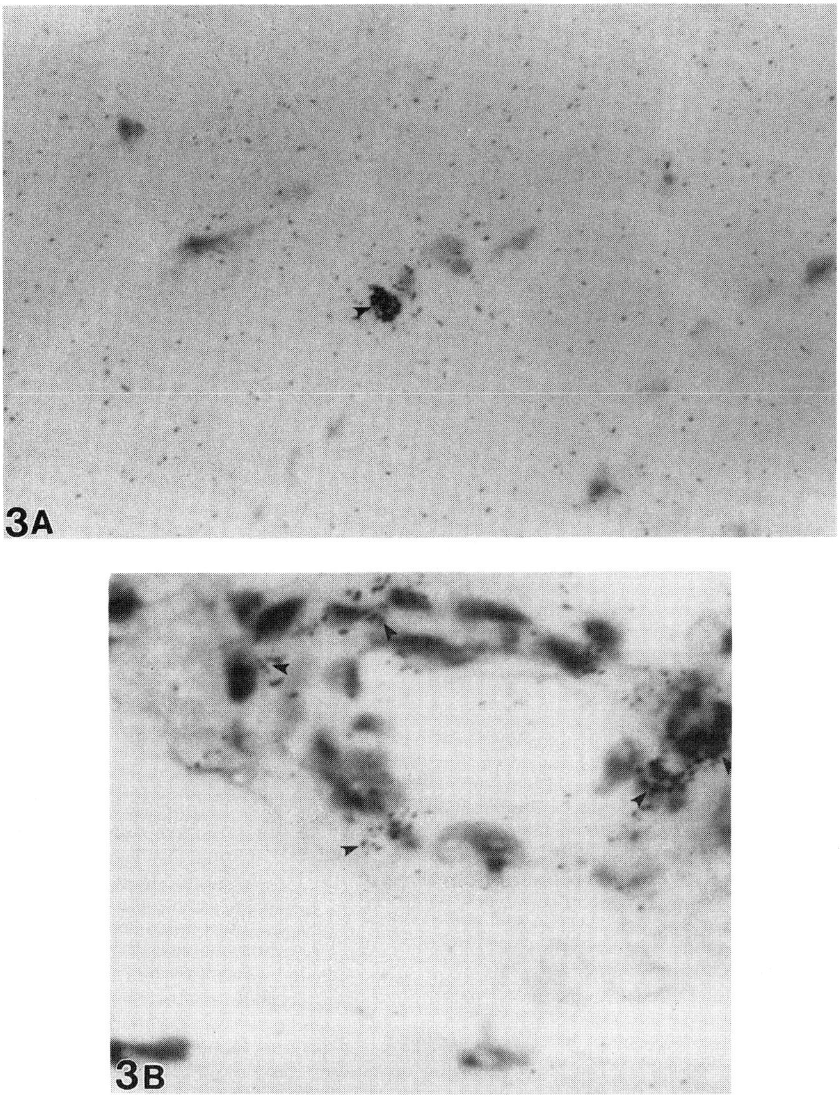

Figure 10.3 *In situ* hybridization shows HIV RNA signals, as hybridization granules, with occasional scattered endomysial (A) or perivascular (B) cells (× 480)

In HIV myopathy, therefore, there is no evidence of persistent infection of the muscle fibres by the virus or integration of the HIV proviral genome within the muscle DNA. Similar observations have been made in transgenic mice transfected with the HIV proviral genome. These mice showed no signs of myopathy and, in contrast with other tissues, such as skin, gut, or brain, in which HIV proviral DNA was detected, no HIV-positive signals were

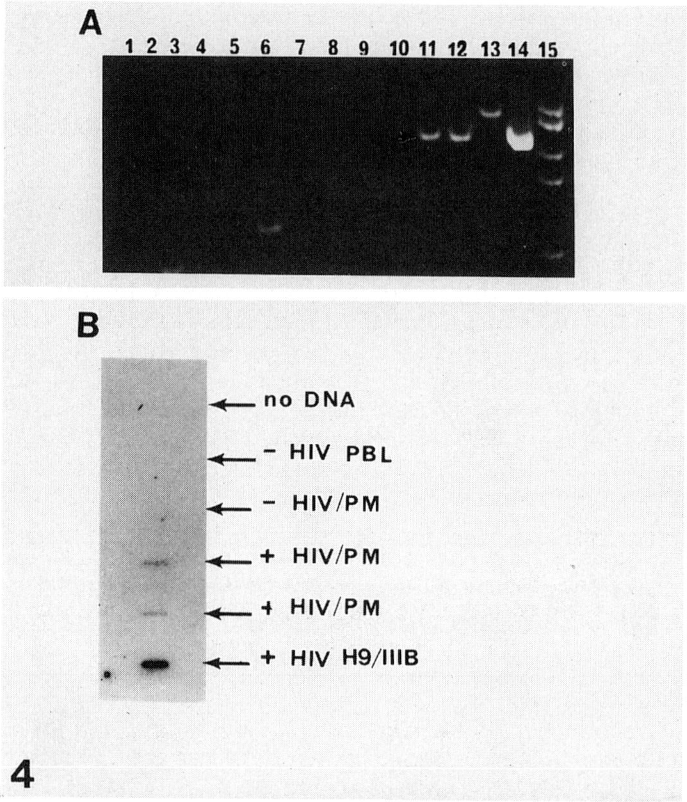

Figure 10.4 Characterization of amplified DNA product after the polymerase chain reaction using HIV *pol* primers. A. Amplified DNA from patients with HIV myopathy resolved in acrylamide gel is stained with ethidium bromide. The lanes represent DNA extracted from normal HIV-negative lymphocytes (lane 2), patients with HIV myopathy (lanes 3–12), DNA extracted from a muscle of an HTLV-I-positive but HIV-negative patient for internal retroviral control (lane 13), and from HIV-positive (H9/IIIB) lymphocytes (lane 14). Lane 1 represents water and no DNA, and lane 15 represents low-range DNA molecular weight markers (281, 271, 254 and 213 bp). Note positive amplified DNA signals in only two patients with HIV myopathy (lanes 11 and 12) and the HIV-positive control lymphocyte (lane 14). The signal in lane 13 is from a patient with HTLV-I infection and probably represents cross-reactivity with an HTLV-I DNA fragment. B. Slot-blot hybridization of denatured amplified DNA, hybridized with a ^{32}P-labelled *pol* HIV probe. Amplified DNA products are shown from the HIV-negative lymphocytes (−HIV PBL), the HIV-negative patient with polymyositis (−HIV/PM), the two HIV-positive patients with polymyositis (+HIV/PM) (represented in lanes 11 and 12 in panel A) and the HIV-positive lymphocytes (+HIV H9/IIIB). Note positive hybridization signals only in the muscles from the two HIV-myopathy patients and in the HIV-positive control lymphocytes

noted in muscle[48,53]. In spite of all the above, however, a transient, acute and non-persistent intramuscular (intermyofibrillar) infection, capable of altering the expression of normal muscle antigens and triggering a secondary autoimmune attack, cannot be excluded. In such a case, a hypothetical intermyofibrillar infection could result in endomysial inflammation, which may become self-sustaining as the host cannot mount the expected antiviral response and down-regulate the inflammatory reaction.

Infection of cultured human muscle with HIV and HIV-infected autologous lymphocytes

To demonstrate whether HIV is capable of infecting human muscle, we established human myoblasts and myotubes in tissue culture from healthy muscles obtained during routine diagnostic biopsies. These cultures were experimentally infected and transfected with a high concentration (5×10^5 infectious units) of intact HIV or HIV proviral DNA construct[53]. The infected and transfected cultures were monitored by assays for reverse transcriptase and p24 antigen and with PCR. After 2 months, the cultured myotubes remained morphologically intact and identical to the non-infected control cultures. The supernatant was negative for reverse transcriptase and p24 antigen. The PCR also failed to amplify HIV-specific signals in the DNA extracted from the muscle cultures.

In another series of experiments, we infected human muscle myotubes with homologous, interleukin-2 (IL-2)-activated and HIV-infected peripheral blood lymphocytes and monocytes to determine whether muscle infection can be mediated by infected lymphocytes. Up to 10% of the lymphocytes applied to these cultures were infected, as determined by immunocytochemistry using antibodies to gp41 and p24 antigens. After 6 weeks in culture, and in spite of clear attachment of the lymphocytes to the myotubes (Figure 10.5), no infection of the muscle cells was noted. This was based on the absence of cytopathic effect, the absence of p24 antigen in the supernatant and the negative reverse transcriptase activity (Figure 10.5B) after the first week. DNA extracted from the myotubes after 6 weeks did not amplify the HIV viral genome using PCR and specific primers. These observations indicate that human muscle in culture is resistant to infection not only with intact HIV, but also with HIV-infected homologous lymphoid cells, and argue against, but do not exclude, the possibility that HIV can cause a persistent infection of the muscle.

Immunopathogenesis

Because HIV myopathy has clinical and histological similarities with polymyositis in HIV-negative patients, in which autoimmune mechanisms have been implicated, we used immunohistological techniques to compare muscle biopsies from 19 patients with HIV myopathy and five HIV-negative patients with polymyositis[47]. Muscle specimens were stained with a variety of monoclonal antibodies against lymphocyte subsets, macrophages, natural killer (NK) cells, MHC class I and II antigens and interferon (IFN) α and γ. The predominant inflammatory cells within the endomysial infiltrates were $CD8^+$ T cells ($48.9 \pm 7.6\%$ of the total cells) and macrophages ($38 \pm 4.7\%$), which surrounded or invaded healthy, non-necrotic muscle fibres (Figure 10.6 and Table 10.2). The majority of the $CD8^+$ cells are cytotoxic T cells,

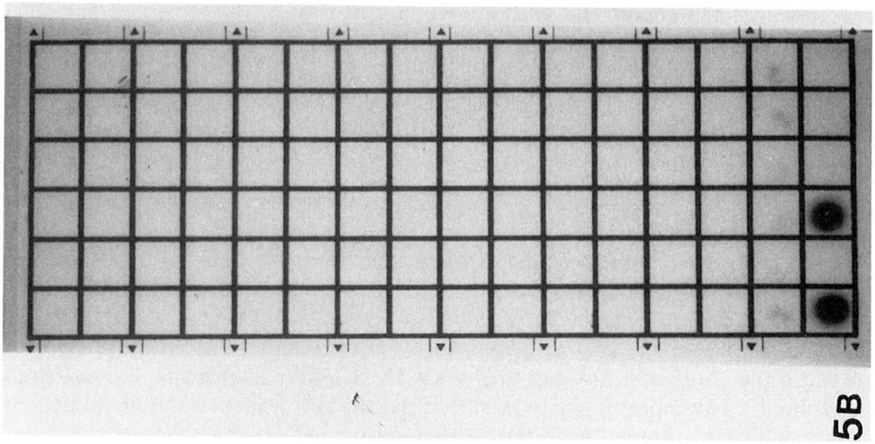

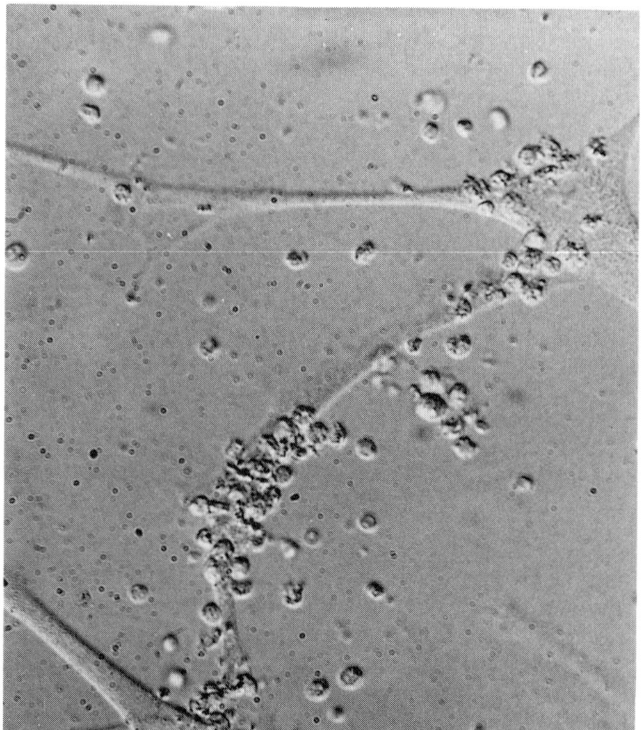

Figure 10.5 HIV-infected lymphocytes are shown in culture with homologous myotubes (A). No infection of the muscle was observed, as evidenced by the absence of a cytopathic effect (A) and negative reverse transcriptase (B). Positive activity in B (left wells) is due to the initially applied HIV-positive lymphocytes

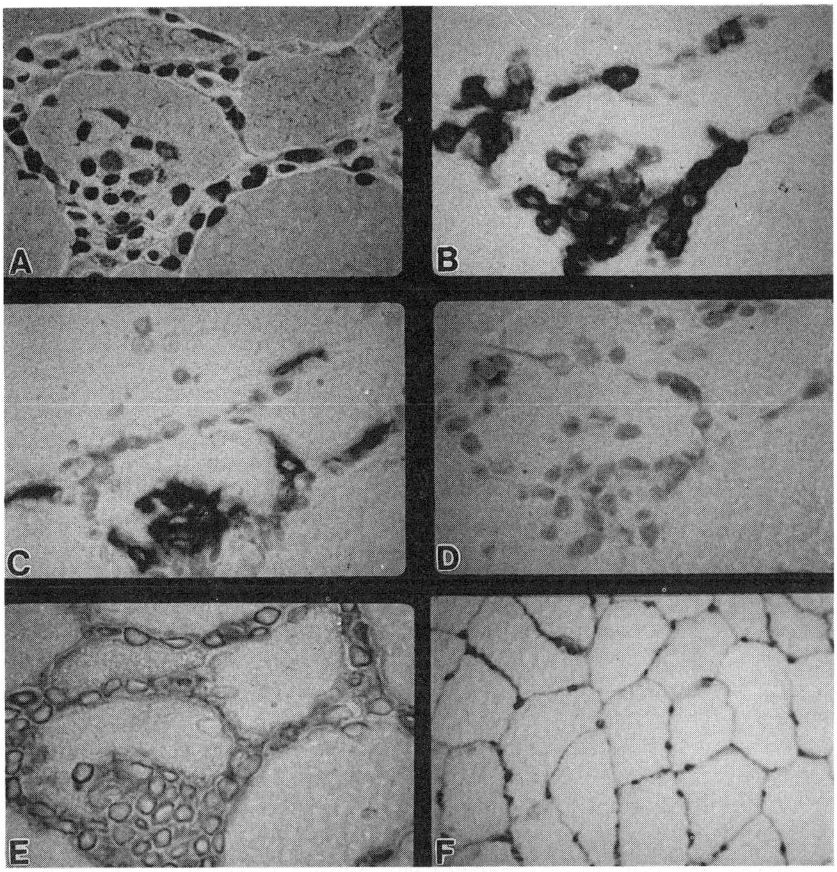

Figure 10.6 **Transverse frozen serial sections of a muscle biopsy specimen from a patient with** HIV-associated polymyositis. Sections were stained with haematoxylin and eosin (A) and with monoclonal antibodies to CD8 (B), macrophages (C), CD4 (D), and MHC-I antigen (E and F). A cluster surrounding a muscle fibre consists of $CD8^+$ cells (B) and macrophages (C). $CD4^+$ cells (D) are sparse. Sarcolemma and surrounding cells strongly express MHC-I antigen in the proximity of inflammation (E) and in areas remote from inflammation (F). (Avidin–biotin immunoperoxidase technique counterstained with methyl green; A-E, $\times 480$; F, $\times 280$)

not naïve or suppressor cells, because very few of them were $2H4^+$. The $CD4^+$ cells accounted for $12.6 \pm 3.2\%$ of the total number of cells (Table 10.2). Because the CD4 marker is expressed on macrophages[47], the true number of endomysial T4-positive cells (calculated by subtracting the acid phosphatase-positive macrophages from the $CD4^+$ cells) did not exceed 4–5% of the total. Many of these macrophages surrounded healthy, non-necrotic muscle fibres, even in the early phases of muscle invasion, indicating that some of these cells may not be scavenger cells but rather primary immune effector or antigen-presenting cells that play a role in mediating the muscle fibre injury. NK cells and B cells accounted for less than 1% of the endomysial cells. No positive cells expressing interleukin-2 were present to suggest recent

Table 10.2 Endomysial mononuclear cell infiltrates in clusters in patients with retrovirus-related polymyositis

	HIV polymyositis	*HTLV-I polymyositis*	*Polymyositis*
Total cells	966	1276	973
Mean number	193 ± 91	213 ± 110	194 ± 105
CD8+ (%)	49 ± 7.6	41 ± 6.2	50.4 ± 5.7
CD4+ (%)[b]	12.6 ± 3.2[c]	32 ± 7.3	21.1 ± 4.2
M5+ (%)	38 ± 4.7[c]	26 ± 3.3	27.9 ± 5.4
B cells (%)	≤ 0.1	≤ 1.0	≤ 0.1
NK cells (%)	≤ 1.0	≤ 1.0	≤ 1.0

[a]Three different cell clusters were counted in each of five patients with HIV polymyositis, HTLV polymyositis and seronegative polymyositis
[b]Corresponds to the total of T4+ cells and CD4+ macrophages that express the CD4 marker
[c]Significant difference ($p < 0.001$, unpaired t test) for comparison with HIV-negative polymyositis
[d]Significant difference ($p < 0.05$, unpaired t test) for comparison with HIV-negative polymyositis

activation of T cells. Interferon was not immunolocalized[47]. The MHC class II antigen was present only in the macrophages and mononuclear cells, but rarely in the sarcolemma of the muscle fibres. By contrast, the MHC class I antigen was expressed in the sarcolemma of almost all of the muscle fibres, regardless of their proximity to the clusters of lymphoid cells (Figure 10.6), in a pattern identical to that described in HIV-negative polymyositis[54]. This indicates that the recognition of the putative muscle antigen by the CD8+ cytotoxic T cells is restricted to the MHC class I antigen. Because viral antigens were not present in the muscle fibres, the CD8+ cytotoxic T cells surrounding the sarcolemma are not virus-specific but rather are sensitized against previously unidentified muscle fibre antigens. Although destruction of virus-specific and MHC-restricted cytotoxic T cells can theoretically be responsible for viral persistence by allowing the infected muscle fibres to escape immunological surveillance[55], there is no evidence that HIV persists within the muscle, as discussed earlier.

Other factors

As HIV infection progresses, immune dysregulation gives way to frank immunosuppression, setting the stage for direct muscle infection by opportunistic pathogens. Although rare, infection of the muscle can occur in the course of disseminated infection with the opportunist organisms *Cryptococcus neoformans*[17], *Toxoplasma gondii*[16], *Mycobacterium tuberculosis*[56,57] and *Mycobacterium avium intracellulare*[17,58]. We have not seen cytomegalovirus within the myofibrils in our muscle biopsy specimens, but we have seen non-caseating granuloma in the muscles of two patients, who had myalgia, fatigue, and muscle weakness (reference 5, and MC Dalakas, unpublished observations).

Other contributing myotoxic factors include vitamin deficiencies relating to the long-standing infection and poor nutrition, the induction of type II muscle fibre atrophy due to disuse, prolonged immobilization, or muscle wasting related to systemic sepsis or bacteriotoxins and myocytotoxicity due to the plethora of antibacterial, antiparasitic, antifungal, or antiviral drugs used to treat the underlying illnesses. Elevated levels of cachectin, a macrophage-derived factor, or tumour necrosis factor, arising directly from HIV infection or other co-infections, is found in patients with AIDS[59] and may contribute to the muscle wasting syndrome by interfering with lipoprotein lipase activity or other aspects of lipid metabolism. Contrary to one report[60], we feel that the HIV wasting syndrome does not represent an inflammatory myopathy but rather type II muscle fibre atrophy due to the factors mentioned earlier.

MYOPATHY ASSOCIATED WITH HUMAN T CELL LYMPHOTROPIC VIRUS TYPE (HTLV-I)

The human T cell lymphotropic virus type I (HTLV-I) has been linked not only to T cell leukaemia in adults but also to polymyositis and tropical spastic paraparesis (TSP)[61–64]. In Jamaica, HTLV-I is endemic, with a 7–18% prevalence of HTLV-I antibody positivity in the healthy population[61]. However, IgG anti-HTLV-I antibodies were found in up to 85% of Jamaicans with polymyositis, which indicates that the association is not due to chance. In Kagoshima, Japan, the prevalence of HTLV-I infection was significantly higher in patients with histologically proven polymyositis (27.5%) than in the general population (11.6%)[62].

In patients who are positive for HTLV-I, polymyositis may occur alone or together with TSP[63,64]. Although myelopathy associated with HTLV-I is frequently reported in Japan, polymyositis appears less prevalent in Japanese who are positive for HTLV-I, which suggests that genetic susceptibility of the host may be a confounding factor for the development of muscle disease. Myositis associated with HTLV-I has been seen in Haitians and, rarely, in native Americans[64]. Sera and muscle biopsies from patients with polymyositis or dermatomyositis have been negative for HTLV-I and HTLV-II antibodies, as determined by enzyme-linked immunosorbent assay[65] and for HTLV-I or HIV-I viral genome, as determined by PCR in the extracted DNA from the muscle tissue[66].

The initial symptoms in polymyositis related to HTLV-I infection are muscle weakness and elevated serum creatine kinase levels[61]. The muscle biopsy shows a brisk perimysial or interstitial inflammatory response with muscle fibre necrosis and phagocytosis (Figure 10.7). In two patients with TSP who had elevated creatine kinase levels and in four HTLV-I-positive patients with T cell leukaemia, some of whom had elevated creatine kinase but no other signs of myopathy, muscle biopsies showed features of denervation (MC Dalakas: unpublished observations).

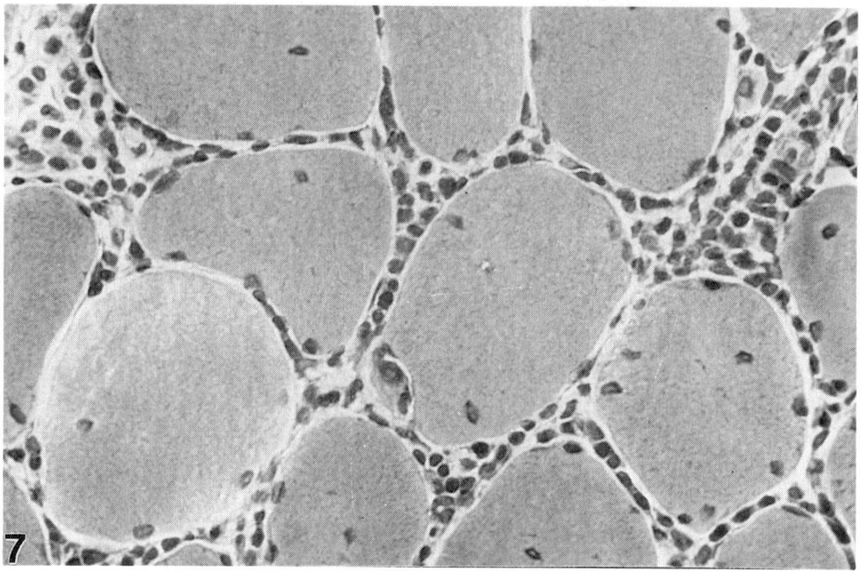

Figure 10.7 Cross-sections of a muscle biopsy specimen from a patient positive for HTLV-I, who had muscle weakness and elevated serum creatine kinase. Perivascular inflammation and inflammatory cells surrounding mostly healthy muscle fibres ($\times 680$)

Pathogenesis of HTLV-I myositis

We have also performed studies similar to those described above in patients with HTLV-I myositis. Immunocytochemical studies on muscle biopsy specimens using antibodies to HTLV-I viral proteins showed viral antigens only in occasional $CD4^+$ infiltrating perimysial lymphoid cells but not within the muscle fibres[67]. Similar findings were reported in the muscle biopsies from Japanese patients infected with HTLV-I[62]. The only study in which *in situ* hybridization showed HTLV-I particles within the muscle fibres of a patient co-infected with HIV and HTLV-I[67], has not been reproduced. We amplified viral sequences in only some of serial 10 μm sections of muscle biopsy specimens from four patients with HTLV-I myositis (Figure 10.8). As the virus was not found within the muscle fibre (by means of immunocytochemistry), we suspect that these amplified products probably represent infected lymphoid cells rather than infected muscle fibres. To determine whether integrated HTLV-I sequences are present within the myonuclei and the satellite cells, we searched for viral sequences in the DNA extracted from the muscle cultures established from biopsies of four patients. We were unable to detect HTLV-I-specific amplification bands within the genomic DNA (Figure 10.8). In addition, PCR-confirmed HTLV-I-positive peripheral blood lymphocytes, applied to homologous myotubes, did not cause cytopathic effect (Figure 10.9) and the virus did not integrate within the DNA of the myotubes (Figure 10.8)[68].

The primary endomysial cell in polymyositis associated with HTLV-I

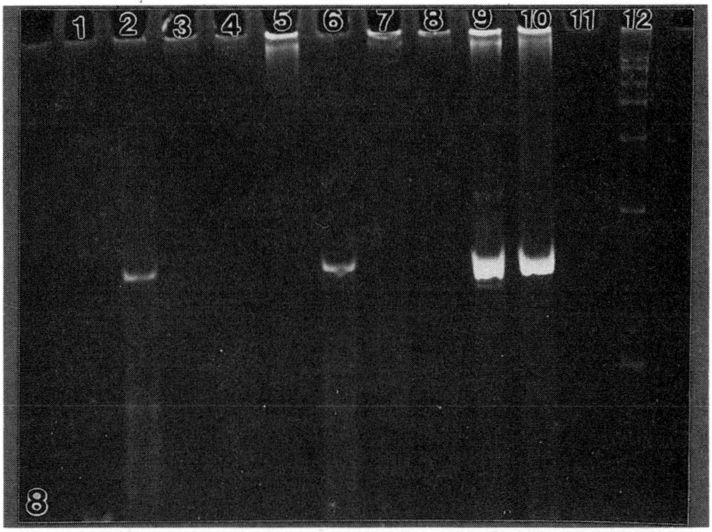

Figure 10.8 Amplification performed by PCR using specific HTLV-I *pol* primers in the DNA (1,5) or RNA (2,6) extracted from the muscle biopsies of two patients (1–4 one, 5–8 the other) with HTLV polymyositis, and the DNA extracted from their respective myotubes in cultures before (3,7) and after (4,8) co-cultivation with their homologous lymphocytes. Amplified HTLV-I products were found only in the RNA extracted from the muscles (2,6) and in the DNA extracted from their lymphocytes (9,10). Lane 11 represents water and 12 shows low-range DNA molecular weight markers (281–213 bp)

infection was the $CD8^+$ cytotoxic T cell, which along with macrophages invaded or surrounded healthy, non-necrotic and MHC-I antigen-expressing muscle fibres (Figure 10.10A,B). A T cell-mediated and MHC-I antigen-restricted cytotoxic process, similar to that noted in HIV myopathy and in retrovirus-seronegative polymyositis[45,66], is also the main immunopathological mechanism underlying the myopathy associated with HTLV-I infection. In contrast with HIV polymyositis however, HTLV-I infection is characterized by more frequent endomysial $CD4^+$ cells, as shown by double immunocytochemistry performed on the same section (Figure 10.11).

Four muscle biopsies from HTLV-I-positive patients with leukaemia but without clinical or histological signs of myopathy showed a marked expression of MHC class I antigen (Figure 10.12), probably induced by circulating lymphokines or cytokines released during the chronic persistent viral infection. The MHC-I expressing muscle fibres could recognize viral antigens or present endogenous self antigens to cytotoxic T cells and render the muscle susceptible to T cell-mediated destruction, as proposed by Honfeld[69].

MYOPATHY ASSOCIATED WITH HUMAN FOAMY RETROVIRUS

Transgenic mice carrying the *bel* region of the human foamy retrovirus (HFV), under the transcriptional control of its own long terminal repeat,

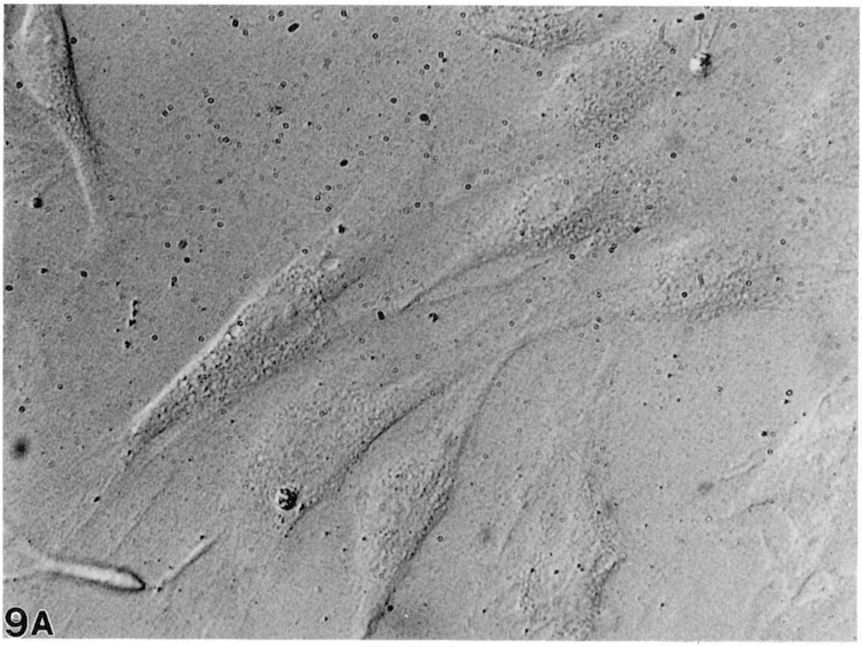

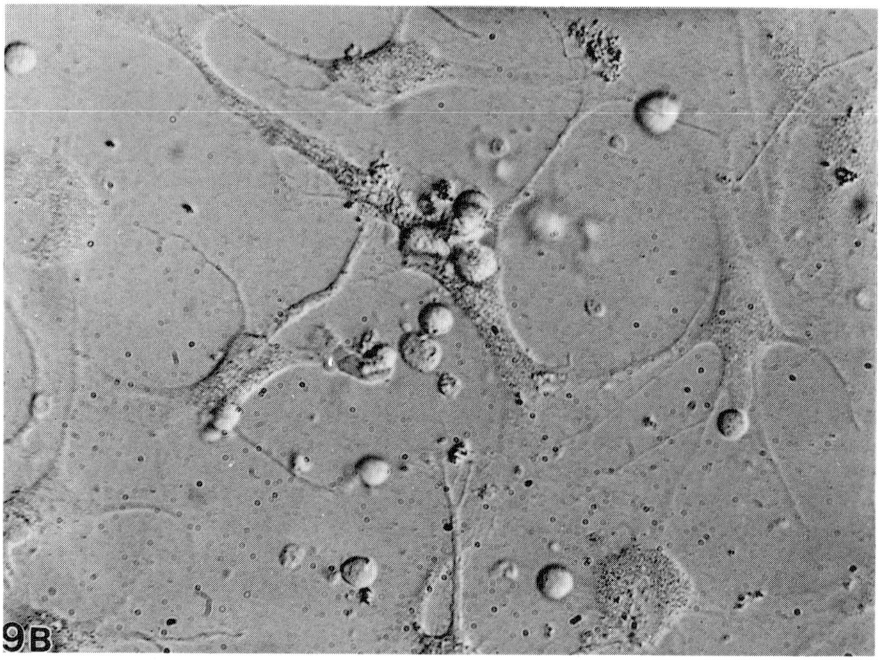

Figure 10.9 Myotubes from a muscle biopsy of an HTLV-I-positive patient infected with the virus isolated from his own lymphocytes (A), and co-cultured with autologous HTLV-I-positive lymphocytes (B). The myotubes were resistant to infection and no cytopathic effect was noted

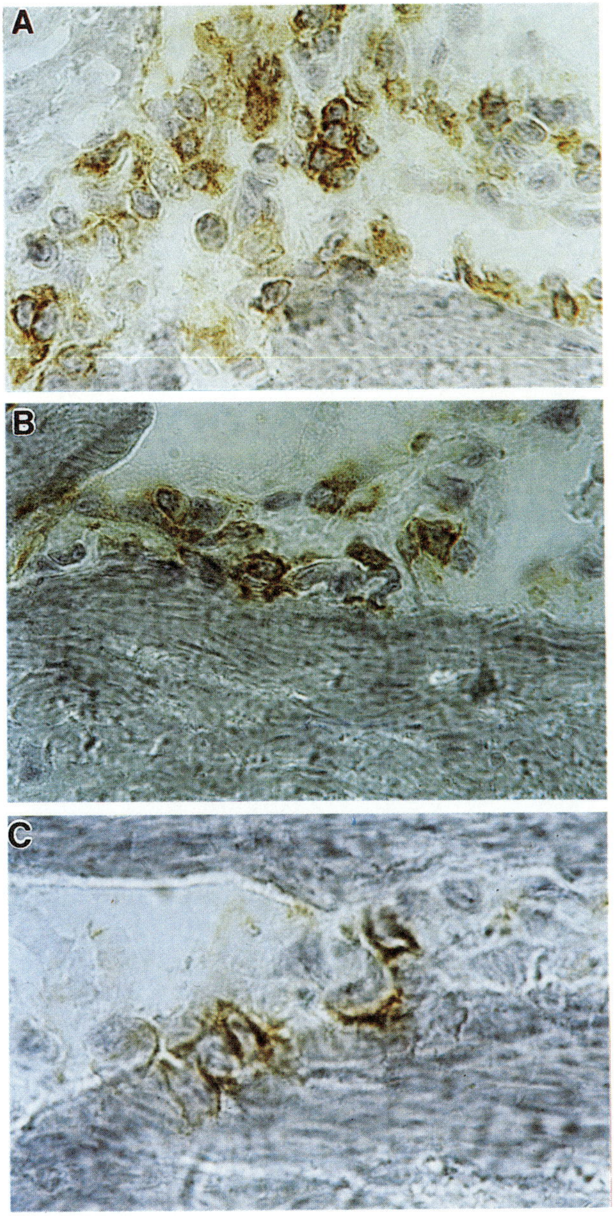

Figure 10.10 Two muscle fibres from an HTLV-positive patient with polymyositis stained for CD8$^+$ cells. The CD8$^+$ cells attach to the healthy muscle fibres (A,B). At higher magnification (C), extensions of the CD8$^+$ cells are seen to penetrate the basal lamina. MHC-I expression was strongly expressed in the muscle fibres even away from the inflammation (not shown)

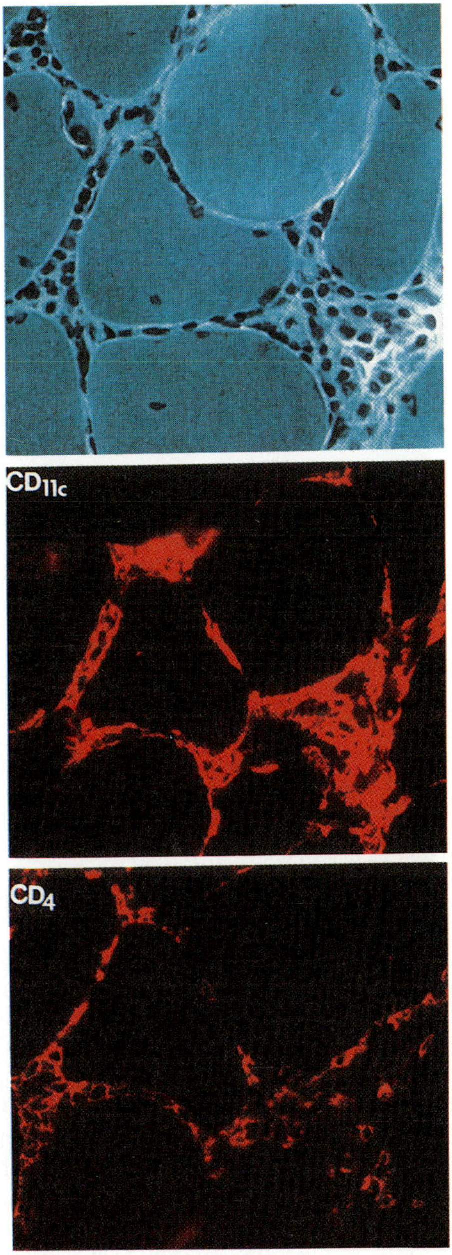

Figure 10.11 Double immunocytochemistry of an endomysial infiltrate from a muscle biopsy specimen of a patient with HTLV-I PM. Section is stained for trichrome (top), CD11c (for T cell, centre) and CD4 cells (bottom). Note that a number of the infiltrating T cells express the CD4 marker. (The majority of the lymphocytes are however CD8$^+$ cells, (see Figure 10.10))

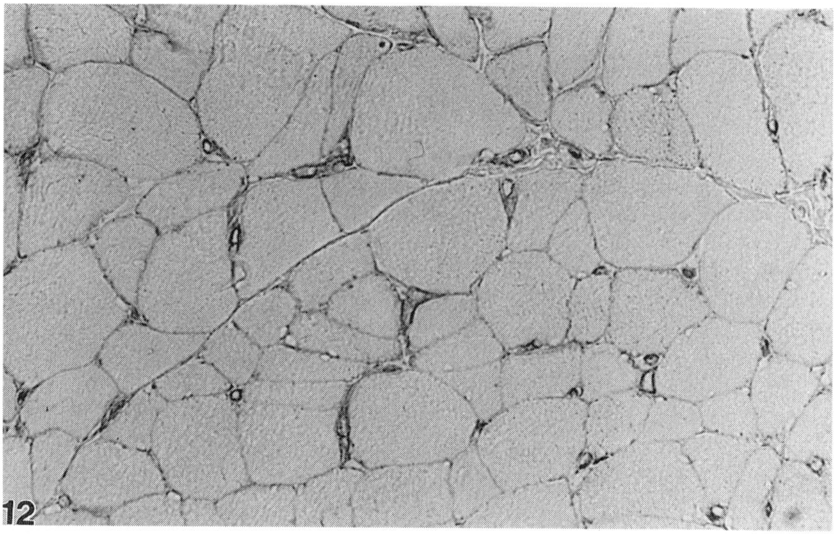

Figure 10.12 Frozen section of a muscle biopsy from a patient with HTLV-I infection and T cell leukaemia who did not have clinical or laboratory signs of a myopathy shows some neurogenic features and type II fibre atrophy. All muscle fibres, however, express MHC-I antigen

express the transgene in the striated muscle and exhibit a destructive myopathy[70]. The majority of the viable muscle fibres express viral RNA before degenerative features develop, which suggests that HFV is directly responsible for the myopathy. Of interest is the fact that *bel*-1 has homology with the *tat* and *tax* proteins of the HIV-I and HTLV-I respectively, the two other retroviruses associated with myopathy.

MYOPATHY ASSOCIATED WITH THE SIMIAN RETROVIRUS TYPE I (SRV-I) AND SIMIAN IMMUNODEFICIENCY VIRUS (SIV)

The simian retrovirus type I (SRV-I), which is similar to the Mason Pfizer monkey virus, infects monkeys and can cause immunodeficiency, Kaposi's sarcoma and polymyositis that is histologically identical to the human disease[71,72]. The infected animals experience muscle weakness, muscle wasting and elevated creatine kinase levels. The muscle biopsy shows perivascular and interstitial inflammation with phagocytosis and muscle fibre necrosis. Immunocytochemistry shows viral antigens only in the endomysial lymphocytic infiltrates, and not within the muscle fibres[71,72]. However, SRV-I is capable of infecting muscles in tissue culture, as determined by assays of reverse transcriptase in the supernatant, without exerting a cytopathic effect on the muscle[71]. Another simian retrovirus, the simian immunodeficiency virus (SIV) which is closely related to HIV, can also cause immunodeficiency, encephalopathy, and lymphopenia. We studied two monkeys with SIV, one of which had severe inflammatory myopathy which was histologically identical to the human disease (MC Dalakas, M Gravell, unpublished observations).

IMPLICATIONS AND SIGNIFICANCE OF RETROVIRUSES IN THE AETIOLOGY OF POLYMYOSITIS

The immunopathological characteristics of HIV and HTLV-I-associated myositis are similar to those of patients with polymyositis and inclusion-body myositis in whom the search for all viruses has failed[24–26,42,66,73]. The types and subtypes of the endomysial inflammatory cells are also remarkably similar in all three conditions (Table 10.2). It seems, therefore, that a T cell-mediated and MHC class I antigen-restricted cytotoxic process is a common final pathogenetic mechanism in all patients with polymyositis, regardless of whether the disease has been triggered by a known virus. The muscle fibres expressing MHC class I antigens do not seem to recognize viral antigens, but they may present endogenous self antigens to cytotoxic T cells and render the muscle fibre susceptible to a T cell-mediated destruction. The virus need not be present nor must it persist within the muscle fibre, but it may persist in other parts of the body and in other cells, as is the case for microglia, macrophages and $CD4^+$ cells in the circulation or the lymphoid organs. In the setting of such a persistent infection, cytokines or lymphokines secreted by the retrovirus-positive circulating or endomysial lymphoid cells may expose normally hidden or newly surfacing muscle antigens against which there is no self tolerance, allowing autoaggressive cytotoxic T cells to invade muscle fibres[5,24]. Furthermore, sarcolemmal proteins share common regions of homology with retroviral sequences[74,75], which may allow circulating anti-retroviral antibodies to cross-react with muscle proteins. This may result in a stable antigen–antibody complex that serves as a muscle neoantigen, leading to self sensitization. Consistent with this hypothesis of molecular antigenic mimicry is the observation that antibodies to ribonucleoproteins found in the serum of some HIV-negative patients with polymyositis share common antigens with retroviral proteins coded for by the *gag* and *pol* genes[74,75].

The association of five different retroviruses with inflammatory myopathies prompted us to look for retroviral proteins in the serum from HIV-negative patients with inflammatory myopathies. Western blotting showed that human sera variably recognize at least two proteins of HIV, HTLV-I and HTLV-II[75]. This reactivity was especially prominent in patients with inclusion body myositis. Furthermore, DNA extracted from the same muscle biopsies gave specific amplification products with HTLV-I primers for the *gag*, *env*, *tax-rex*, and *pol* genes[75]. These products may represent endogenous retroviruses, widely present within the human DNA[76], which can become pathogenic, leading to polymyositis if partially transcribed and translated into functional gene products or, if mutated, may become infectious or immunogenic. Retroviruses, therefore, may be the leading candidate viruses in the cause of inflammatory myopathies.

MYOPATHY ASSOCIATED WITH AZT THERAPY

Before 1986, when AZT (zidovudine) was introduced for the treatment of AIDS[77], the incidence of HIV myopathy was low, and myopathy was considered a rare clinical complication of HIV infection. Over the last few years, however, an increasing number of patients receiving long-term AZT therapy have developed myopathic symptoms that generally improve when the drug is discontinued[78–81]. Several studies have now unequivocally demonstrated that AZT is capable of inducing a unique mitochondrial DNA-depleting myopathy, attributable to its mitochondrial toxicity[20–23,82]. AZT is myotoxic not only in HIV-positive patients but also in cultures of normal human muscle and in normal rats given AZT[83–85].

Myopathy may develop in up to 30% of adults treated with long-term (> 12 months), high-dose (> 1200 mg daily) AZT[22,86]. Although cumulative drug dose may be an important determinant[23], we have observed the disorder in adults treated exclusively with the newer, low-dose regimens for early stage disease[86]. The clinical features of AZT myopathy include proximal muscle weakness, myalgia, predominantly in the thighs and calves and often exacerbated by exercise, and elevation of creatine kinase levels, which may also be worsened by exercise. Weight loss and elevated serum lactate may herald the presence of AZT myopathy[86]. The electromyogram shows myopathic units like those seen in patients with HIV myopathy. AZT myopathy improves when the drug is discontinued. The myalgia resolves rapidly, often within 2 weeks, but the weakness improves more slowly. Patients with severe weakness (MRC grade 3 or below) improve but may not fully recover, underscoring the need for an early diagnosis[87].

HIV myopathy is clinically similar to AZT myopathy. Without specialized diagnostic testing, such as muscle biopsy[5–7,20–22,26] or magnetic resonance spectroscopy (MRS)[88,89], the only clinical way of distinguishing AZT from HIV myopathy is by stopping the drug and monitoring for clinical improvement, manifested as increased strength, decreased muscle pain and reduction in serum creatine kinase. While elevations of CK levels usually accompany both HIV and AZT myopathy, we have seen patients with histologically severe AZT myopathy and normal CK levels (MC Dalakas, unpublished observations). Serum CK level alone is not, therefore, a reliable screening test for AZT myopathy.

The unique features that distinguish AZT myopathy from that due to HIV are seen in histological studies. Muscle specimens of AZT-treated patients show prominent, numerous fibres with 'ragged-red' features in trichrome-stained preparations, indicative of abnormalities in the muscle mitochondria[20–23] (Figure 10.13A-B). Although these fibres may resemble the ragged-red fibres seen in the muscles of patients with mitochondrial myopathies[20,23], they usually have subsarcolemmal or central granular accumulations next to single, longitudinal or circumferential, 'red-rimmed cracks' or pale granular degeneration with 'cracks' filled with neutral fat (Figure 10.12). The combination of these findings, which represent various stages of mitochondrial dysfunction and depletion of mitochondrial DNA, defines what we have now called the 'AZT fibre'[5,7,42]. Some of these fibres are small and angulated,

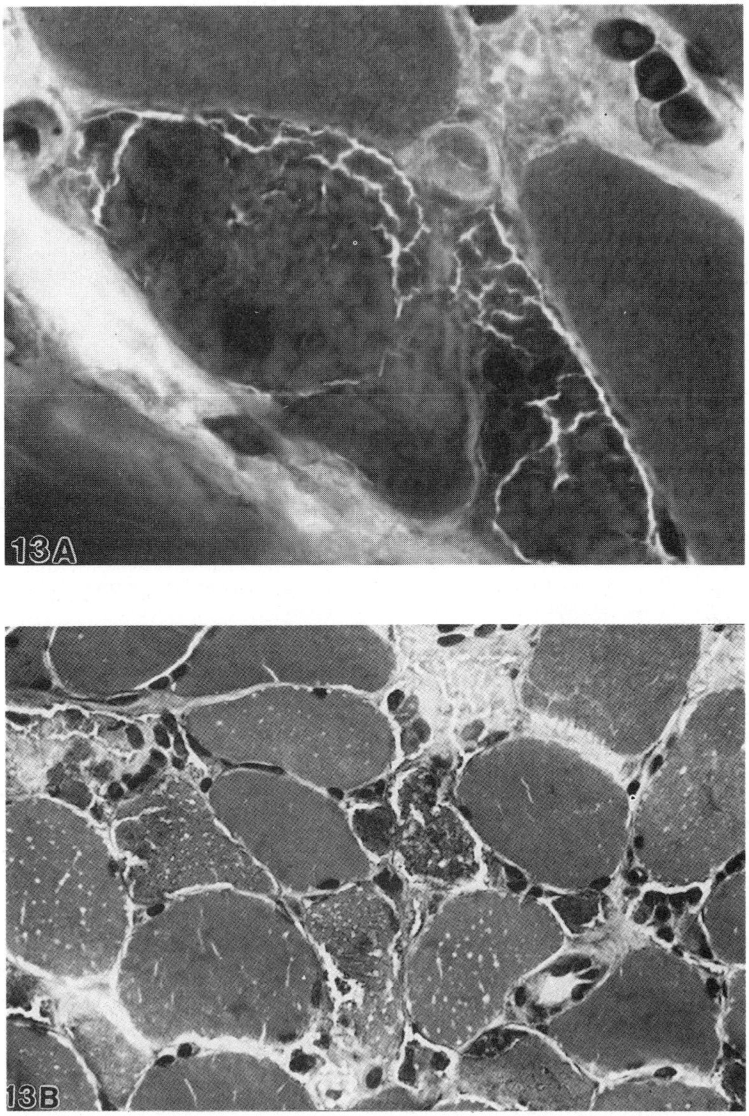

Figure 10.13 Transverse frozen sections of muscle biopsy specimens from patients with AZT myopathy. A. Two 'ragged-red' fibres, corresponding to proliferation of mitochondria (trichrome, × 800) are noted; B: Numerous AZT fibres ('cracked' fibres with granular degeneration, or 'washed-out' fibres) (trichrome, × 420). Arrowheads indicate rods. Within these cracks there is accumulation of neutral fat (not shown)

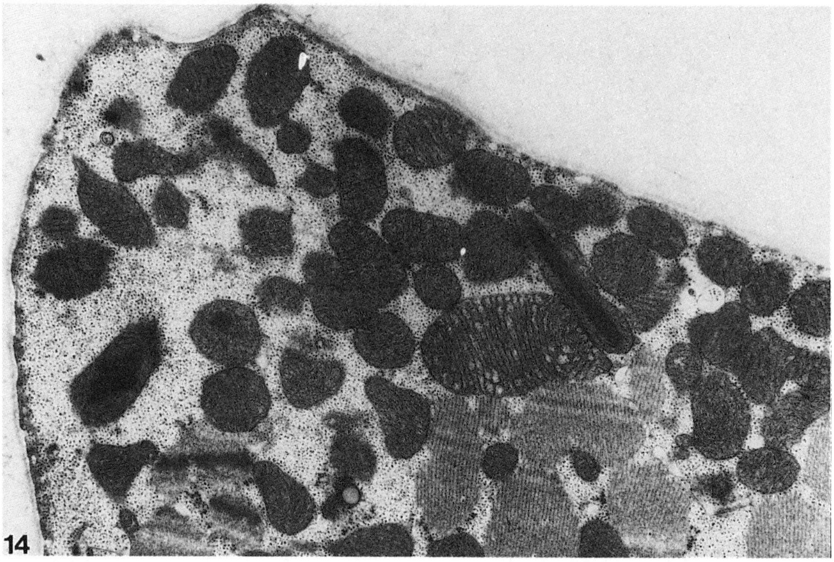

Figure 10.14 Electron microscopy of an AZT myopathy muscle fibre shows proliferation of mitochondria of various sizes and with abnormal cristae

some are large or of normal size and others contain rods, irregular cytoplasmic bodies and vacuoles (Figure 10.12A). These changes are fully or partially reversible with the discontinuation of AZT, as demonstrated by the noticeable improvement in the cytoarchitecture of the muscle fibres and the marked reduction in the number of AZT fibres in repeat muscle biopsy specimens obtained from several of our patients. Electron microscopic studies have confirmed the presence of abnormal mitochondria, which are ubiquitous throughout the muscle, even in fibres that appear normal on light microscopy[86] (Figure 10.14).

Immunocytochemical studies performed on muscle biopsy specimens, using antibodies to single- and double-stranded DNA, have shown severe depletion of immunostainable mitochondrial DNA[29], whereas Southern blots of the extracted muscle mitochondria showed up to 80% reduction in mitochondrial DNA; this is reversible on withdrawal of the drug[82].

Mitochondrial dysfunction in AZT myopathy can be confirmed *in vivo* using $[^{31}P]$magnetic resonance spectroscopy ($[^{32}P]$MRS), a non-invasive method for assessing muscle metabolism. Marked phosphocreatine depletion with slow recovery after exercise has been observed by us and others[88,89].

The pronounced reduction in mitochondrial DNA agrees with the finding that *in vitro* AZT is readily incorporated into the mitochondrial matrix, resulting in termination of the DNA chain[90]. Sequentially, this results in compensatory proliferation of mitochondria, structural abnormalities and impaired function by inhibiting the expression of cytochrome b messenger RNA and affecting oxidation–phosphorylation coupling, as well as activity of the complex I + III of the mitochondrial respiratory chain. Of interest is

Table 10.3 Distinction between HIV myopathy and AZT myopathy

	HIV myopathy	*AZT myopathy*
Clinical symptoms and signs		
Proximal muscle weakness	+	+
Myalgia	+	++
Myopathic electromyogram	+	+
Elevated creatine kinase	+	+
Onset of myopathy after AZT therapy	N/A	~12 months
Muscle biopsy findings		
Inflammation	++	0 → +
Rods	Rare	+++
Cytoplasmic bodies	Rare	+++
'Ragged-red' fibres	Absent	+++
Immunocytochemistry		
Primary endomysial cells surrounding muscle fibres	$CD8^+$ cells, macrophages	$CD8^+$ cells, macrophages*
MHC-I antigen in muscle fibres	Present	Present
Virology		
HIV antigen within muscle fibres	Absent	Absent
HIV antigen in endomysial lymphoid cells	Rarely present	Rarely present
HIV antigen in cultured myotubes	Absent	Absent
Molecular studies and DNA immunocytochemistry		
Muscle mitochondrial DNA	Normal	Reduced
Immunostainable mitochondrial DNA	Normal	Reduced
Therapy		
Response to prednisone	Yes, in some cases	?
Response to NSAID	Possible	Possible
Response to discontinuation of AZT	N/A	Yes

AZT, azidothymidine; NSAID, non-steroidal anti-inflammatory drug
*The degree of inflammation is less pronounced than in HIV myopathy

the fact that *in vitro*, dideoxycitidine (ddC) does not inhibit γ-polymerase as efficiently as does AZT[90], perhaps accounting for the ddC's apparent lack of myotoxicity (MC Dalakas, unpublished observations).

Muscle specimens from patients with AZT myopathy exhibit various degrees of endomysial inflammation characterized by lymphocytes (mostly $CD8^+$ cells) and macrophages, but the inflammation is less severe than that seen in HIV myopathy[5–7,22,23]. MHC class I antigen expression is also prominent on the muscle sarcolemma. In many patients therefore, a T cell-mediated and MHC class I-restricted cytotoxic process related to the underlying HIV infection appears to co-exist with AZT toxicity; this may persist even after the drug is stopped[22]. The clinical, histological and molecular differences between AZT myopathy and HIV myopathy are summarized in Table 10.3.

HIV-RELATED PERIPHERAL NEUROPATHIES

Peripheral neuropathies (Table 10.4) usually develop in a stage-specific fashion in HIV-infected adults[1,2,4,7,91,92]. Guillain–Barré syndrome (GBS)

Table 10.4 HIV-related peripheral neuropathies in adults and children

Guillain–Barré syndrome (GBS)
Chronic inflammatory demyelinating polyneuropathy (CIDP)
Mononeuritis multiplex
Ganglioneuronitis
Lumbosacral polyradiculoneuropathy, often due to CMV
Painful sensory axonal neuropathy
Nucleosides (ddI, ddC) neuropathy

Table 10.5 Clinical features of HIV-related peripheral neuropathies

	GBS	*CIDP*	*Polyradiculitis*	*PSN*
Stage of disease	Early	Early	Late	Late
Onset	Acute	Subacute	Subacute	Subacute
Course	Resolution (spontaneous or with treatment)	May be relapsing	Progressive	Progressive
Pain	Rare	Rare	Occasional	Marked
Weakness	Marked	Moderate to marked	Marked	Mild or absent
CSF protein	Markedly elevated	Markedly elevated	Elevated	Normal to mildly elevated
CSF pleocytosis	Lymphocytic	Lymphocytic	Polymorphonuclear	Absent or mild lymphocytic
EMG/NCS	Demyelinating features	Demyelinating features	Polyradiculoneuropathy	Axonal features
Other	Respiratory compromise		Sphincters involved	
Treatment	Plasmapheresis, intravenous immunoglobulins, steroids	Same as GBS	Gancyclovir	Symptomatic

GBS: Guillain–Barré syndrome; CIDP: chronic inflammatory demyelinating polyneuropathy; PSN: painful sensory neuropathy

and chronic inflammatory demyelinating polyneuropathy (CIDP), both dysimmune demyelinating peripheral nerve disorders, may occur early in the infection or may be the presenting manifestation of unsuspected HIV infection[1,2,4,91,92] (Table 10.5). The only difference between HIV-negative GBS or CIDP and the HIV-associated condition is that patients with the latter often have pleocytosis in the spinal fluid. Sural nerve biopsy shows segmental demyelination with often perivascular and, rarely, endoneurial inflammation (Figure 10.15). One case of HIV-related GBS in a child has recently been reported[93] and we are aware of another HIV-infected child who developed classic features of CIDP (MC Dalakas, unpublished observations). Other, less common, peripheral neuropathies that may develop in early-stage HIV infection include acute ganglioneuronitis coincident with seroconversion[94] and mononeuritis multiplex[1] (Table 10.4). The clinical features characteristic for each of these neuropathies are listed in Table 10.5.

The most common neuropathy in AIDS patients is a painful sensory axonal neuropathy which, according to some studies, may affect up to 70%

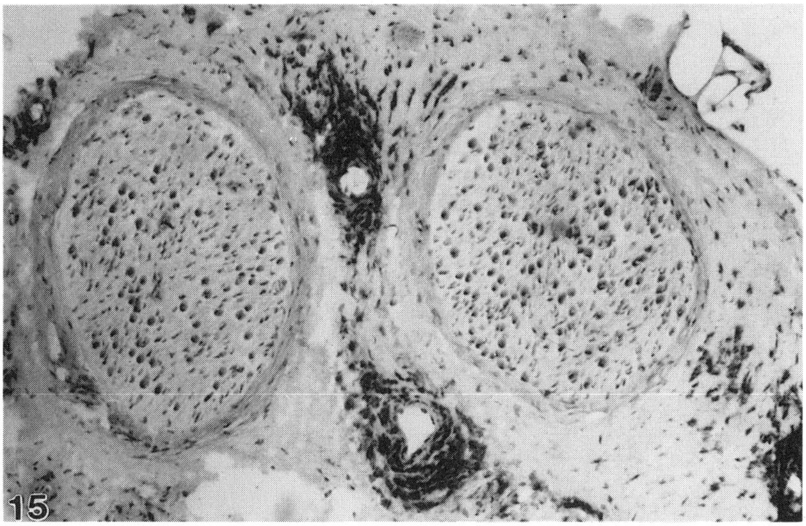

Figure 10.15 Cross-section of a sural nerve biopsy from a patient with HIV polyneuropathy stained with antibodies to T cells (CD11c) shows brisk perivascular inflammation with a few endoneurial positive cells

of adults with later-stage HIV infection[19]. Painful axonal neuropathy can also complicate therapy with dideoxyinosine (ddI) or ddC[7,95–97] and may represent the cumulative effect on the peripheral nerves of various endogenous or exogenous neurotoxins produced as a result of a multisystem disease and dysfunction of many organs. Despite the relative lack of motor involvement, severe neuropathic pain in such patients can be disabling. Pain may be so uncomfortable that even light stimuli, such as contact with sheets, is intolerable. Clinical findings include distal pansensory loss or reduced sensation, areflexia and, in advanced cases, distal weakness.

Electrodiagnostic and pathological studies clearly indicate that peripheral nerve pathology is nearly ubiquitous in AIDS patients, whether or not there is clinical evidence of peripheral neuropathy[14,15,19,98,99]. While clinical experience, supported by a small cross-sectional study including electrodiagnostic testing, has suggested that axonal neuropathy does not occur in children[100], two children with a clinical symptomatology consistent with AIDS-neuropathy were recently reported[101]. Sural nerve biopsy is consistent with axonal degeneration without signs of inflammation.

Another neuropathy seen in later-stage HIV infection, is the lumbosacral polyradiculoneuropathy, affecting roots and sensory ganglia, which is often related to cytomegalovirus (CMV) infection[1,2,4,102,103]. CMV polyradiculoneuropathy presents with lower extremity muscle weakness, sacral and distal paraesthesias, areflexia and atrophy, mostly of the legs, associated with sphincteric dysfunction resembling a cauda equina syndrome. The spinal fluid may show pleocytosis and harbours CMV, which can be detected by culture or cytological examination. CMV inclusions are often found within

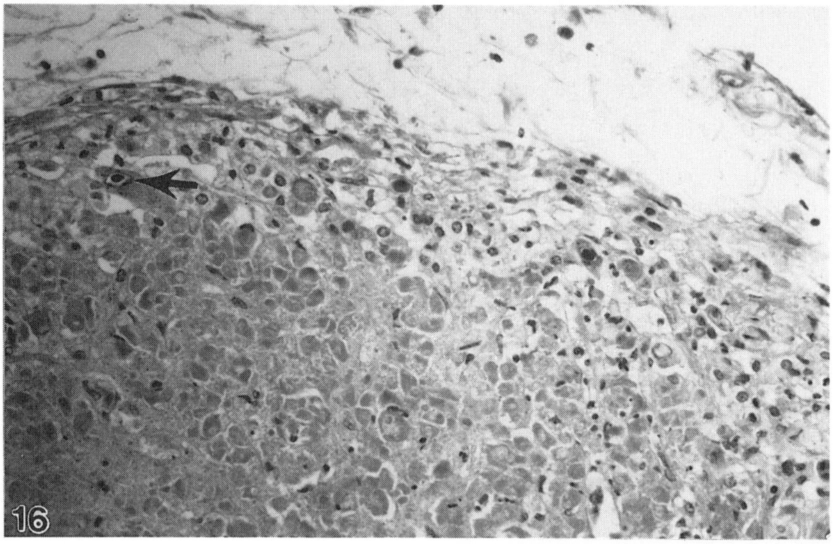

Figure 10.16 Cross-section of a root from a patient with HIV polyneuropathy stained with haematoxylin and eosin. CMV inclusions are noted within the Schwann cells (arrow)

the Schwann or endothelial cells at autopsy (Figure 10.16). The disease is thought to represent reactivated CMV infection of nerve root, rather than primary infection. This may explain why this neuropathy has not yet been described in children with AIDS, despite their frequent infection with CMV[104]. Recognition is important: anti-CMV therapy with gancyclovir may be life-saving[105].

Although AZT is myotoxic, the two other antiretroviral drugs, ddC and ddI, cause a dose-dependent reversible axonal painful sensory neuropathy[96–98]. Animal studies suggest that ddC may be primarily toxic to the myelin sheath, while the axonal damage is secondary[106]. The major feature which distinguishes a ddI- or ddC-related painful neuropathy from the painful sensory axonal neuropathy of AIDS is that the latter tends to be progressive while the nucleoside-related peripheral neuropathies tend to improve when the drugs are discontinued[7,96–98]. Another clinical feature of nucleoside neuropathy is 'coasting', or worsening of symptoms for a period of time after the drug is discontinued, followed by clinical improvement[7,107,108]. It is interesting that epidemiological studies and clinical experience have not implicated AZT as a peripheral neurotoxin[109]. Whether specific structure–function relationships dictate nucleoside neuro- or myotoxicity is uncertain, but this would have obvious implications for the development of new antiretroviral agents that lack neurotoxic potential. Dideoxynucleoside-related peripheral nerve toxicity has not yet been seen in children, even when higher doses are used.

Pathogenesis of peripheral neuropathies in HIV infection

The possible mechanisms include direct viral infection, immune alterations triggered by the viral illness, complications of antiretroviral therapy, sequelae of chronic illness or a combination of all the above.

HIV has been cultured from the peripheral nerve[15,110] and we have amplified HIV RNA from sural nerve biopsies of two patients. There is no convincing evidence, however, that the neuropathy results from direct infection of the peripheral nerve with the virus. Our own immunocytochemical studies using double-label techniques on sural nerve biopsies have shown that HIV is present only in rare endoneurial macrophages, and not within the Schwann cells or the axons (Figure 10.17). Immunocytochemistry shows that the endoneurial infiltrates in the sural nerve biopsies from such patients consist mostly of macrophages, while $CD8^+$ cells are sparse and $CD4^+$ cells are absent (Figure 10.18). There is also strong expression of MHC class I and HLA-DR antigens in Schwann cells, endothelial cells or macrophages, as shown in serial sections (Figure 10.18A–D). The role of the activated macrophages and their recognition of putative nerve antigen(s) is, however, currently unknown. It is possible that systemic viral infection or rare HIV-infected endoneurial lymphoid cells release lymphokines and cytokines that expose new antigens against which there is no self-tolerance, generating a tissue-specific autoimmune attack in a mechanism similar to that described earlier for the HIV myopathy. Proliferating macrophages may play a major role as immune effector cells or as sensitized cytotoxic cells mediating demyelination, similar to that which occurs in HIV-negative Guillain–Barré syndrome. The frequency of anti-myelin or GM1-specific autoantibodies in the serum of these patients is similar to that seen in HIV-negative patients with demyelinating polyneuropathies (MC Dalakas, unpublished observations).

As HIV infection progresses, immune dysregulation gives way to frank immunosuppression, setting the stage for direct infection by opportunistic organisms such as CMV, that may be harboured by Schwann cells as described earlier (Figure 10.16). Peripheral nerves also become sensitive to the effects of the systemic illness, neurotoxins, lymphokines or cytokines; this may account for the painful neuropathy. Antibiotics, particularly antimycobacterial and chemotherapeutic agents, are also known peripheral neurotoxins. If multiple medical insults contribute to the cause of AIDS-related painful sensory neuropathy[98], the rarity of this neuropathy in children with AIDS might be explained by the shorter incubation period of HIV infection in children compared to adults[104], shorter survival and less exposure to neurotoxic agents such as drugs or alcohol before seroconversion.

TREATMENT

Myopathies

Patients with mild myopathic symptoms and signs that are not functionally limiting can be monitored by serial examinations and CK determinations. Many of these patients will remain stable and not require specific therapy.

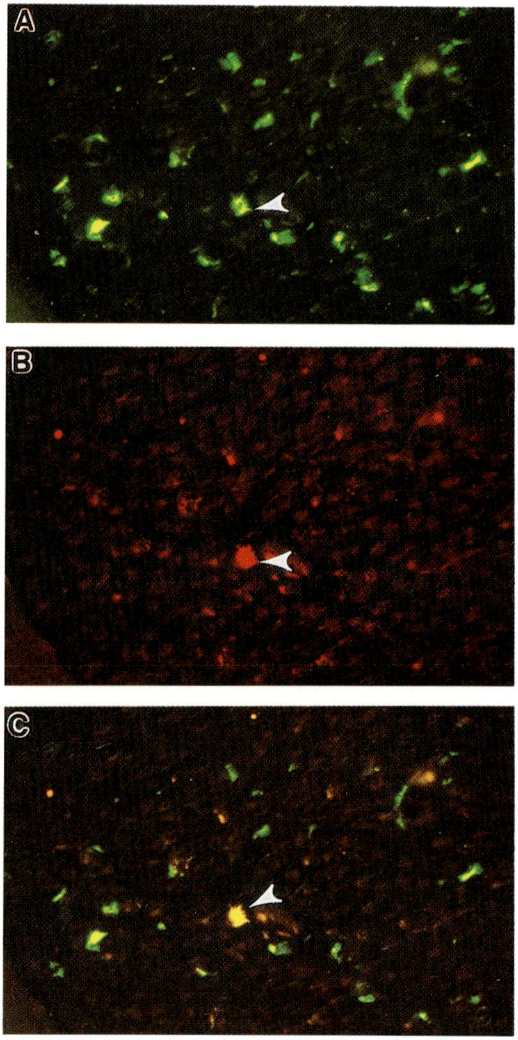

Figure 10.17 Double immunofluorescence of a nerve biopsy from a patient with CIDP dually immunostained for macrophages (A) visualized with green fluorescence and HIV p41 antigen (B), visualized with red fluorescence. There is proliferation of macrophages (A). One of the macrophages is HIV-positive (C), as confirmed by its yellow-orange colour (arrow) (C), produced by superimposition of the green (A) on the red fluorescence (B)

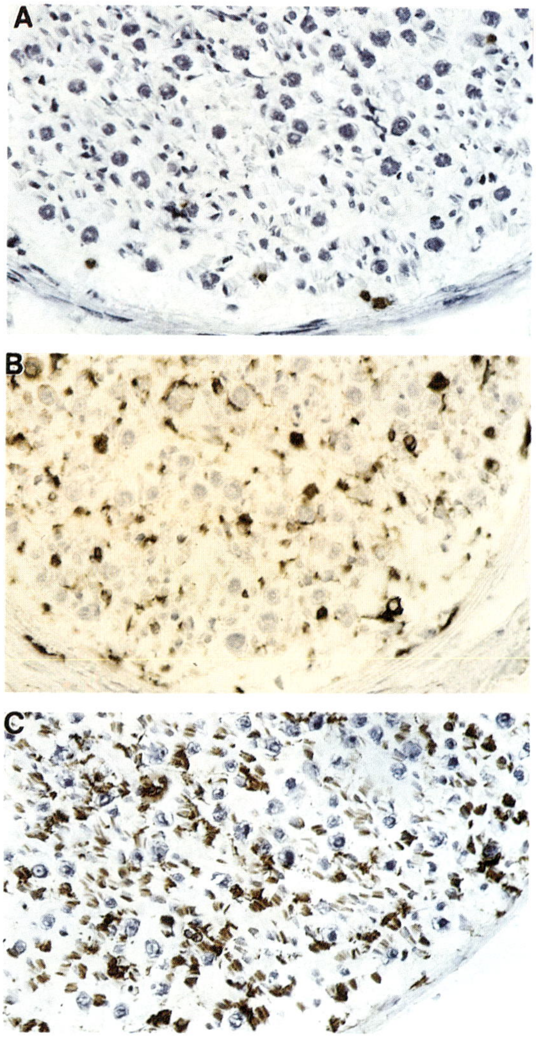

Figure 10.18 Serial sections of a nerve biopsy from a patient with HIV-CIDP stained for $CD8^+$ cells (A), macrophages (B), and DR (C). Only two $CD8^+$ cells are seen within the nerve fascicle (A). Most of the lymphoid cells present in the endoneurial parenchyma are macrophages (B). There is also strong expression of DR (C) and MHC-I (not shown)

Non-steroidal antiinflammatory drugs (NSAIDs) may be useful in managing myalgia.

Patients with HIV myopathy not taking AZT may benefit from treatment, although the drug has been reported to worsen the myopathy[111]. In patients already receiving AZT or those who do not improve with AZT, prednisone 1 mg/kg/day may be tried, slowly tapering following the regimen described for seronegative polymyositis[24–26]. In such patients, however, we favour treatment with high-dose intravenous immunoglobulin at 2 g/kg divided over 2–4 days, a regimen we have used successfully in seronegative inflammatory myopathies (MC Dalakas, unpublished observations).

Although intravenous immunoglobulin has not been studied prospectively in HIV myopathy, it is an attractive therapy because it avoids the side-effects associated with steroids and further immunosuppression. Currently, intravenous immunoglobulin is our recommended treatment of choice for HIV myopathy, although controlled studies have not been conducted to document its efficacy.

AZT myopathy often improves if the dose of AZT is reduced, with or without complete cessation of the drug. Improvement generally begins within 1–2 months and may be incomplete, even when the drug is stopped permanently. Alternative antiretroviral therapy with ddI or ddC may be other options. Two of our patients with clinically suspected AZT myopathy improved clinically on ddI, and two others with histologically proven AZT-myopathy improved clinically and histologically, one after change to ddI and the other after change to ddC (M Dalakas, unpublished observations).

In patients taking AZT who are unable or unwilling to undergo biopsy, NSAID with or without reduction of AZT is suggested. If disabling myopathy persists, AZT should be withheld and another antiretroviral agent substituted if possible. If functionally significant myopathy persists after 4–8 weeks without AZT, the myopathy is probably a primary inflammatory myopathy requiring either a short course of prednisone or intravenous immunoglobulin. Such clinical guesswork can be avoided if examination includes a muscle biopsy, a procedure we recommend for all HIV-infected patients whose clinical picture suggests myopathy. If biopsy is not available, it is advisable to intervene in a stepwise fashion whenever possible so that therapeutic responses can be clearly determined.

Patients with histological signs of type II muscle fibre atrophy should receive supportive care, with particular attention to physical therapy and mobilization. In all patients with myopathy, it is important to remember that CK is a marker for muscle disease and not a clinical endpoint. Thus, it is essential to monitor strength as well as CK level. Normal CK levels, while comforting to the physician, mean little if significant weakness persists[24–26].

There is general agreement regarding the management of pyomyositis[40,41]. All patients should receive intravenous antibiotics active against *S. aureus* (anti-staphylococcal penicillin or vancomycin) pending results of blood and abscess cultures. While most patients will recover with antibiotics alone, surgical incision and drainage may be required, particularly for later-stage infection. A high index of suspicion for secondary abscesses must be maintained because these may also require surgical intervention. Patients should be closely monitored for evidence of sepsis.

Neuropathies

Demyelinating neuropathies improve with immunomodulatory therapies such as intravenous immunoglobulin or plasmapheresis. Steroids may be considered for treatment of CIDP[1–7]. Intravenous immunoglobulin is our treatment of choice because it augments rather than suppresses immune function and has been effective in both children and adults with seronegative GBS or CIDP. In GBS, respiratory function may need to be monitored in an intensive care unit, and mechanical ventilatory support considered if vital capacity falls below 1 litre.

Gancyclovir appears to be effective in CMV-related polyradiculoneuropathy[105]. The role of foscarnet, recently approved for CMV retinitis, in this disorder remains to be determined. Painful sensory neuropathy can be disabling because of intractable pain, even though muscle weakness may be minimal. Tricyclic antidepressants, non-steroidal anti-inflammatory drugs, anticonvulsants (carbamazepine and phenytoin), narcotic analgesics and topical capsaicin in various combinations provide some relief from neuropathic pain, though symptomatic management of this condition is a notoriously difficult clinical problem.

References

1. Dalakas MC, Pezeshkpour GH. Neuromuscular complications of AIDS. Muscle Nerve. 1986;9:92.
2. Dalakas MC, Pezeshkpour GH. Neuromuscular diseases associated with human immunodeficiency virus infection. Ann Neurol. 1988;23S:38.
3. Dalakas MC, Pezeshkpour GH, Gravell M, Sever JL. Polymyositis in patients with AIDS. J Am Med Assoc. 1986;256:2381.
4. Dalakas MC, Wichman A, Sever JL. AIDS and the nervous system. J Am Med Assoc. 1989;261:2396.
5. Dalakas MC. Retrovirus-related muscle diseases. In Engel AG, editor. Myology. Harper and Row, In press.
6. Dalakas MC, Illa I. HIV-associated myopathies. In: Pizzo A, Wilfert CM, editors. Pediatric AIDS: The Challenge of HIV Infection in Infants, Children and Adolescents. Baltimore: Williams and Wilkins; 1991:420–9.
7. Jay CA, Dalakas MC. HIV-associated myopathies and neuropathies. In: Pizzo A, Wilfert CM, editors. Pediatric AIDS: The Challenge of HIV Infection in Infants, Children and Adolescents. Baltimore: Williams and Wilkins; 1994:559–73.
8. Simpson DM, Bender AN. Human immunodeficiency virus-associated myopathy: analysis of 11 patients. Ann Neurol. 1988;24:79.
9. Stern R, Gold J, DiCarlo EF. Myopathy complicating the acquired immune deficiency syndrome. Muscle Nerve. 1987;10:318.
10. Lange DJ, Britton CB, Younger DS, Hays AP. The neuromuscular manifestations of human immunodeficiency virus infections. Arch Neurol. 1988;45:1084.
11. Gonzales MF, Olney RK, So YT, *et al.* Subacute structural myopathy associated with human immunodeficiency virus infection. Arch Neurol. 1988;45:585.
12. Mahé SA, Chabin E, Fendler JP. Acute rhabdomyolysis coincident with primary HIV infection. Lancet. 1989;2:1454.
13. Piette AM, Tusseau F, Vignon D, *et al.* Acute neuropathy coincident with seroconversion for anti-LAV/HTLV-III. Lancet. 1986;1:852.

14. Mah V, Vartavarian LM, Akers M-A, Vinters HV. Abnormalities of peripheral nerve in patients with human immunodeficiency virus infection. Ann Neurol. 1988;24:713–17.
15. de la Monte SM, Gabuzda DH, Ho DD, *et al.* Peripheral neuropathy in the acquired immunodeficiency syndrome. Ann Neurol. 1988;23:485–92.
16. Gabbai AA, Schmidt B, Castelo, Oliveira ASB, Lima JGC. Muscle biopsy in AIDS and ARC: analysis of 50 patients. Muscle Nerve. 1990;13:541–4.
17. Wrzolek MA, Sher JH, Kozlowski PB, Rao C. Skeletal muscle pathology in AIDS: an autopsy study. Muscle Nerve. 1990;13:508–13.
18. Groopman JE. Zidovudine intolerance. Rev Infect Dis. 1990;12(Suppl.5):S500–6
19. So YT, Holtzman DM, Abrams DI, Olney RK. Peripheral neuropathy associated with acquired immunodeficiency syndrome: prevalence and clinical features from a population-based survey. Arch Neurol. 1988;45:945–8.
20. Dalakas M, Pezeshkpour GH. AZT-induced destructive inflammatory myopathy with abnormal mitochondria (DIM-Mi): study of seven patients. Neurology. 1989;39(Suppl.1):152.
21. Dalakas M, Illa I, Pezeshkpour GH, Laukaitis J. Can we distinguish AZT-induced myopathy from that due to HIV? Neurology. 1990;40(Suppl.1):414.
22. Dalakas MC, Illa I, Pezeshkpour GH, Laukaitis JP, Cohen B, Griffin JL. Mitochondrial myopathy caused by long-term zidovudine (AZT) therapy. N Engl J Med. 1990;328:1098.
23. Mhiri C, Baudrimont M, Bonne G, *et al.* Zidovudine myopathy: a distinctive disorder associated with mitochondrial dysfunction. Ann Neurol. 1991;29:606.
24. Dalakas MC (ed.). Polymyositis and Dermatomyositis. Stoneham, Massachusetts: Butterworth; 1988.
25. Dalakas MC. Inflammatory myopathies. Curr Opin Neurol Neurosurg. 1990;3:689.
26. Dalakas MC. Polymyositis, dermatomyositis and inclusion-body myositis. N Engl J Med. 1991;25:1487.
27. Baguley E, Wolf C, Hughes GRV. Dermatomyositis in HIV infection. Br J Rheumatol. 1988;27:493.
28. Gresh JP, Aguilar JL, Espinoza LR. Human immunodeficiency virus (HIV) infection-associated dermatomyositis. J Rheumatol. 1989;16:10–1397.
29. Pezeshkpour GH, Illa I, Dalakas MC. Ultrastructural characteristics and DNA immunocytochemistry in HIV and AZT-associated myopathies. Hum Pathol. 1991;22:1281.
30. Dalakas MC, Pezeshkpour GH, Flaherty M. Progressive nemaline (rod) myopathy associated with HIV infection. N Engl J Med. 1987;317:1602.
31. Gabello A, Martinez-Martin P, Guitterrez-Rivas E, Madero S. Myopathy with nemaline structures associated with HIV infection. J Neurol. 1990;237:64.
32. Engel AG, Gomez MR. Nemaline (Z disk) myopathy: observations of the origin, structure and solubility properties of the nemaline structures. J Neuropathol Exp Neurol. 1967;26:601.
33. Yamaguchi M, Robson RM, Stromer MH, Dahl DS, Oda T. Actin filaments from the backbone of nemaline myopathy rods. Nature. 1978;271:266.
34. Reyes MG, Tal A, Abrahamson D, Schwartz M. Nemaline myopathy in an adult with primary hypothyroidism. Can J Neurol Sci. 1986;13:117.
35. Comi G, Medaglini S, Galardi G, *et al.* Subclinical neuromuscular involvement in acquired immune deficiency syndrome. Muscle Nerve. 1986;9:665.
36. Younger DS, Hays AP, Uncine A, Lange DJ, Lovelace RE, DiMauro S. Recurrent myoglobinuria and HIV-seropositivity: incidental or pathogenic association? Muscle Nerve. 1989;12:842.
37. Wessel HB, Zitelli BJ. Myasthenia gravis associated with human T cell lymphotropic virus type-III infection. Pediatr Neurol. 1987;3:238.
38. Nath A, Kerman RH, Novak IS, Wolinsky JS. Immune studies in human immunodeficiency virus infection with myasthenia gravis: a case report. Neurology. 1990;40:581.
39. Martini L, Vion P, LeGangneux E, Grandpierre G, Becquet D. AIDS and myasthenia gravis: an exceptional association. Rev Neurol. 1991;147:392.
40. Schwartzman WA, Lambertus MW, Kennedy CA, Goetz MB. Staphylococcal pyomyositis in patients infected by the human immunodeficiency virus. Am J Med. 1991;90:595.
41. Widrow CA, Kellie SM, Saltzman BR, Mathur-Wagh U. Pyomyositis in patients with the human immunodeficiency virus: an unusual form of disseminated bacterial infection. Am J Med. 1991;91:129.
42. Dalakas MC. Inflammatory and toxic myopathies. Curr Opin Neurol Neurosurg.

1992;5:645–54.

43. Valone FH, Payan DG, Abrams DI, Goetz EJ. Defective polymorphonuclear leucocyte chemotaxis in homosexual men with persistent lymph node syndrome. J Infect Dis. 1984;150:267.
44. Engel AG, Emslie-Smith AM. Inflammatory myopathies. Curr Opin Neurol Neurosurg. 1989;2:695.
45. Arahata K, Engel AG. Monoclonal antibody analysis of mononuclear cells in myopathies. I. Quantitation of subsets according to diagnosis and sites of accumulation and demonstration and counts of muscle fibers invaded by T cells. Ann Neurol. 1984;16:193.
46. Engel AG, Arahata K. Monoclonal antibody analysis of mononuclear cells in myopathies. II. Phenotypes of autoinvasive cells in polymyositis and inclusion body myositis. Ann Neurol. 1984;16:209.
47. Illa I, Nath A, Dalakas MC. Immunocytochemical and virological characteristics of HIV-associated inflammatory myopathies: similarities with seronegative polymyositis. Ann Neurol. 1991;29:474.
48. Lamperth L, Illa I, Dalakas MC. *In situ* hybridization in muscle biopsies from patients with HIV-associated polymyositis (HIV-PM) using labeled HIV-RNA probes. Neurology. 1990;40(Suppl.1):121.
49. Leon-Monzon M, Lamperth L, Dalakas MC. Search for HIV proviral DNA and amplified sequences in the muscle biopsies of patients with HIV-polymyositis. Muscle Nerve. 1993;16:408–13.
50. Chad DA, Smith TW, Blumenfeld A, Fairchild PG, DeGirelami U. Human immunodeficiency virus (HIV)-associated myopathy: immunocytochemical identification of an HIV antigen (gp41) in muscle macrophages. Ann Neurol. 1990;28:579.
51. Hantai D, Fournier JG, Vazeux R, Collin H, Baudrimont M, Fardeau M. Skeletal muscle involvement in human immunodeficiency virus infection. Acta Neuropathol. 1991;81:496.
52. Leon-Monzon MEL, Dalakas M. Detection of HIV in muscle and nerve biopsies by DNA-amplification techniques. Neurology. 1991;41(Suppl.1):376.
53. Lamperth L, Vicenzi E, Dalakas M. Infection and transfection of human muscle by HIV or HIV proviral-DNA construct. Neurology. 1991;41(Suppl.1):211.
54. Emslie-Smith AM, Arahata K, Engel AG. Major histocompatibility complex class I antigen expression, immunolocalization of interferon subtypes, and T cell-mediated cytotoxicity in myopathies. Hum Pathol. 1989;20:224.
55. Oldstone MBA. Molecular anatomy of viral persistence. J Virol. 1991;65:6381.
56. Pouchot J, Vinceneux, Barge J, Laparre F, Boussougant Y, Michon C. Tuberculous polymyositis in HIV infection. Am J Med. 1990;89:250–1.
57. Johnson SC, Stamm CP, Hicks CB. Tuberculous psoas muscle abscess following chemoprophylaxis with isoniazid in a patient with human immunodeficiency virus infection. Rev Infect Dis. 1990;12:754–6.
58. Wrzolek MA, Rao C, Kozlowski PB, Sher JH. Muscle and nerve involvement in AIDS patient with disseminated Mycobacterium avium intracellulare infection. Muscle Nerve. 1989;12:247–9.
59. Lähdevirta J, Maury CPJ, Teppo AM, Repo H. Elevated levels of circulating cachectin/tumour necrosis factor in patients with acquired immunodeficiency syndrome. Am J Med. 1988;85:289.
60. Simpson DM, Bender AN, Farraye J, Mendelson S, Wolfe DE. HIV wasting syndrome may represent a treatable myopathy. Neurology. 1990;40:535.
61. Morgan OS, Rodgers-Johnson P, Mora C, Char G. HTLV-I and polymyositis in Jamaica. Lancet. 1989;2:1184.
62. Higuchi I, Nerenberg M, Yoshimine K, *et al.* Failure to detect HTLV-I by *in situ* hybridization in the biopsied muscle of viral carriers with polymyositis. Muscle Nerve. 1992;15:43.
63. Goutreau G, Karpati G, Carpenter S. Inflammatory myopathy in association with chronic myelopathy in HTLV-I seropositive patients. Neurology. 1988;8(Suppl.):206.
64. Evans BK, Gore I, Harrell LE, Arnold T, Oh SJ. HTLV-I associated myelopathy and polymyositis in a U.S. native. Neurology. 1989;39:1572.
65. Madden DL, Mundon FK, Tzan NR, *et al.* Serologic studies of MS patients, controls, and patients with other neurologic diseases: Antibodies to HTLV-I, II, III. Neurology.

1988;38:81–4.
66. Leff RL, Love LA, Miller FW, *et al.* Viruses in the idiopathic inflammatory myopathies: absence of candidate viral genomes in muscle. Lancet. 1992;339:1192–5.
67. Wiley CA, Nerenberg M, Cros D, Soto-Aguilar MC. HTLV-I polymyositis in a patient also infected with the human immunodeficiency virus. N Engl J Med. 1989;320:992.
68. Dalakas MC, Leon-Monzon M, Illa I, Rodgers-Johnson P, Morgan O. Immunopathology of HTLV-I-associated polymyositis (HTLV-PM): studies in 6 patients. Neurology. 1992;42(S):301–2.
69. Goebels N, Michaelis D, Wekerle H, Hohlfeld R. Human myoblasts as antigen-presenting cells. J Immunol. 1992;149:661–7.
70. Bothe K, Aguzzi A, Lassmann H, Rethwilm A, Horak I. Progressive encephalopathy and myopathy in transgenic mice expressing human foamy virus genes. Science. 1991;253:555.
71. Dalakas MC, London WT, Gravell M, Sever JL. Polymyositis in an immunodeficiency disease in monkeys induced by a type D retrovirus. Neurology. 1986;36:569.
72. Dalakas MC, Gravell M, London WT, Cunningham G, Sever JL. Morphological changes of an inflammatory myopathy in rhesus monkeys with simian acquired immunodeficiency syndrome. Proc Soc Exp Biol Med. 1987;185:368.
73. Leon-Monzon M, Dalakas MC. Absence of persistent infection with enteroviruses in muscles of patients with inflammatory myopathies. Ann Neurol. 1992;32:219–22.
74. Rucheton M, Graafland H, Fanton H, Ursule L, Ferrier P, Larsen CJ. Presence of circulating antibodies against gag-gene MuLV proteins in patients with autoimmune connective tissue disorders. Virology. 1985;144:468.
75. Illa I, Leon-Monzon M, Dalakas MC. Retroviral sequences in patients with polymyositis, dermatomyositis and inclusion-body myositis. Neurology. 1992;42(S):302.
76. Shih A, Misra R, Rush MG. Detection of multiple, novel-reverse transcriptase coding sequences in human nucleic acids: relation to primate retroviruses. J Virol. 1989;63:64.
77. Yarchoan R, Klecker RW, Weinhold KG, *et al.* Administration of 3′-azido-3′-deoxythymidine, an inhibitor of HTLV-III/LAV replication, to patients with AIDS or AIDS-related complex. Lancet. 1986;1:575.
78. Bessen LJ, Greene JB, Louie E, Seitzman P, Weinberg H. Severe polymyositis-like syndrome associated with zidovudine therapy of AIDS and ARC. N Engl J Med. 1988;318:708.
79. Gorard DA, Henry K, Giloff RJ. Necrotising myopathy and zidovudine. Lancet. 1988;1:1050.
80. Panegyres PK, Tan N, Kakulas BA, *et al.* Necrotising myopathy and zidovudine. Lancet. 1988;1:1050.
81. Helbert M, Fletcher T, Peddle B, Harris JRW, Pinching AJ. Zidovudine-associated myopathy. Lancet. 1988;2:689.
82. Arnaudo E, Dalakas M, DiMauro S, Schon EA. Depletion of muscle mitochondrial DNA in AIDS patients with zidovudine-induced myopathies. Lancet. 1991;337:508.
83. Dalakas MC, Lamperth L, Dagani F. Abnormal muscle mitochondria induced by AZT in vitro and in an animal model: morphological, enzymatic and oxygen-consumption studies. Neurology. 1991;41(S):375.
84. Lamperth L, Dalakas MC, Dagani F, Anderson J, Ferrari R. Abnormal skeletal and cardiac muscle mitochondria induced by zidovudine (AZT) in human muscle in vitro and in an animal model. Lab Invest. 1991;65:742–51.
85. Lewis W, Papoian T, Gonzalez B, *et al.* Mitochondrial ultrastructural and molecular changes induced by zidovudine in rat hearts. Lab Invest. 1991;65:228.
86. Jay C, Ropka M, Hench K, Grady C, Dalakas M. Prospective study of myopathy during prolonged low-dose AZT: clinical correlates of AZT mitochondrial myopathy (AZT-MM) and HIV-associated inflammatory myopathy (HIV-IM). Neurology. 1992;42(S):145.
87. Chalmers AC, Creco CM, Miller RG. Prognosis in AZT myopathy. Neurology. 1991;41:1181.
88. Weissman JD, Constantinitis I, Hudgins P, Wallace DC. 31P magnetic resonance spectroscopy suggests impaired mitochondrial function in AZT-treated HIV-infected patients. Neurology. 1991;41:519–623.
89. Soueidan S, Sinnwell T, Jay C, Frank J, McLaughlin A, Dalakas M. Impaired muscle energy metabolism in patients with AZT-myopathy: a blinded comparative study of exercise 31P magnetic resonance spectroscopy with muscle biopsy. Neurology. 1992;42(Suppl.3):146.
90. Simpson MV, Chin CD, Keilbough SA, Lin T-S, Prusoff WH. Studies on the inhibition of mitochondrial DNA replication of 3′-azido′-3-deoxythymidine and other dideoxynucleoside

analogs which inhibit HIV-1 replication. Biochem Pharmacol. 1989;38:1033.
91. Cornblath DR, McAuthur JC, Kennedy PGE, Witte AS, Griffin JW. Inflammatory demyelinating peripheral neuropathies associated with human T-cell lymphotropic virus type III infection. Ann Neurol. 1987;21:32–40.
92. Parry GJ. Peripheral neuropathies associated with human immunodeficiency virus infection. Ann Neurol. 1988;23(Suppl):S49–53.
93. Raphael SA, Price ML, Lischner HW, Griffin JW, Grover WD, Bagasra O. Inflammatory demyelinating polyneuropathy in a child with symptomatic human immunodeficiency virus infection. J Pediatr. 1991;118:242–5.
94. Elder G, Dalakas M, Pezeshkpour G, Sever G. Ataxic neuropathy due to ganglioneuritis after probable acute human immunodeficiency virus infection. Lancet. 1986;2:1275–6.
95. Lambert JS, Seidin M, Reichman RC, *et al.* 2′,3′-dideoxyinosine (ddI) in patients with the acquired immunodeficiency sydrome or AIDS-related complex: a phase I trial. N Engl J Med. 1990;322:1333–40.
96. Merigan TC, Skowron G, Bozzette SA, *et al.* Circulating p24 antigen levels and responses to dideoxycytidine in human immunodeficiency virus (HIV) infections: a phase I and II study. Ann Intern Med. 1989;110:189–94.
97. Dubinsky RM, Yarchoan R, Dalakas M, Broder S. Reversible axonal neuropathy from the treatment of AIDS and related disorders with 2′,3′-dideoxycytidine (ddc). Muscle Nerve. 1989;12:856–60.
98. Fuller GN, Jacobs JM, Guiloff RJ. Subclinical peripheral nerve involvement in AIDS: an electrophysiological and pathological study. J Neurol Neurosurg Psychiatry. 1991;54:318–24.
99. Chavanet P, Solary E, Giroud M, *et al.* Infraclinical neuropathies related to immunodeficiency virus infection associated with higher T-helper cell count. J Acquired Immune Deficiency Syndrome. 1989;2:564–9.
100. Koch TK, Koerper MA, Wesley AM, Lewis EM, Weintrub PS, Bredesen DE. Absence of an AIDS-related peripheral neuropathy in children and young adult hemophiliacs (abstract). Ann Neurol. 1989;26:476–7.
101. Belman AL. AIDS and pediatric neurology. Neurol Clin. 1990;8:571–603.
102. Eidelberg D, Sotrel A, Vogel H, Walker P, Kleefield J, Crumpacker CS. Progressive polyradiculopathy in acquired immune deficiency syndrome. Neurology. 1986;36:912–16.
103. Behar R, Wiley C, McCutchan A. Cytomegalovirus polyradiculoneuropathy in acquired immune deficiency syndrome. Neurology. 1987;37:557–61.
104. Falloon J, Eddy J, Wiener L, Pizzo PA. Human immunodeficiency virus infection in children. J Pediatr. 1989;114:1–30.
105. Miller RG, Storey JR, Greco CM. Ganciclovir in the treatment of progressive AIDS-related polyradiculopathy. Neurology. 1990;40:569–74.
106. Feldman D, Brosnan C, Anderson TD. Ultrastructure of peripheral neuropathy induced in rabbits by 2′,3′-dideoxycytidine. Lab Invest. 1992;66:75–85.
107. Kieburtz KD, Seidlin M, Lambert JS, Dolin R, Reichman R, Valentine F. Extended follow-up of peripheral neuropathy in patients with AIDS and AIDS-related complex treated with dideoxyinosine. J Acquired Immune Deficiency Syndrome. 1992;5:60–4.
108. LeLacheur SF, Simon GL. Exacerbation of dideoxycytidine-induced neuropathy with dideoxyinosine. J Acquired Immune Deficiency Syndrome. 1991;4:538–9.
109. Bozzette SA, Santangelo J, Villasana D, *et al.* Peripheral nerve function in persons with asymptomatic or minimally symptomatic HIV disease: absence of zidovudine neurotoxicity. J Acquired Immune Deficiency Syndrome. 1991;4:851–5.
110. Ho DD, Rota TR, Schooley RT, *et al.* Isolation of HTLV-III from cerebrospinal fluid and neural tissues of patients with neurologic syndromes related to the acquired immunodeficiency syndrome. N Engl J Med. 1985;313:1493–7.
111. Berger JR, Shebert, Gregorios JB. Exacerbation of HIV-associated myopathy by zidovudine. AIDS. 1991;5:229–30.

Index

Immunology and Medicine Series

1. A.M. McGregor (ed.). *Immunology of Endocrine Diseases.* 1986 ISBN: 0-85200-963-1
2. L. Ivanyi (ed.). *Immunological Aspects of Oral Diseases.* 1986 ISBN: 0-85200-961-5
3. M.A.H. French (ed.). *Immunoglobulins in Health and Disease.* 1986 ISBN: 0-85200-962-3
4. K. Whaley (ed.). *Complement in Health and Disease.* 1987 ISBN: 0-85200-954-2
5. G.R.D. Catto (ed.). *Clinical Transplantation: Current Practice and Future Prospects.* 1987 ISBN: 0-85200-960-7
6. V.S. Byers and R.W. Baldwin (ed.). *Immunology of Malignant Diseases.* 1987 ISBN: 0-85200-964-X
7. S.T. Holgate (ed.). *Mast Cells, Mediators and Disease.* 1988 ISBN: 0-85200-968-2
8. D.J.M. Wright (ed.). *Immunology of Sexually Transmitted Diseases.* 1988 ISBN: 0-74620-087-0
9. A.D.B. Webster (ed.). *Immunodeficiency and Disease.* 1988 ISBN: 0-85200-688-8
10. C. Stern (ed.). *Immunology of Pregnancy and its Disorders.* 1989 ISBN: 0-7462-0065-X
11. M.S. Klempner, B. Styrt and J. Ho (ed.). *Phagocytes and Disease.* 1989 ISBN: 0-85200-842-2
12. A.J. Zuckerman (ed.). *Recent Developments in Prophylactic Immunization.* 1989 ISBN: 0-7923-8910-7
13. S. Lightman (ed.). *Immunology of Eye Disease.* 1989 ISBN: 0-7923-8908-5
14. T.J. Hamblin (ed.). *Immunotherapy of Disease.* 1990 ISBN: 0-7462-0045-5
15. D.B. Jones and D.H. Wright (eds.). *Lymphoproliferative Diseases.* 1990 ISBN: 0-85200-965-8
16. C.D. Pusey (ed.). *Immunology of Renal Diseases.* 1991 ISBN: 0-7923-8964-6
17. A.G. Bird (ed.). *Immunology of HIV Infection.* 1991 ISBN: 0-7923-8962-X
18. J.T. Whicher and S.W. Evans (eds.). *Biochemistry of Inflammation.* 1992 ISBN: 0-7923-8985-9
19. T.T. MacDonald (ed.). *Immunology of Gastrointestinal Diseases.* 1992 ISBN: 0-7923-8961-1
20. K. Whaley, M. Loos and J.M. Weiler (eds.). *Complement in Health and Disease, 2nd Edn.* 1993 ISBN: 0-7923-8823-2
21. H.C. Thomas and J. Waters (eds.). *Immunology of Liver Disease.* 1994 ISBN: 0-7923-8975-1
22. G.S. Panayi (ed.). *Immunology of Connective Tissue Diseases.* 1994 ISBN: 0-7923-8988-3
23. G. Scadding (ed.). *Immunology of ENT Disorders.* 1994 ISBN: 0-7923-8914-X